CM0126187?

No. 143 / 500

HARDY TREE

J. WARWICK SWEENEY

HARDY TREE

A DOCTOR'S BIBLE

BRACKETPRESS
MMXIX

This story involves the biochemical messages within the
human brain and a doctor's consideration of them.
It involves memory, learning and love,
the greatest of these is love.
All characters were born, variously suffered and triumphed.
All are now dead.
This is their story and dedicated to them.

A note on *Hardy Tree*, its structure and ways it can be read

There are two previously untold stories split by their numbered chapters, odd (1, 3, 5 ...) and even (2, 4, 6 ...). You can read the first story (odd numbers) and then start the second story (even numbers). Alternatively, read the chapters in their conventional sequence.

The first part (odd numbers) is arguably more significant because it helped make the second part (even numbers) possible. If you are interested in an autonomous approach to doctoring that sprang from a wish to heal not medicalise you may enjoy a young doctor's approach to life. The second story deals with the same doctor and his treatment of an unfulfilled literary genius for heroin dependency. Late in the doctor's life he had developed a knack for knowing when to inject and when to talk. Both stories interlock in a variety of ways.

Contents

Introduction – J. Warwick Sweeney — xi
Editor's Note — xxxi
Foreword – Andrew J. Lees — xxxiii
Acknowledgements — xliii

1. Rampside — 1
2. London, April 1956 — 21
3. From Science to Séance — 41
4. Siamese Fighting Fish and Ulysses — 65
5. Leave Well Alone — 89
6. 99 Cromwell Road — 107
7. TB — 139
8. Dent Meets Benway — 157
9. Death Before Dishonour — 177
10. Buffoons Talking Bollocks — 201
11. St Pancras, Poor Law Infirmary, 1918 — 221
12. Waking Suggestion — 243
13. Drunks — 277
14. Silent Waiting — 297
15. Eugenics — 311
16. Riding Stang — 331
17. Savages — 351
18. When Lee Became Burroughs — 375

Introduction

J. WARWICK SWEENEY

I hope you enjoy *Hardy Tree* and its stories but there is a purpose to it all. It tells the tale of a doctor. It is analogue not digital. It reminds us of an age when a doctor's appointment was a consultation, a dialogue of mutual benefit. As we anticipate medical transactions by app and delivery of our pills by drones, maybe this should give pause for thought. Is there a connection between the rise in psycho-social disorders and the inexorable drive for efficiency? Are doctors losing sight of their ability to heal?

My interest in these and other themes has probably always been with me, since the principal character of *Hardy Tree* is my maternal grandfather, John Yerbury Dent. He was a doctor in the old style similar to Peter Sassall, John Berger's character in *A Fortunate Man*. This is a rural depiction of the urban Dent. Both doctors were stoic, inventive and discreetly loyal but there was something in Dent not evident in Sassall. I was reminded of this when I recalled meeting John Mortimer, author and barrister. All three men embodied compassion but Dent and Mortimer were infused with a political sensibility. This surfaced as a universal mission to champion the causes of those less fortunate than themselves. Mortimer was a true socialist, one who became increasingly irate with the faux version at Westminster. Towards the end of his life he recognised that New Labour, with a neo-liberal agenda, betrayed many things that both he and Dent had fought for:

> What is sad is the feeling of having waited so long for a powerful Labour government, which would improve social

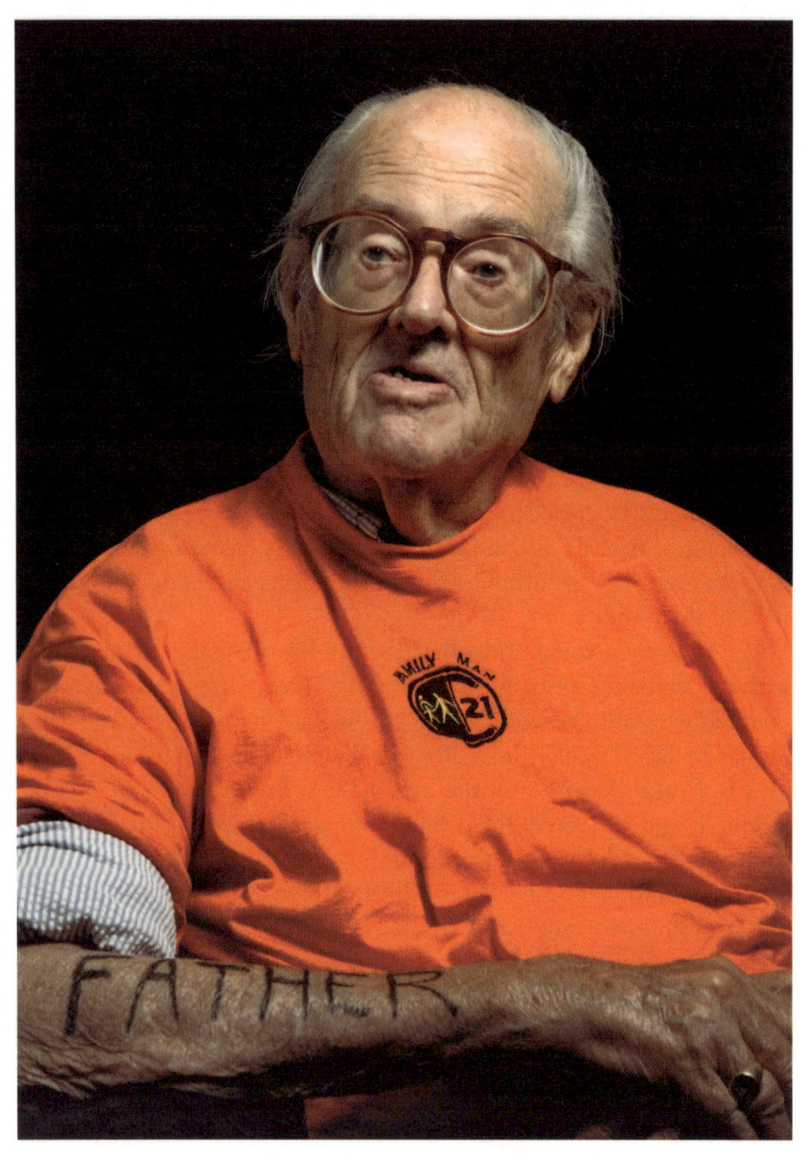

John Mortimer (1924–2009), father, family man, defender of free speech and advocate of penal reform as espoused by the Howard League. [photo: JWS]

justice, care for public services, nurture the arts, and protect civil liberties, only to get one of whose ideas of justice can be dictated by focus groups and last week's headlines.[1]

Today, as social disparities widen, it isn't difficult to recognise the consequences of that betrayal: more displaced people, homelessness, overcrowded classrooms, debt, poverty, the erosion of public services and exponential rise in the psycho-social conditions: the depressions, anxieties and addictions. That last point is relevant to Dent because he became known as a pioneer of addiction therapies and identified the link between anxiety and drug dependency. His purpose was to improve his and thereby our understanding of these debilitating phenomena. He failed in his wider mission because addiction and its allied conditions are a modern scourge that affects everybody either directly or indirectly. Drug abuse in the US alone is estimated to cost $820 billion per year and the annual global deaths from addiction are comparable to the total number murdered throughout the Holocaust. But in terms of individual treatments Dent was successful. My initial aim therefore was to explore both his failure and success and whether we can learn anything from his life and work. In this regard I was helped by the fact that Dent had been a prodigious writer completing several papers, books, articles and broadcasts. Much of this resides within the public domain. The exceptions are his memoirs and some correspondence.

Some years ago my interest took a turn due to a circumstantial meeting with a doctor who was involved in Dent's line of work. This led to another meeting with a leading voice in the world of addiction therapies and molecular research. I was ushered into a room to confront a man who couldn't have looked more disinterested, more bored. He hadn't heard of Dent but knew about apomorphine, the drug Dent had used to help relieve people of their anxieties and depressions.

'Apomorphine,' he said, stifling a yawn, 'Don't you mean aversion therapy?'

I had spent my life wandering the Earth taking photographs and knew nothing about brain science. To say I felt out of my depth would be an understatement. However, I did know that within the world of medical research apomorphine had a notorious reputation based on its vomiting side-effect and its ludicrous association with 'cures' for homosexuality. This disrepute had proven to be a barrier to Dent and research 70 years ago. I looked into the eyes of the so-called 'progressive' voice of neuroscience and wondered where all this was leading.

'No,' I blustered, 'Dent was quite clear about that. Apomorphine was not an aversion therapy, but,' I stressed, 'even if there is an aversive reaction, isn't aversion the flip-side to reward?'

The neuroscientist suddenly lit up. He seemed enthused, even moderately excited and rushed out of the room! He returned with a colleague telling her *she* had to hear what *I* was saying. I was not ready for this. They were the experts; they should have been telling me what to think.

At that moment I realised that medicine and particularly the thorny area of addiction is a fearfully convoluted business. The chasm between the 1950s world in which the autonomous Dent worked and the one of today is probably unbridgeable. Part of me feels sorry for modern health-care professionals who are bound by guidelines and red tape that Dent would have laughed at and thrown in the bin. And this realisation brought me back to the earlier theme of unfettered neoliberalism, the toxic political culture that so drove John Mortimer to distraction.

Trying to understand addiction is confounding enough; those neural mechanisms we'd die without but lead some of us to destruction. Given the rapacious demands of liberal free market economics, I sense that even if someone did provide a 'cure' there'd still be the battle with a political establishment that defines policy based on interests not efficacy. I met other addiction specialists. Some claimed apomorphine did not work or that obviously it had been 'superseded'. I raised the issue of patient choice and asked them if they knew how apomorphine had been used. They did not and I have yet to meet any doctor who has been able or willing to interpret and relate Dent's approaches to a problem which year on year gets worse. I wondered

INTRODUCTION

if for some, and in light of the damning evidence, their 'specialism' isn't a peculiar form of denialism, a symptom of what they themselves have enabled within a 'pill a day' culture. Privately, after a few drinks, some doctors do confess that the ruthless drive for efficiency has led to epidemics of the very conditions they are powerless to prevent: the anxieties, depressions and addictions. As I dug deeper it was dawning on me that Dent's struggle, far from being a closed episode relegated to the dusty annals of British medical history, was in point of fact highly symbolic of the failures to deal with all the systemic ills of neoliberalism, medical or otherwise. No wonder Mortimer had been apoplectic with a Blair government that introduced a 24-hour drinking culture and casino capitalism. As for the antinomian Dent he was better off out of it. He wanted to heal people not turn them into comatose customers.

Turn the clock back eighty years and it was clear that some could see what was coming. Dent, I learned, moved on the fringes of a milieu of writers and intellectuals, many of whom blended their nascent understanding of psychology with Fabianism. Writers like Shaw, Wells, Huxley and Orwell all shared an awareness of the conditioning techniques expounded at length in Dent's first book, *The Human Machine* (Gollancz, 1936). This is a book of broad strokes encompassing amongst other matters an appreciation of human evolution, sex, hypnotism, behaviour, environment, pain and will. Here it appears to anticipate the internet:

> We react much more to the symbol than to the thing itself, and our most important environment consists of our fellow men and what we learn from them. This is what is known as our conversational or symbolic environment [...] Civilisation has consisted of the regulation and mitigation of our external environment and the development of our conversational contacts. We have become less and less affected by the tamed forces of nature while our environment of words has become ever more important. Man dates his origin from the

invention of speech. [...] The electrical and photographic communication of words will make our civilisation not only universal but homogeneous. The human race cannot remain the same after these inventions; and those that adapt... will be those that continue to exist.

– J. Y. Dent *The Human Machine*,
(1936) Victor Gollancz (UK) / Alfred Knopf (US)

In light of the current furore over algorithmically linked databases and 'rigged' voting intentions, these were prescient words. But Dent also sensed that this global homogeneity would trigger a corresponding rise in anxiety. Today as information is spread faster than individuals can think, we react before we understand. Cue the soundbite and fake news, the froth on the surface pretending to tell us about the ocean underneath, its vastness, complexity and depth. It cannot. We need experts but also our faith in them to lead us out of the wilderness. Instead, we have more and more crude manipulators of fear and prejudice endorsed by a superficial media. How many Blairs, Bransons and Murdochs does it take to lose an ecosystem, medicalise an emotion, get a Brexit, a Trump? Social cohesion is breaking up before our eyes in direct proportion to the global spread and inculcation of anxiety. Dent was the first doctor to explore these links and their relationship with addiction. This is from the introduction of his second book:

Because anxiety is almost universally treated by the taking of alcohol and other drugs it is impossible to write a book about anxiety without at the same time dealing with the action of these drugs and with the addictions they so frequently produce. It is equally true that no book on addiction would be complete without a large part of it being devoted to anxiety; for addiction is only a special form of anxiety.

– J. Y. Dent *Anxiety and its Treatment*
(1955) 3rd ed., Skeffington, London.

INTRODUCTION

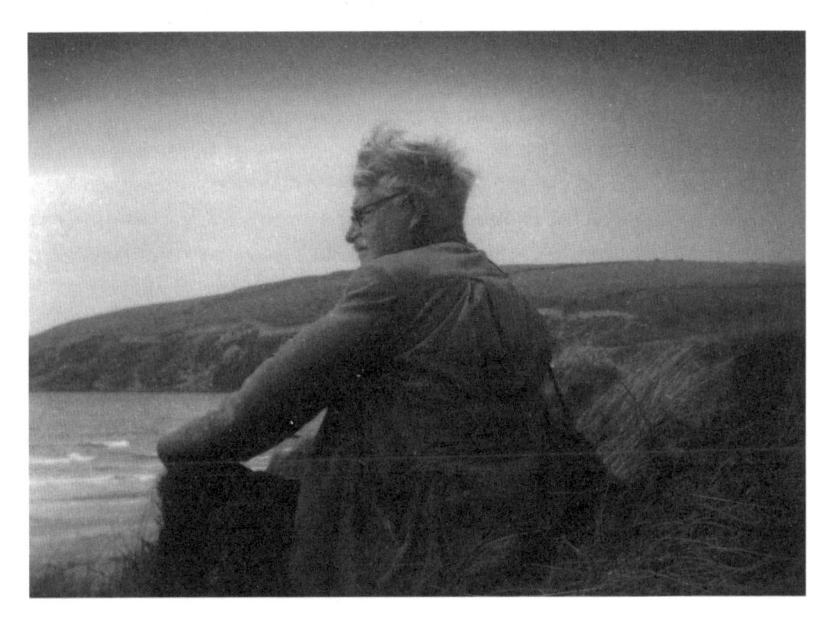

John Yerbury Dent (1888–1962) wrote: 'The human machine responds to three main environments; the internal, external and conversational…. All our behaviour is an automatic resistance to stimuli just as a fish's movements are directed against the current in which it swims.' [photo: Jane Yerbury Sweeney]

Dent was successful at allaying anxiety, but understanding how hasn't been straightforward. I did know, however, that like many of my ancestors, Dent was a raconteur. Whether any storyteller knows it or not, the flow of the human voice may distract the neurasthenic mind permitting it the opportunity to realise unforseen possibilities. This is neuroscience at its most benign. In the old days this facility by doctors was known as 'bedside manner' but neglected nowadays by the overworked GP who eyes the clock after six minutes of appointment. These encounters often end with a prescription of drugs. For the psycho-social 'diseases' these drugs may suppress the natural flow of emotion. They may also create the belief that there is something wrong when there isn't and worst of all, they may drown you altogether in a pharmaceutical soup. Dent's yarns couldn't do that. They chased away demons and bought time so the 'worried well' could find their own path to sustainable healing...and healing matters.

Dent certainly enjoyed talking...and listening to his patients. He believed it an essential part of his job: that every treatment should be tailored to the individual. Today's 'one size fits all' approach he'd consider inimical to the unique character and spirit of everyone. Today the systemic commodification of the patient has turned the beauty of many into the ugliness of pharmaceutical dependence. Dent's creation of a space where the individual's organism repaired, where his or her anxieties could melt and fears fade to nothing was partly why his patients revered him and why neuroscience that ignores this dimension of healing and its interlock with cognition, memory and learning appears so brainless. I am reminded of William Blake's barbed monotype *Newton*, exposing the hubristic materialist trying to outdo Nature. Blake's creation could just as easily be a modern neuropharmacologist tinkering with molecules but ignoring the truth under his nose.

So there it is. *Hardy Tree* amongst other stuff is simply passing down the wisdom of my forebears:

> If you do not prescribe your patient anything you won't be doing him any harm, but if you make him laugh you may be doing him some good.
> – Dr Harry Yerbury Dent, Dent's father.

Dent had a laugh that burst like a thunderclap. Both his parents sprang from strong oral traditions which helped his facility with words. However, by the first half of the twentieth century he'd stepped into a conflicting medical paradigm, one of pharmaceutical intervention. By accident he discovered that apomorphine ($C_{17}H_{17}NO_2$), an off patent drug, quickly relieved patients of their anxieties. This distracted them from the endless cycle of depression and substance abuse. He continued to evolve his approach but quickly found himself out of step with the next emerging paradigm, the current one, of mainte-

INTRODUCTION

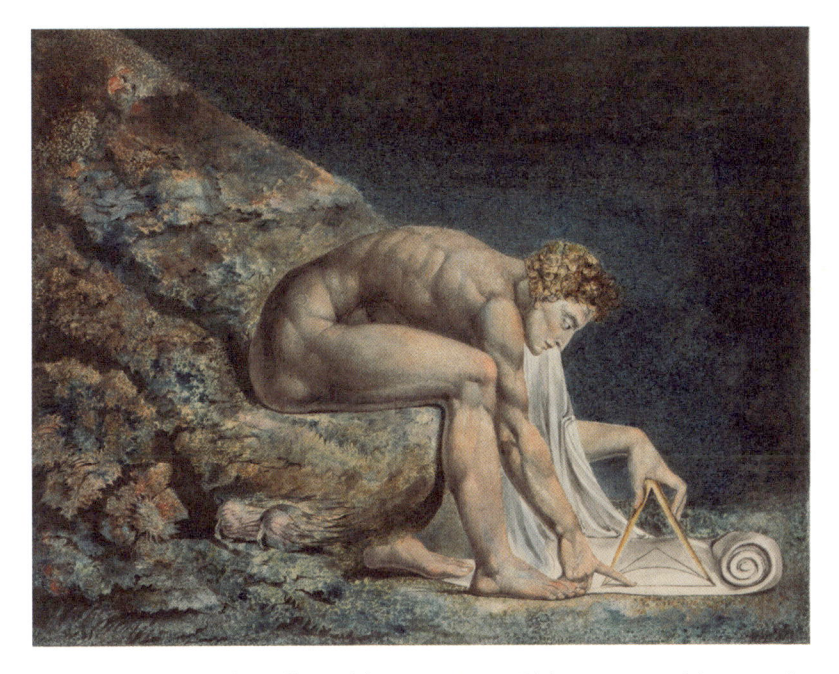

Newton, circa 1795 by William Blake (1757–1827). Blake was a true visionary and arch critic of all forms of formal education which he regarded as inimical to the artistic and creative impulse. [©Tate, London 2018]

nance therapies and dependency on prescription endorsed by multinational corporations with more power than governments.

As I dug I discovered that Dent's appeal for more research into the use of apomorphine was undermined by some very strange assumptions. For instance some molecular biologists appear to have bought into the fallacy that Dent was only interested in a 'bio-chemical interpretation of disease' concluding that he ignored the psycho-social dimensions. Let us be clear, Dent was an advocate of both psychology and pharmacology. This is emphasised in his book *Anxiety and its Treatment* where he explains the stages of addiction from mild to compulsive and his preference for the psychotherapist's or 'synthesist's' approach over the analyst's couch, (p.102). At a symposium he famously remarked; "If there's anything wrong with alcoholics, it's too many psychiatrists". Elsewhere, he explores the benefit of non interference by any medicine, even the pluses of placebo, but also makes clear his interest in talk therapy. He wrote:

> The memory of an unkind or frightening statement lasts longer than the memory of pain. Psychology cannot and should not take the place of medicine and surgery but neither of these can afford to scorn psychological help. I am more and more convinced of the power of the word.
> – *Medici Libris – A Doctor's Bible – Revelation*

This is critical to understanding why Dent was successful even with those at the compulsive end of the addiction spectrum. Contrary to the one-eyed view of Dent's 'bio-chemical obsession' he was in fact an holistic practitioner and to this day neuroscience has only looked at apomorphine through the wrong end of the microscope. This wasn't painting by numbers, every patient had to be individually assessed. To understand this better I built a website:

www.apomorphineversusaddiction.com

and later decided to unravel the treatments given to one of his patients with any information I could find. I chose William Seward Burroughs (1914–97) the celebrated American author because he and his associates had quite a lot to say on the matter. Burroughs had also, as I discovered later, preserved the nurse's Day and Night Reports compiled during his visits to West London in 1956 and 1958 and currently part of the Berg collection, New York Public Library.

Another reason I chose to explore Dent's approach to healing as exemplified by his treatment of Burroughs is because in an effort to unpick the conundrums surrounding addiction social commentators

INTRODUCTION

often cite Burroughs as if he is the oracle. This is odd because he was hardly an expert and in respect of apomorphine also emphasised the bio-chemical while down playing the psycho-social dimensions. I sympathise with his position for various reasons but the unquestioning way others have participated in a lousy game of Chinese whispers could be one of the worst dimensions of celebrity culture. Burroughs was a fetishist and was clever enough to realise that in a trivialising society a few easy hooks were all that was required to garner attention. A further reason I chose to look at Dent's handling of Burroughs is that it is an untold story and the obvious deduction that Dent had not just a profound influence on Burroughs' health but also on his literature. Even a superficial reading of Burroughs's magnum opus, *The Naked Lunch* (1959), demonstrates that Dent's influence on his patient was hardly limited to injections of apomorphine. This isn't surprising as many dimensions of their lives are curiously interchangeable.

Burroughs is an important writer, of that there can be no doubt. His influence has spanned not just one generation but three; the Beats, Hippies and Punks. Nowadays, however, he's defined as a cold-eyed renegade whose reputation is largely based on the notoriety of his drug taking, sexuality and crime. I wondered if this didn't demean him. Surely if people understood better his critical visits to London in the 1950s when arguably he turned his life around then a more complex and interesting figure would emerge? This intrigued me because, after all, so many artists, writers and musicians are cut short by the heady cocktail of dopaminergic deregulation, genius and the bottle. There are simply too many cases to name. Olivia Laing, for instance, in *The Trip to Echo Spring* (2013) specifically traces the lives of six twentieth-century American writers driven to varying degrees of destruction by addiction. But Burroughs survived to die an old man of Letters. Why? Are we disproportionately fascinated by those whose lives end in undiluted tragedy? The silence surrounding the recovery of any celebrity may tell us more about ourselves than we're willing to acknowledge.

If I thought researching Burroughs was going to be easy after

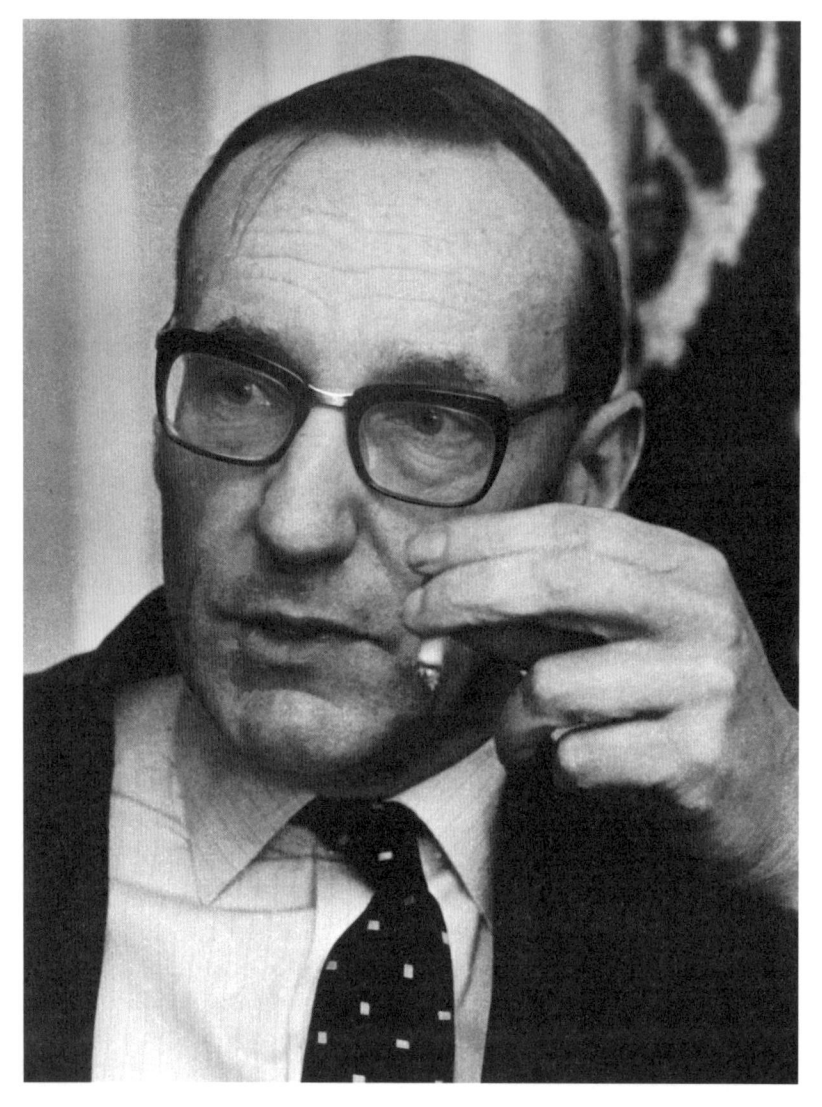

William Seward Burroughs (1914–1997) was a primary figure of the Beat Generation and a postmodernist writer whose influence is considered to have affected a range of popular culture as well as literature. [photo: Graham Keen]

INTRODUCTION

medical orthodoxy I was in for a shock. Nobody who professed to know Burroughs seemed very interested in any interpretation other than their own. I approached a few individuals but their eyes glazed over. Some seemed very anxious to return me to the familiar facets of Burroughs everyone's heard about. This reaction amused me because it was precisely due to Dent's refusal to accept lazy narratives that he treated drug dependants in the first place. I was reminded of the French physiologist Claude Bernard's cute remark: *'It is what we think we know that prevents us from learning'*. It seems this is a characteristic which we can all exhibit from time to time.

Discouraged, I attended talks, lectures and book launches. At one there was an elaborate celebration about a writing technique called 'cut-up' that had been a boon to Burroughs' creativity similar to I Ching as used by John Cage in music. Amongst a small group this turned into a discussion which went round and round like a hamster in a wheel.

'Did you know,' I asked, feeling like a heretic, 'that it was with his London doctor that Burroughs first confronted the random collision of words?'

'No,' I was told, 'it was with Brion Gysin, the experimental artist,' to which the rest of the group nodded in what Burroughs might have described as 'the academic manner'.

Sometime later I met Oliver Harris, the pre-eminent Beat scholar and Professor of American Literature. He nails part of the problem:

> The mythic narrative of Beat legends has either been told and retold, taken up by generation after generation of fascinated and uncritical listeners, or it has been critically ignored, dismissed as an essentially false and empty story. Rarely has this narrative been subjected to close textual or historical analysis.[2]
> – Oliver Harris, *"Virus-X": Kerouac's Visions of Burroughs*

From my perspective *'mythic'* Burroughs is a barrier to knowledge. It has become a rut in the road, driven deeper by each reiteration

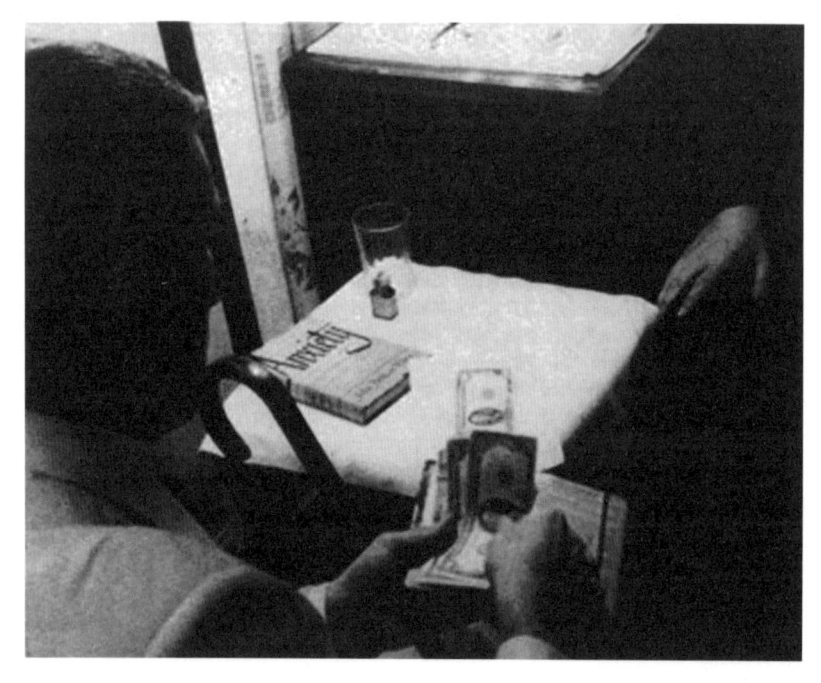

A still from the collaborative film *The Cut-ups* (1966) by Antony Balch which features a consultation between a doctor and his patient. John Yerbury Dent understood that language was the primary conditioning tool and used it as an aid to counter-conditioning. Burroughs, who always paid his dues alludes to this by placing Dent's *Anxiety* book on the table between him and Brion Gysin. Popular culture tells us the originator of the 'cut-up' technique was Gysin but the genesis of this idea was medical not artistic. [image: Antony Balch]

connecting those crumbling edifices, cock and bull. As I re-read *The Naked Lunch* I also availed myself of various critical reviews from the period. Mary McCarthy, in a piece entitled 'Dejeuner sur l'herbe'[3] (1963), recognised that what stood out as original in Burroughs' work was its 'scientific bent', its 'biochemistry, anthropology and politics', three themes that had dominated Dent's own work and writing. Other commentators have been intrigued by the sudden moral flowering in Burroughs and wondered from where a previously prosaic writer

INTRODUCTION

suddenly grew a moralising backbone? Indeed. In fact so sharp is this transformation one passage almost reads like a dictation from *Quaker Faith and Practice*. *The Naked Lunch*, so the cliche goes, refers to that frozen moment when you see what is on the end of your fork. Oddly and despite libraries of analysis, the only thing that has never been put on a fork is the treatment that arguably made its writing possible. I was also told that if my premise that Dent had influenced Burroughs' writing was correct then Burroughs would have said so. Burroughs, despite being constrained by the conventions of medical confidentiality, did. It is just that nobody has been willing or bothered to interpret it. Myth has become fundamentalism.

Around this time I had the good fortune to meet Andrew Lees, Professor of Neurology at UCL. In a successful career Andrew has used apomorphine to provide symptomatic relief of Parkinson's disease. When I met him I wasn't feeling very well having just fallen 150 feet off a cliff in Snowdonia. He seemed curious. 'What had that been like?' he asked. I told him that, in mid-air, you might expect to go rigid with fear. In fact, the opposite happened: I had relaxed.
'You fell like a baby?' he suggested.
'Yes, I suppose so.'
'Then you have insight.' He smiled.
What Andrew was hinting at is the brain's extraordinary power to intercede on our behalf. That in a split second it can shut down our consciousness, our 'front brain', and rely on 'back brain' pathways. In a peculiar way I was confronting, through an extraordinary experience, a further dimension of Dent's appreciation of neurology, that the real power house of the brain is not our executive side, the cortex, but the back brain limbic pathways. Since that day Andrew has become a friend and a hugely significant figure in my determination to peel back the layers of this particular onion, the mysteries surrounding addiction, apomorphine and how we heal.

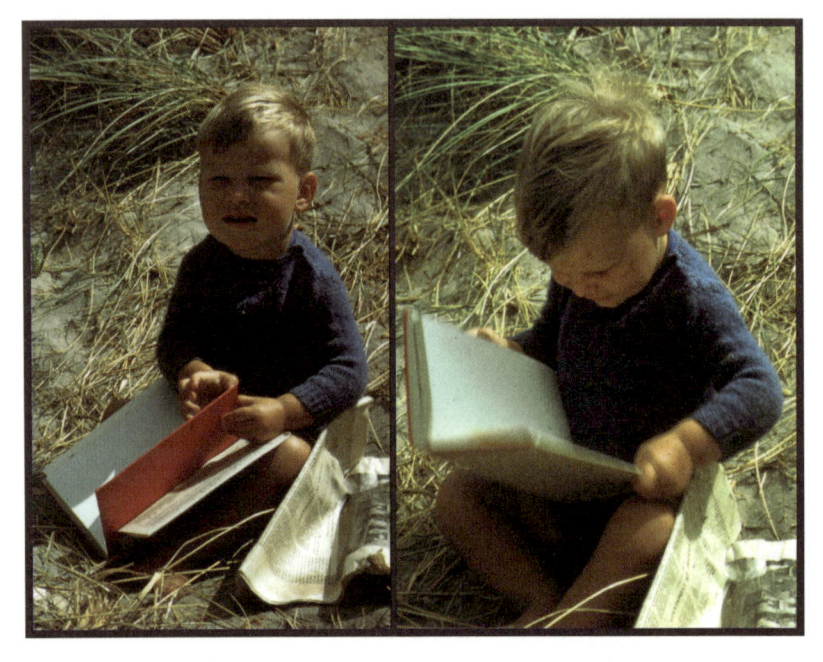

This is me aged three, the annotated caption reads: 'Warwick, "reading"'. In truth I was just aping my environment inhabited by 'book worms'. My grandfather endorsed the game with a photo, a simple example of psychological encouragement and typical of him, his character and doctoring. With influence like this I had little chance of bibliophobia. [photos: J.Y. Dent]

Burroughs had been similarly intrigued. He had wanted to be a doctor and liked the idea that science should inform art. However, this exchange, like neural pathways, should be a two-way street. Burroughs' treatment, 'apomorphine modus Dent', certainly helped him in a multitude of inter-connected ways. Regrettably myth foments more easily than understanding, particularly when research involves science rather than the easy hooks of soap opera. On a recent walking tour in Soho that promised to provide insight into 'Burroughs' London' I witnessed a small gathering of the cognoscenti outside a random '23' numbered doorway. '23' is the prime number constantly referred to by

INTRODUCTION

Burroughs after apomorphine but not before. It was as though this chin-stroking fraternity was waiting for the door to be opened by Burroughs himself. As an exercise in futility this was on a par with trying to extract sunbeams from cucumbers, but in light of the deeper truth of Burroughs' visits to London during the 1950s this fetishizing has become a sad, reductive farce.

In mitigation it must be acknowledged that Burroughsian mythology surrounding his recovery from opiate addiction has been predicated on the fallacy that apomorphine was a 'cure'. This was cultivated early on by the Beats, and Burroughs, in the midst of much personal disarray, may have been swept along by what amounted to a PR exercise. It certainly suited the Beats and radical counter-culture to peddle the idea that Pharma withheld a cure for drug addiction. This was an easy narrative to set alongside the backdrop of corrupt corporate interests and covert military presence in various parts of the world involved in narcotic production. This unholy alliance persists to this day so I have some sympathy with this view. But apomorphine was never a 'cure' as both doctor and patient knew and anybody who has referred to it as such without qualification has not added to the sum of human knowledge. This does not mean that apomorphine wasn't biochemically remedial, but to isolate it from every other dimension of Dent's methods and Burroughs' experiences is unhelpful. There are some extremely thick tomes on the life and times of William S. Burroughs. It almost amounts to an industry. They contain references to Dent that betray a lack of scrutiny and the use of the word 'cure' has often been used as the end of argument rather than the beginning of discussion. Given that Burroughs said that he had no claims to call himself a writer prior to apomorphine, then the existing narrative, a sketch drawn on water, makes little sense and helps nobody.

In April 1956, Burroughs, knocking on Death's door, was sent to knock on Dent's. This was 1950s London, a society cowed by a

HARDY TREE

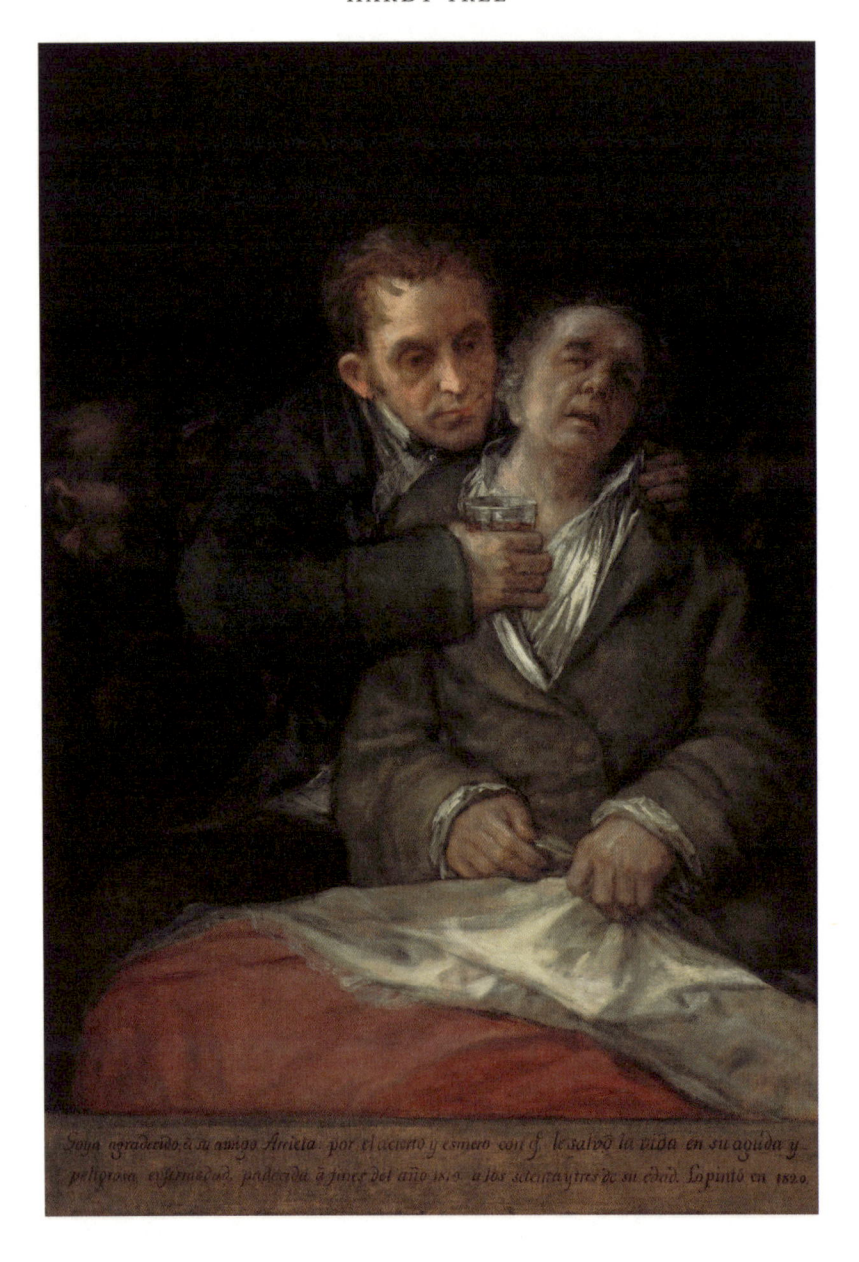

[xxviii]

INTRODUCTION

repressive establishment promising the gallows for murder and, as Alan Turing discovered, chemical castration for homosexuality. Burroughs must have been horrified. Every living memory collected told me that Dent would have none of it. We could not afford to be too serious about anything, particularly society's precious sensibilities, its grotesque, nit-picking snobbery. However, Dent was up against it. His illustration, for instance, of the ills of prohibition, over-diagnosing and over-prescribing were rarely taken seriously, with consequences which continue to blight society. His consolation was kindred spirits who wandered in from nowhere but left going somewhere. In that respect the mythologising around Burroughs, the gaping hole in his canon, demeans not only the writer but Beat culture itself. With his progressive ideas on treatment, his knowledge of geo-politics, control, language and the law and his transgressive views on taboo and sex, Dent was arguably more Beat than the Beats. Bizarrely these and other dimensions of Burroughs's 'cure' have remained in the closet. The irony is extraordinary, the implications tragic.

Even before Dent got through to Burroughs there were only three-hundred registered opiate addicts in the whole of the UK. Today you may find this number within every small town. In fact we are now told that every form of addiction, anxiety and mental illness is out of control. This inculcation of a cradle-to-grave society dependent on global Pharma has happened under the sinister shadow of rampant capitalism: fast food, pharmacy and gambling outlets on every high street. As Dent said, *'everything is environment'*, yet we find ourselves increasingly under the thumb of unethical corporations, spineless

[opposite] *Self-Portrait with Dr Arrieta*. Francisco Goya (1746–1828) and William Burroughs were equally suspicious of doctors. This shared conviction was eventually confounded by their respective doctor's style of hands on compassion. Goya paid his homage in oil, Burroughs consistently did the same in words.
[©Bridgeman Images, 2018]

governments and spin, our individual potentialities ever harder to realise against the endemic toxicity of a lab-rat culture upheld by pecuniary values and bugger all else.

Dent lived life as he saw it and ended up that curious embodiment of someone able to combine ethics and empathy with science and understanding. He was not religious about his Quakerism, preferring atheism, but hoped everyone could be free to enjoy his or her potential. You could not spend five minutes in his company without realising that this was his primary purpose as both man and doctor.

Nowadays it may be too late for society to embrace any form of collective empiricism let alone Dent's. This would depend on real world settings designed to aid decision making by patients. The focus should be ethical outcomes with the neglected concept of abstinence its target. By necessity this would involve support by every ministry, medical agency, practitioner, research initiative and trial. Indeed everything devoted to solving the causes of sickness and not the treatment or maintenance of symptoms. As life became art the antithesis of this ideal was parodied by Burroughs in *The Naked Lunch*, a reaction to an experience of healing as relevant today as when it was written. It is my belief that both patient and doctor would want to encourage a deeper awareness of this understanding as their friendship was built on trust between equals.

J. Warwick Sweeney
1st June 2018

References
1. John Mortimer, 'The Summer of a Dormouse' review *The Guardian*, Robert McCrum, 2000.
2. Oliver Harris, '"*Virus-X*": Kerouac's Vision of Burroughs' in J. Skerl (Ed.) *Reconstructing the Beats* (New York: St. Martin's Press), 2004.
3. Mary McCarthy, 'Dejeuner sur l'Herbe', *New York Review of Books*, 12 February 1963.

Editor's Note

I met Warwick by chance in London in March 2017. I was looking for proofreading and editing work, and Warwick had a partially written manuscript in need of an editor.

Despite having done an English Literature degree, I had only vaguely heard of Burroughs before meeting Warwick, and many of the themes and issues discussed in *Hardy Tree* were equally new to me. Fortunately, this seemed to be what Warwick wanted. As I read the early drafts of each chapter I was moved by the parallel stories of a doctor and his patient and a young doctor's struggle against injustice.

Some challenges were posed at the start by the staggered timeframe and at one point I drew up a timeline to keep track of events. I enjoyed receiving revised drafts and reading new passages, and getting a sense of how the book would fit together when all the chapters were completed. The preface was perhaps the section which underwent the most changes, following a tempering of Warwick's passionate polemics, and I love how it brings the themes of the book together in a moving and succinct way.

Throughout the book's pages there are many memorable characters and moments, but two scenes which have particularly stayed with me are both ones in which Dent sits with a patient, taking the time to listen, to talk and to empathise, as he does many times in the book. The first is a powerful scene involving a reading of *The Rime of the Ancient Mariner,* and the second is a quieter scene taking place in the gardens of St Pancras, overlooking a monument designed by the author Thomas Hardy.

I hope you enjoy reading *Hardy Tree* as much as I have.

– Antje Rex

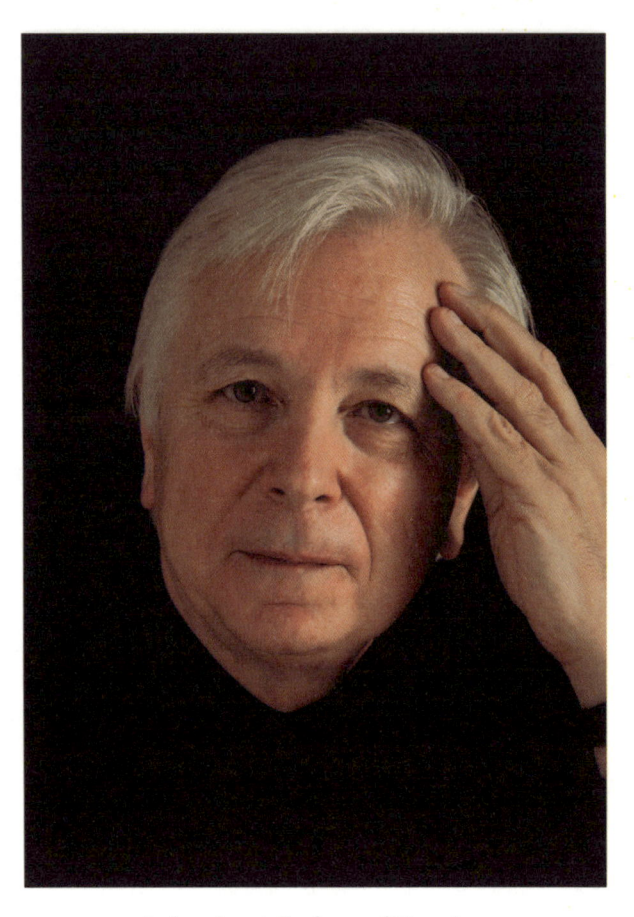

Andrew Lees is Professor of Neurology
at the National Hospital, Queen Square, London and UCL.
In 2011 Andrew became the world's most
highly cited Parkinson's researcher.

Foreword

A. J. LEES

During my final year of medical apprenticeship at The London Hospital, Whitechapel I entered into a Mephistolean pact with William Seward Burroughs. The 'Pope of Dope' agreed to leave me alone until I had qualified provided I paid attention to what he had written about bad doctoring, dangerous scientists and institutional corruption. Later he became an invisible mentor in my quest to find a cure for the shaking palsy.

In April 1956 William Burroughs had arrived in London hooked on synthetic opioids. It was his good fortune to be referred on to Dr John Yerbury Dent, a medical practitioner who had gained a reputation for the treatment of alcohol dependence. When Burroughs arrived in West London he was at the end of the line and desperate for a quick fix for his junk sickness. Previous detoxication attempts in Tangiers had all ended in failure. At their first meeting Dent persuaded Burroughs to be admitted for treatment to his clinic for apomorphine treatment.

Apomorphine was first synthesised in the middle of the nineteenth century by Matthiesen and Wright two English chemists working at St Bartholomew's Hospital by heating opium with hydrochloric acid in anaerobic conditions. Despite its structural similarities to morphine it had negligible narcotic properties but was a potent emetic. It was first used by veterinary scientists to treat behavioural vices in farm animals and then introduced into medicine as a treatment for acute poisoning. It was later employed as a sedative, a treatment for palpitations, chorea and hysterical seizures and at the beginning of the twentieth century it had been used to treat delirium tremens. In France up until the 1970s it was marketed as a treatment for sexual deviation including homosexuality and later was licensed in Europe and the United States as a treatment of erectile dysfunction under the trade name of Uprima.

Dent's two nurses injected apomorphine into Burroughs every two hours round the clock. He was also permitted heroin injections and alcohol during the first two or three days of acute opioid withdrawal and given very small doses of insulin. Dent also used suggestion to reinforce the pharmacological effects of the drug. Within a week his patient was 'clean' and ready for discharge. Before Burroughs left London he continued to see Dent who made it clear that the onus of travel beyond a tomorrow free of pain and junk lay firmly on his patient's shoulders.

On 3 August four months after Burroughs had left 99 Cromwell Road he wrote to Dent from Venice:

> Dear Doctor,
> Thanks for your letter. I enclose that article on the effects of various drugs I have used. I do not know if it is suitable for your publication. I have no objection to my name being used.
> No difficulty with drinking. No desire to use any drug. General health excellent. Please give my regards to Mr...... I use his system of exercises daily with excellent results.
> I have been thinking of writing a book on narcotic drugs if I could find a suitable collaborator to handle the technical end.
> Yours truly,
> William Burroughs

Opioid withdrawal and apomorphine facilitated Burroughs' dream recall, retrieval of the lost subconscious and formative memories and created a vividness in his perception that is reflected in some of the phantasmagorical imagery that bears a remarkable similarity with Bulgakov's *Master and Margarita* and Coleridge's opium fuelled word hoards. Burroughs became a champion of the 'junk vaccine' and hoped to get the 'shrinks' at the Federal Medical Center in Lexington interested in the treatment. Much later he wrote that without Dr Dent's help he would never have managed to assemble the contents of *Naked Lunch*. Apomorphine remained a Schedule 2 drug in the State of California until 2010 (drugs with established medical use but with a high potential for abuse, with use potentially leading to severe psychological or physical dependence). Although ending up on a methadone programme, Burroughs wrote that maintenance therapy was like treating an alcoholic with whisky and that apomorphine was a far better approach.

Five years after Dent's death apomorphine was shown to stimulate dopamine receptors in the brain but despite growing evidence apomorphine treatment faded away as its last advocates in Scandinavia and Switzerland died or retired. Science had confirmed Dent's hunch that apomorphine was a metabolic stimulant with actions on the hindbrain and that it was not an aversive therapy for addiction like antabuse. Despite mounting evidence that the dopamine pleasure and reward circuits may be an important final common pathway in the neurobiology of addiction by the late 1970s apomorphine had disappeared from its last strongholds of Scandinavia and Switzerland.

By this time the honeymoon period of L-DOPA was long over and many of my patients were experiencing a chaotic roller coaster ride, which some of them incorrectly attributed as a tolerance to their medication. Through the 1980s I intensified my search for a cure for this incapacitating 'on off syndrome' that was ruining lives. I re-read *Deposition: Testimony Concerning a Sickness* where Burroughs had described the 'algebra of need' and how apomorphine had helped him kick heroin. A few nights later the structural formula of apomorphine floated by me in a dream.

This triggered a series of experiments at the Middlesex Hospital,

Mortimer Street first on myself and then on volunteers with Parkinson's disease that now looking back I consider my most lasting achievement in medicine. Delivery of apomorphine by a mini-pump smoothed out the patients' oscillations and returned their independence. A man who was barely able to walk or speak for six hours each day told me that apomorphine had turned the clock back five years. Not long after our paper had been published in *The Lancet* apomorphine returned once again to the British Pharmacopoeia.

It was around this time that I was contacted by two of Doctor Dent's daughters, Ann Rubinstein and Jane Sweeney. On our first meeting Ann handed me a copy of her father's book *Anxiety and its Treatment* first published in 1940 and an article written by one of his patients, the Macmillan publisher Alan Maclean which began:

> I'd heard of an eccentric elderly doctor called John Dent who was said to offer a swift chemical treatment with no psychiatric strings. He'd successfully treated the film director Anthony Asquith, the uncle of Mark Bonham-Carter, who'd been observing my drinking habits with increasing alarm. At least he didn't sound like the pin-striped proprietor of some expensive torture chamber with panoramic views across London from Harrow-on-the-Hill. So I rang him up and got my head bitten off. When I mentioned Asquith's name he said he didn't discuss his patients. Who was I? and What did I want? I said help was what I wanted and that at last seemed to be the right answer.
>
> Dent opened the door in his braces. Short, portly, shaggy white hair and moustache to match, he wore a Savage Club tie loosely knotted halfway down his front. He looked like an old dog... and had 'the loudest laugh of any man in London'.

I joined Ann and Jane in their campaign to encourage more research into addiction and a re-investigation of their father's notion that very anxious people were particularly susceptible to substance dependence. Echoing Dent, Burroughs had drawn comparisons between the need of diabetics for insulin and junkies for dope. There were also similarities between the treatment approaches we were using to help Parkinson's disease and those our colleagues in endocrinology were using to help brittle diabetics. Unfortunately the highly conservative and politicised world of drug addiction remained unresponsive to our campaign despite the fact that the success rate in the treatment of alcoholism remained low and the use of methadone as maintenance therapy was involved in the death of hundreds of heroin addicts.

Twenty years later I met two of their children Warwick Sweeney and Antonia Rubinstein, both of whom were as passionate as their mothers had been about the lack of progress in the management of alcoholism and drug addiction. Warwick told me, 'For me it goes much deeper still. I am interested in the politics of addiction. I also share my grandfather's taste in literature. All his books filled my home growing up, Sterne, Swift and Wells. Everything is environment. It was inevitable that he rubbed off on me.'

Antonia later confided in me over a drink at the Groucho Club in Soho that within the family Warwick was considered John Dent reincarnate, sharing both many of his views and his physical appearance.

When I was writing *Mentored by a Madman: The William Burroughs Experiment* I entered into an intense and fruitful epistolary exchange with Warwick and learned a great deal about his grandfather, some of which I included in my own fanatasia. In a world where inebriety was a shameful weakness, gay sex a criminal offence and abortion illegal Dent had been prepared to treat individuals at the point of need using a 'Robin Hood' business model to run his practice before the National Health Service was founded.

Despite his lack of political nous and distaste for public office he had also served dutifully as the Secretary of the Society for the Study of Addiction from 1944–47 and was in the middle of a second term of office when he treated William Burroughs. He had also been the

Editor of the *British Journal of Inebriety* since 1941 (now the *British Journal of Addiction*).

He believed strongly that the British Government's decision to severely restrict medical practitioners using heroin to treat addiction was wrong. In 1955 he wrote:

> ...if doctors are forbidden to prescribe heroin or prevented from obtaining it very soon they will not be able to treat their patients except with medicines prescribed from Whitehall, or the American Bureau of Mr Anslinger [the first commissioner of the US Treasury Department's Federal Bureau of Narcotics and an advocate of the prohibition and criminalisation of drugs].

If alive he would also have condemned the 1968 policy change that put an end to the unique 'British system' that had allowed GP's to keep addicts away from dealers by prescribing them hard drugs.

I feel sure he would also have supported the work of the Welsh psychiatrist John Marks whose prescription of heroin on a Home Office licence in his drug dependency clinic in Widnes between 1982 and the early nineties markedly reduced crime, prostitution and drug related deaths including those from AIDS on Merseyside. His harm reduction approach also reduced the actual number of addicts and killed off the pyramid selling schemes. Marks received support and protection from prominent members of the Drugs Squad including Bing Spear, the Chief Inspector of the Government's Drug Inspectorate, but eventually the Government manoeuvred him out and like Dent's apomorphine his successful experiment was expunged from the history books.

Both men were at the end of the line when Burroughs consulted Dent. Burroughs was hooked on junk and unable to write while Dent was denigrated by his profession as a maverick. Almost all Burroughs' previous consultations with doctors had been disappointing. The New York psychiatrists who had misdiagnosed him with paranoid schizophrenia and then tried to straighten him out with Freudian analysis and hypnotherapy were well meaning frauds while the 'croakers' who had supplied him with dope on the upper west side of Manhattan were no better than drug pushers. Dent and Burroughs were both iconoclasts with a strong distaste for consumerism and globalisation. They fed on one another, exchanged stories and discussed subjects of mutual interest like the Maya civilisation and cats. Although Dent's approach to Burroughs was formal it was fraternal and less patronising or unequal than most of the consultations he had experienced up until then. Most importantly Dent's approach was non-judgemental. The two men shared a fierce integrity and brutal honesty as well as a moral indignation at the vested interests of corporations, drug cartels and Big Pharma that profited from stoking anxieties. Dent was also a good writer who had published two books so was in a position to advise and encourage Burroughs in his writing.

In the end Burroughs, at a pivotal moment in his life, came to trust and like Dent.

Anyone who has read Willliam Burroughs' books will know that they are full of frightening doctors who epitomise power and control. The amoral Doctors Benway and and Lymph in *Naked Lunch* may have been Burroughs' revenge for the corruption that he felt defined contemporary doctorhood.

Then there is Dr Tetrazzini who starts his list by throwing a scalpel across the room into the patient and then making his grand entrance like a ballet dancer. The discovery of a tumour throws him into a temper 'fucking undisciplined cells' he snarled advancing on his target like a matador.

Whether Dent ever told Burroughs medical anecdotes is unknown but Underhill the incompetent honorary visiting surgeon at Dudley Guest Hospital during Dent's training has close similarities to both Benway and Tetrazzini:

> Underhill peered into the man's abdomen.
> 'NOW, what's this, eh?'
> 'A kidney, sir?' suggested Dent, astounded at what was unfolding.

'Are we sure?'

'Quite sure.'

'And this?'

'The other kidney, sir, most definitely,' said Dent. Dalton cursed under his breath.

'So, this is the appendix?'

'No, sir,' said Dalton wearily, 'I think you'll find that that is the spleen.'

'The spleen. Good God! What the devil's it doing here?!'

'There's the appendix,' indicated Dalton, pointing to a perfectly healthy organ.

'But can we be sure? London?'

'There's no doubt about it, sir; Dalton is correct, that is the appendix.'

'Wonderful, SO, my boy, we've located the offender and now the punishment. We'll cut the blighter out, right out! Save this poor man, in the nick of time by the look of it. Scissors. SCISSORS, Nurse, come a-long!'

Burroughs was hypochondriacal, adept at self-medicating and frequently advised his friends and acquaintances on medical matters. His relationship with doctors was complex and ambiguous. He saw himself as a sort of healer among his associates and had enrolled for a medical degree at the University of Wien in the hope of one day becoming a psychiatrist.

Much of John Dent's medical career occurred before the formation of the National Health Service. Doctors had far more power and professional freedom than is the case today. The main pre-occupation of the General Medical Council was with breaches of confidentiality rather than medical mistakes or incompetence. Dent was prepared to break convention if his conscience told him he was doing the right thing. He was a charismatic persuasive force for good and also a cute judge of what he could get away with. He believed in what he did and also why he was doing it and there can be no doubt that this rubbed off on his anxious and addicted patients who desperately wanted and needed him to succeed.

Driven by opportunist Members of Parliament, a series of scandals and the media, doctors now find they face opprobrium and a degree of regulation that is neither logical nor necessary. Growing distrust of the medical profession has led to a number of undesirable complications including an increasing reluctance by patients to accept 'a wait and see' approach often leading to over-investigation. 'Do no harm' has been replaced by 'Watch your back, cover your ass and harm be damned'. A growing disrespect for medical science and the institutions of medicine has also encouraged alternative practitioners, government officials and the fourth estate to feel comfortable attacking doctors even to the point of perversely further undermining medical care. The new breed of NHS doctor will be well trained in communicating but only able to provide formal, contractual services, from an agreed menu of options, as requested by the consumer patient. Creativity and imagination will be displaced by a system of smiling doctors working to protect their contractually defined interests rather than rebelling against the indignities of disease.

In the current climate and despite his reputation as being one of the 'best around' for treating alcoholics Dent would have been given a hard time by the new incumbents at the Home Office. His use of diminishing doses of heroin during the acute withdrawal phase would have probably involved him going for a period of retraining ('brainwashing by "The Maudsley Mafia"' as he would have called it) and he would be forced to submit to a paper mountain of mind numbing red tape.

Alcoholism kills millions of people every year and iatrogenic synthetic opioid dependence has reached epidemic proportions in parts of the United States yet Western governments continue to shy away from investigating alternative non-maintenance approaches to the management of addiction. Although John Yerbury Dent was considered an outdated fossil by the new medical establishment his ability to communicate on an equal footing with his patients about their illnesses and its management and his willingness to go that extra distance if he felt it was in his patients' interest put many of them to shame. He also merits posthumous fame, even though he would never have sought it, for his early warning of how medicine was in danger of being corrupted into an instrument of social control, a view shared and promulgated in *Naked Lunch* by his most famous patient William Burroughs. *Hardy Tree* is a book of contemporary relevance. It reminds us that medicine is a calling not a business, and an art not a science.

– A. J. Lees
London, August 2018

Acknowledgements

The episodes in the first part (odd numbers) spring directly from Dent's unpublished memoirs *Medici Libris – A Doctor's Bible* and bequeathed to me. These were copied and edited by Rhoda Brenan who also wrote the letter which concludes the story. To her and her grandson, Nic Cary, I am deeply indebted. Other examples of correspondence included are copied verbatim. In the second part (for the first time in print) all London addresses and even phone numbers are accurate and I have stuck to specific dates and times where possible.

I must devote unreserved thanks to my mother and aunts who apart from being able to corroborate details were also able to offer recollections and insight into how their father may or may not have reacted in certain situations. Of course, family history, private correspondence and personal memories inform both stories but the majority of ideas and the strength of their ethos reside firmly within the public domain.

The main texts are numerous; editorials from the Society for the Study of Addiction, press cuttings, umpteen books, medical reports and scientific papers. Chief among these are several publications by William Seward Burroughs and two by John Yerbury Dent but Alan Maclean's and Patrick Riddell's autobiographies have also contributed.

    Many other agreeable personalities have helped.
    In the beginning there was Christian Brett sending me a samizdat

copy of *APO-33* (Beach Books, 1968) and who has also bookended the project by typesetting *Hardy Tree* with care and imagination. This was followed by a circumstantial meeting with Charlie Lowe a very fine man who opened my eyes to the tortured world of drugs, politics and science.

Thanks to Jim Pennington who with dogged curiosity unearthed some extraordinary and significant 'finds' and also provided the London photographic portrait of Burroughs taken by Harriet Crowder.

I have relied throughout on archival research which is by no means exhaustive particularly as I believe this is an unfinished history. The London Metropolitan Archive, The Black Country Museum, Friend's House, 174 Euston Road, and The Henry W. and Albert Berg Collection at the New York Public Library have all corroborated many details. Burroughs' nurses Mary Gibson and Hannah Mason-Jones whose diligent professionalism and care is evidenced by the 'Day and Night Reports' housed and supplied by the NYPL (Berg) have been critical. Conversations and correspondence with Ian Macfadyen, Oliver Harris, Tim Gluckman, Isabelle Baudron, Dominic Thackray, Jamie Greco and Christian Brett have all offered Burroughsian insight though not necessarily adopted. All opinion and interpretation is mine but wherever possible based on the triangulation of events; interlocking texts, vocabulary, circumstance and memory.

Along the route of neurobiological pathways I have been helped unstintingly and encouraged throughout by neurologist Andrew Lees. His gentle wisdom from the sidelines has helped get the ball over the line. Closer to home, my family. Brother Simon has been a constant ally, Phil and Derek Barker, Andrew Buchanan, Emma Friedmann, Lyn Wait, Antonia Rubinstein and Zac Russell have all contributed and in different ways. Amongst my friends Jonathan Naess and Neil

ACKNOWLEDGEMENTS

Ross have been rock solid sounding boards and, specific to certain chapters or themes, my friendships with Linda Aryaeenia, Chloe Double, Ranjan Balakumaran, Michael Connolly, Robin Lawrence, Gee Vaucher, Lydia Dickie, Penny Rimbaud, Andy McGeeney, Ben Fargen, Cat Duerden, Leonard Winkler and Brian Pearce have been critical and illuminating. To Kathy Whalen at Incline Press for her critical eye. All your acts of kindness, small or large, are highly valued and in some way form part of the whole. Thank you.

Ultimately my deepest gratitude and respect shall remain with all the participants of the story. Men and women who lived, variously suffered and triumphed. All are now dead and this book is dedicated to their memory.

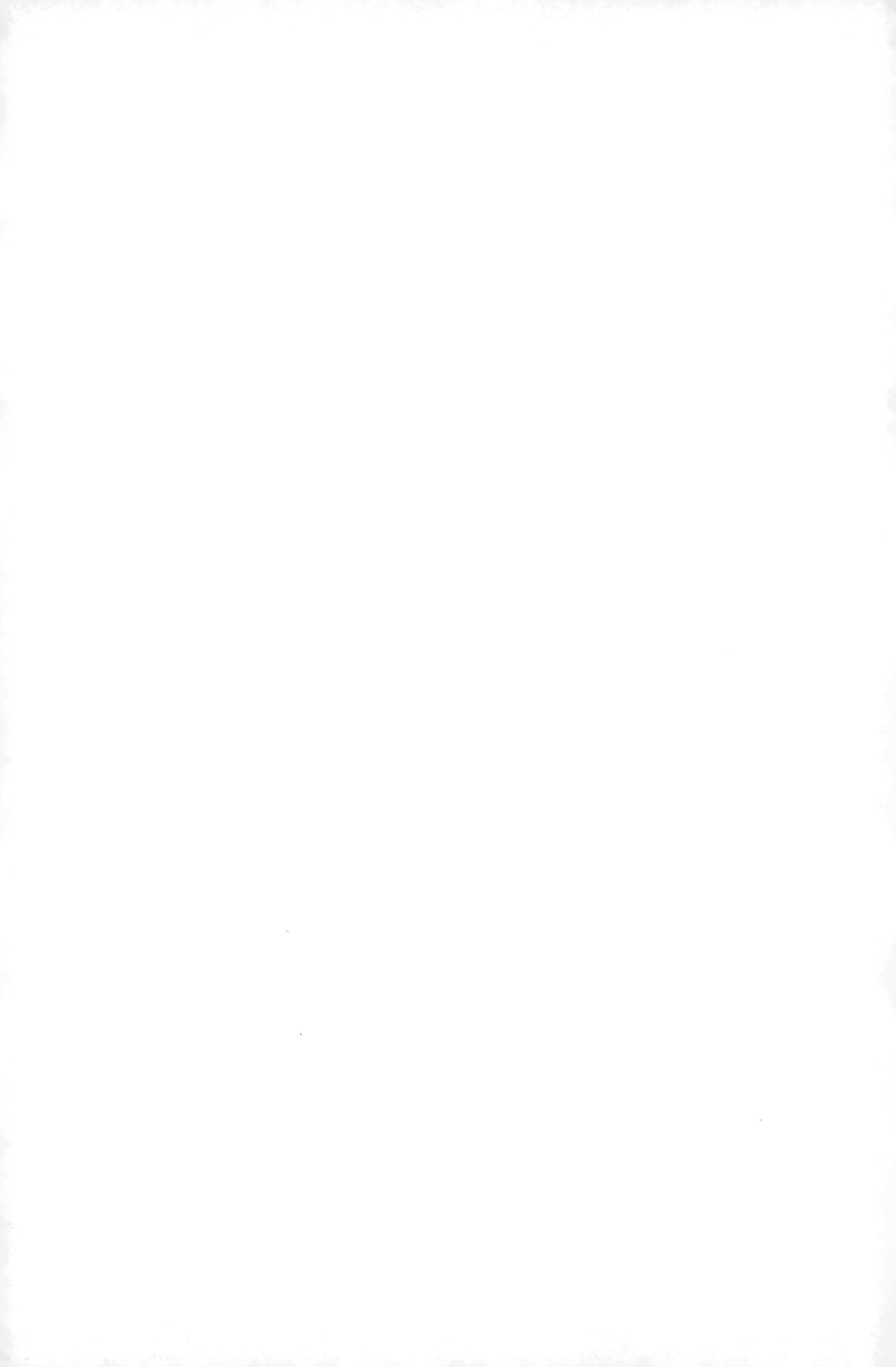

HARDY TREE

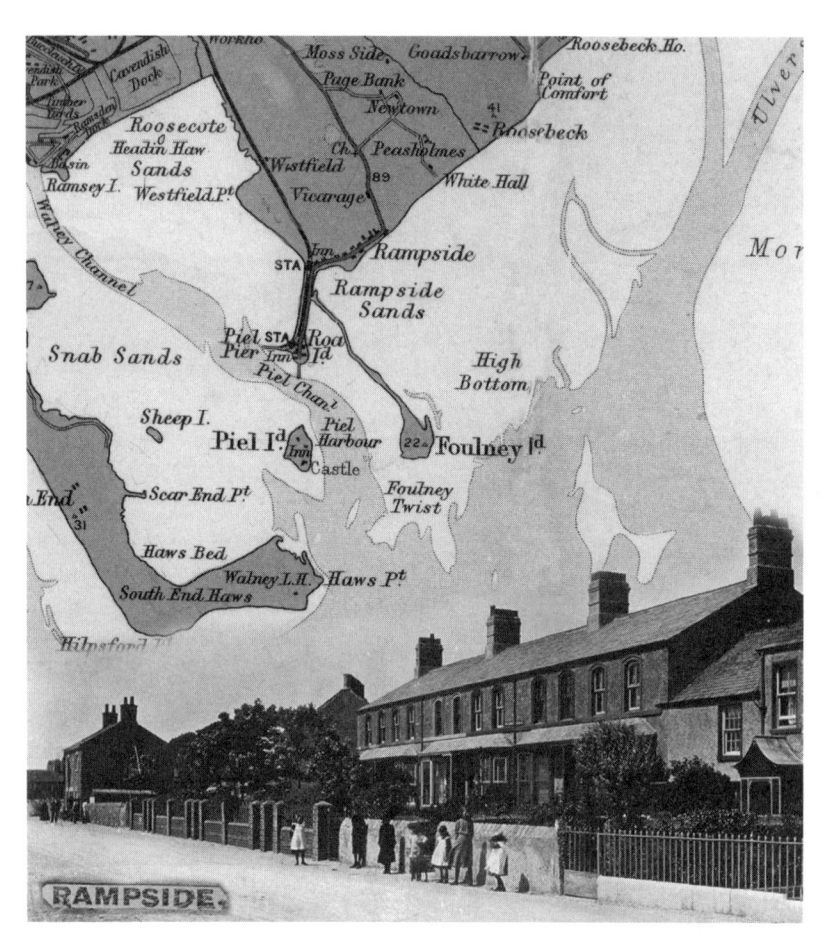

Rampside village lines the northwest rim of Morecambe Bay and overlooks the sedimentary spit and tidal island, Foulney.

I

Rampside

The dripping slate and sandstone figures have turned their backs to the wind. Stirred by sounds of weathering they recall ofttimes when they heard the same in life. Times when, formed of softer materials, they huddled on quaysides longing for boats... and cheered each other with words of solace and hope....

The churchyard is exposed. Its rugged stone wall, buckled by sycamores, rings a lonely church plugged with lime and roughcast. Lower down, across sodden fields, lie two rows of broken-toothed cottages; a thin smile forced out between salt marsh and the gaping expanse of sky and space. This is the borderland between Cumbria and Lancashire and the home of Rampside, a modest, coastal village.

In such a place it is possible to read its history from the physical. The impressions of floods, storms, shipwrecks, even earthquakes offer a trajectory of wonder confined only by the boundary stones of imagination. But if the enormity of this yawning landscape pierced with the cries of migrating birds proves too daunting you can pluck a detail from the shore or hedgerow and peer at it in the shell of your hand; a beetle perhaps...a pebble...a feather. Everything has origins which can help plumb the depths of the past. It is up to us...shallow or deep ...shallow or deep.... Sometimes, the wind seems aware of this mysterious dialogue and suggests clues. It is on nothing more that this story starts, the bright air drawing back the eternal sighs of stage and scene.

Late one afternoon a wayfarer came to Rampside. Pausing, he listened to the pitch of the breeze amid a tangle of buckthorn and tried to match the whistle with his own. Suddenly the cry of a bird silenced him. 'Pee-whit' it shrilled while soaring and plunging overhead seemingly for no other reason than unbridled joy. The traveller marvelled at the bird's tumbling virtuosity... his eyes unable to keep pace with its blissfully mad and helter-skelter flight. 'That bird's riffs and freewheeling majesty highlight my earthbound ways,' he mused, grinning. 'Magical,' he whispered and continued his way along the coast.

As he faded from view a low sun sprinkled its gold dust over waving grass heads and along a stone wall leading to Rampside's Meeting House. Inside, the village elders leant towards one another and discussed whether to add a white-washed bell-tower to the seafarers chapel above the village. The talk was earnest, the views fervently expressed, the billowing tobacco smoke grew dense. They were close to making a momentous decision.

'It could be a life-saving and navigational landmark,' urged one of the most venerated, scratching the back of his hand with his stubbled chin. 'It'd 'elp cocklers and winklers too,' he added to murmurs of approval.

'Aye,' said another, raising his pewter tankard towards the sea, "Oot thar the tide outstrips a runnin' man.'

'A gallopin' 'oss,' declared another, his voice as turbulent as the dark waters in the bay. 'A whole family washed away winklin' last year...'

This comment drew a murmur of remembrance and assent underscored by a tattoo of rapping on the broad oak table.

And so in 1840 the church tower was built. It pleased the community for this was a deed prompted by Christian fellowship and pushed to fruition by benign purpose. Two decades later it was rumoured that the sight of the bell-tower had saved more souls than its Sunday toll. This impiety gathered credence when the congregation started to shrink. At first this was not dwelt upon but by the 1880s it dominated every parish meeting.

'Down again,' grumbled the chief elder.

'St Michael'z too far away. In winter it'za mighty long walk up for some.'

'Ain't 'owt t' do wi' where the church iz,' objected another, wryly, 'itz 'coz the new parson ain't accepted yet.'

RAMPSIDE

This caused a stir and some vigorous pipe smoking.

One of the elders, steadfastly loyal to the previous clergyman, bowed to one side like a skiff in a gale and mumbled to his friend: 'Aye, an' that's cos ee'z nither use nor ornament.'

'Nor ever will be!' agreed his comrade.

The minister in question, Reverend John Park, an impressively tall and erudite man with bushy sideburns, got wind of the mutterings and grew anxious that his sermons had become too priestly, too suggestive of a lofty tone. Knowing the Bible backwards had, early in his career, attracted much admiring notice from his peers, even the occasional visiting academic. However, among Rampsiders, his penchant for Latin and canonical orthodoxy cut no ice. Worse, it had aroused self-doubt that no amount of flattery or nostalgia for his Cambridge days could dispel. The more he worried the more he wrestled with the reasons for his inadequacy. Congregations are notoriously devoted to the previous incumbent, he told himself. He was an 'incomer', after all, all the way from Pennington, near Ulverstone, a full ten miles away. But the main problem, he was starting to appreciate, was that Rampsiders are not easily made and showed no sign of turning. His anxiety was confirmed by every cruel cough and shuffle from the pews and the increasing number of empty places among them. This demonstrated his inability to engage with 'his' flock on *their* terms, but sadly he knew no other way. He persisted with his biblical tone and the congregation continued to dwindle. 'Oh dear!' he lamented, 'I am a trier condemned to failure.' He was close to despair. Then out of the blue a solution came to him, as welcome as summer's first swallow. Putting down the Good Book he dashed from the vicarage to find his elder sister Harriet.

'Please,' he implored, 'if you could listen to my sermon on Saturday and engender within it the common touch.'

What on earth! She wondered, continuing to dust the rolling board. She had never even learnt to read or write so how was it possible that her self-assured and highly educated brother should be asking her for help? And, of all things, with his sermon? Without reacting she took in the clues as if they were ingredients for a recipe. She let them fall between the deep folds of her bright mind. One by one Reason's fingers sifted them till, balanced with her quiet ways, one method stood out. She was pleased with her solution but this would be difficult for it meant standing up to her brother. This was something neither she nor any of their four younger sisters had ever done. She took a deep breath and arranged her argument in apple pie order. Nobody provides a wedding cake without making a few loaves first.

'Well, John,' she started, 'I 'av bin thinkin' aboot me aches an' pains. An' the troop oop that hill ain't gettin' shorter.' Her brother nodded. 'Or easier,' she stressed. He nodded again. 'An' ais sure the girls gi' you all the support they can and will allus do. An' Mary iz practising 'er organ scales, you 'av my word on that.'

'Is she?' asked her brother doubtfully, thinking how everyone felt obliged to tolerate sister Mary's tuneless performances.

'Oh, yes, she iz doin' 'er best,' said Harriet, wincing at a catalogue of discordant memories. 'Probly needs a tad more experience,' she fibbed. 'And Emma. She will continue runnin' the reading school.'

'Yes,' agreed brother John, 'all the children love her stories.'

Harriet thought she should keep her next point to herself, namely, she actually drew no comfort from religion. It was only family unity that forced her to endure the weekly tramp to church; nothing at all to do with the admonishments of sin from that awful creaking pulpit even if the pulpiteer was her religiously devoted brother.

'Well... and?' urged John, a touch of fret in his voice.

'Aye, well,' continued Harriet, leaning against the dresser, 'I know I ain't skollally but if I 'as listened and corrected your words on Saturday...' she hesitated, '...why the 'eck shud I have t' listen back to meself on Sunday?'

'What are you saying, Harriet?' he blurted, trying to deny what he'd heard.

'Wha'oim sayin' John iz, 'elp deserves 'elp,' she said.

'You will be doing God a great service if you make this sacrifice,' he pitched, his voice weakening.

'Never mind 'im,' she said leaning forward and thumping the pastry with the rolling pin. 'I agree to your wishes if you scooze me from attendin'!'

'What?!' John's jaw sagged like an empty clothes line, his sense of fraternal entitlement cut from under him.

'That'z me offer, tek it or leave it.'

A stunned silence was marked by the parlour clock's tick-tockety-tack. Nobody knew what vintage the timepiece was, but its black casing, rough oak boxing and tarnished face suggested it might be as old as time itself. Harriet secretly corrected it twice a day but she'd throw herself in the waves before giving up on her treasured clock.

'An' then, while you're oop there savin' folk from the fires of hell,' she chimed, 'I'll be doon 'ere cookin'. Then we'll 'av 'ot instead o' cold. It'd be mighty welcome in winter, it shall.' Her argument was watertight. She raised her eyebrows in anticipation of the inevitable.

'Well, yes, I suppose so,' mumbled John looking at the floor.

'Settled then,' she grinned and thumped the pastry once more. 'You an' the 'hole family can 'av Sunday lunch 'ere afta. Earthly rewards for angels that ain't flyin' yet.'

He nodded, choosing to ignore Harriet's irreverence. 'Very well,' he coughed. 'We shall all benefit, the blessed congregation and our wonderful family. The Lord be praised for his blessed providence.'

And so it came to be. Every Saturday night as Harriet prepared the Sunday roast with all its fixings, brother John would read her his sermons. Occasionally, she let his pious homilies go but on other occasions her preference for 'tellin' it blunt' would bring him down to Earth with a bump.

'What's that, yer bampot?'

'A reference to Satan.'

'Well, speak plain. Tha knows if y' sayz "beast" folk'll think cows.'

He duly simplified his references while Harriet peeled, boiled and baked. She was in her element; a culinary cloud of flour and steam dispensing common sense as easy as pie. As beneficial as this domestic synod became it also provided Harriet with a new lease of life. She quickly rose to the challenge and occasionally suggested whole themes for sermons. Her sisters would nod knowingly to one another as 'ole' 'Arriet's homespun' rained down from the pulpit. Relative to their learned brother each of his five sisters considered themselves 'unedicated' but Harriet's 'gift o' gab' reflected their shared, no-nonsense approach to life. In any case, with Harriet's advanced age, her being childless and the best cook for miles, they warmed to this arrangement which nowadays might be termed 'community benefit'. The congregation swelled and John Park rapidly became an extremely contented and popular parson with further opportunities to cement his reputation by performing his other duties; part-time lawyer and doctor.

His 'doctoring' was not complicated as he only prescribed one medicine: port. If things got difficult he would write to his youngest sister Daisy's husband for advice. He was a 'real' doctor with a practice in London. Sometimes, though, in emergencies, he was obliged to send for Dr Crank from Ulverstone.

Crank was an enormous man of twenty stone, perpetually red-faced, and always arrived at the homes of the ill in a flurry of consternation. Eased down from his pony and trap he would insist on a hearty lunch while he listened to the patient's list of ailments. The treatment was always the same; port. Indeed, Crank had so much faith in this remedy that he took it himself before, during and after his meal.

'Never fails,' he'd tell his patient.

'But Ize ulready tekkin' it,' would often come the baleful reply.

Crank would interrupt his chewing of a chicken leg and fix the afflicted with a cold stare. 'Well double the dose, man. Try it before bed, warmed with cinnamon and feverfew if you must. You'll be right as rain in a week. That'll be half a guinea.'

One Saturday John Park discussed this state of affairs with Harriet.

'The pity of it is,' he said, 'nobody can call for Crank until they're stocked up with what he likes to dispense and consume.'

'Well, that ain't fair,' indicated his sister.

'Oh? And why is that?'

'Coz only a few in the parish can afford port. Why should only 'em that can buy it get the great and valid attention of Dr Crank, mm?'

'My!' said John, blind to his sister's sarcasm, 'that really is very unfair.'

Harriet thought for a moment.

''Ere, tell you what. Why not put quinine in the port you giv'oot?'

'I'm not with you, Harriet, how would that help?'

'Well, it wunt do owt to port but change its taste. Mek it horrid, like medicine should be.'

'You've lost me, Harriet.'

'Oh dear, yer daft 'ayperth. If the port you give is foul t' taste the man o' 'owse ain't goin' t' drink all of it hisself, is 'ee?'

'An',' prompted Harriet, with a sparkle in her eye, 'this can be the subject o' yer sermun tomorrer. Get yer pen ready.'

'What a good idea! There's Timothy 5:23, Corinthians 9, I think, and…'

'No, John, no!' Harriet clapped her hands in front of her brother's blinking eyes. 'Tell 'em straight, so they know 'ow t' 'elp 'emselves…'

'Yes, of course. I get carried away.'

'And the booty of it iz, Daisy's comin' oop from Smoke later. She'll tek this message back, to 'er 'usband, an orl 'iz doctah friends.' Harriet spread her arms. 'All o' Lunnon town will 'ear aboot it. Sing yer praises, they will.'

'Oh, do you think so?'

Harriet sighed and answered him with a look.

Sister Daisy arrived late with her three-year-old son and, exhausted by the journey, went straight to bed. The next morning she rose late and dashed up to the church, anxious not to miss a moment. She was taken aback to find such a large congregation and that their usual places under the pulpit were taken. Not everything had changed however; Mary's organ playing still reminded her of a novice believing she were Schubert. The singing was worse; a murder of crows believing they were songbirds. After a tortured rendition of 'Rock of Ages' the congregation folded into the pews. A sudden veil of silence descended, prompted by eager anticipation of their week's highlight: the sermon. John Park climbed the rickety steps of the pulpit and stood tall.

'I chose the hymn "Rock of Ages",' he started, 'because I wanted to explore the meaning of the line in the opening verse: *"Be of sin the double cure, cleanse me from its guilt and power"*. You may find this strange but I see a match in those words to the number of troubled souls in the midst of our parish. It is, you see, both the *"guilt"* and the *"power"* of sin that must be recognised for what it is. We must accept that by searching for salvation from our ills we admit temptation. Now I can tell from some of your faces that you are mystified as to where this temptation lies. Well, for illness, for the ache and the lassitude of the mind and body it is the custom to offer the cure of port. I have been tasked many times to conform to this practice of using port as medicine but I ask, is it not true that this practice introduces calamity more intolerable than any disease it fights?'

He paused, believing his words were standing as tall as he.

'So, let us return to that line you sang so delightfully just a minute ago: *"the double cure, cleanse me from its guilt and power"*, because is it not true that wine and spirit provide short lift but eternal agonies? The double cure is the realisation that free from temptation we shall enjoy the full beneficence of the Lord. Our exultant hearts cleansed by temperance, will rejoice in His love.'

John Park beamed down upon the packed rows of his admiring parishioners. At last, he could see the irrefutable evidence of his magnetic and illuminating thoughts. Standing room only and such a golden silence. His face shone like the sun.

'I have noticed, too,' he said firmly, edging towards his sister's parochial themes, 'how the good and happy farmer in the fields hereabouts only grows enough barley to exactly fit his needs and how he is the first to benefit most from such prudent practice. And so, I have decided to continue to dispense port when it be required but with a preference for not prescribing it at all!' John Park paused to straighten his crimson robe. 'So friends, as our cordial parish stands exultant in the brightness of Our Lord's ordained path, hereafter, when medicine be necessary I shall only dispense it mixed with quinine. This, like the contented farmer, will give us a happier, healthier community. Imagine, if you can, two boats that leave from Roa Harbour. One is awash with liquor and the other with honest toil and purpose. Ask yourselves which is most likely to run aground and end up dashed upon the rocks? And which, blameless and free of intoxication, is able to labour upon the waves and return brimful with an abundant harvest dispensing fortune and favour upon us all? To our well-clothed, well-fed and learned families?'

'Hallelujah,' a fisherman cried from the back.

'And imagine the pain I feel when pressed to administer help to the ill and sick who, isolated by a life wasted, must spend their final years in the agonies of shame. A man scarcely able to look another in the eye. And consider the sight of the fallen man when the air is stained with profanity forced to lie amid the rancour of remorse caused by drunkenness. Imagine too the pain visited upon a true man of God having to endure the heckling shriek of ugly laughter from the wanton woman in the city street. These are the things which make a thoughtful man sick at heart. But, worshippers, this is the intolerable practice I am urged to contribute towards with bottles of liquor. It is a remedy for fools which can only accelerate the destruction of Man's true Nature, all his social sensibilities and self-respect.'

There was a rumble of agreement throughout the congregation and two more 'Hallelujahs'.

'And so, in conclusion, be of good heart and stay with your strong constitutions delivered by God and bestowed upon the righteous. No more will I sanction the prescription of port alone unless it be laced with quinine. This will ensure it is only to be used as medicine.'

'God is love' someone cried and John Park welcomed the intervention.

'Yes,' he concluded, raising his palms towards the rafters, 'a good life is a temperate life and the true gateway to heaven. Amen.'

Daisy gulped. She picked up her small son and hurried back down the hill to Harriet. She must get there before the others... and brother John himself.

Daisy burst into the parlour, 'So, John's doin' al reet, after a sticky start?' she gasped.

'Eez holdin' hiz oon, aye,' Harriet replied, attracted to her nephew playing with his Mother's hair ribbon.

'Oh Harriet! Eze doin' better than that! I admit he lost me a bit at the beginning of his sermon, but the rest of it was wonderful. He spoke to the villagers as if he's one of them. The church was packed and people hanging around afterwards chatting about reading school and games for the children, just like old times.'

'I s'pose,' said Harriet, refusing to share her sister's enthusiasm.

Daisy tried to catch her sister's eye but she wasn't playing. She realised that Harriet may have been prepared to help their brother dilute his high church mannerisms but she also knew that Harriet was modest to a fault. Daisy weighed up her options. Like her sister she too could be determined. Furthermore, her years away from home, in London, had eroded some of the blind deference she was expected to have for any man. She decided to press.

'His good ideas are yours, ain't they?' she insisted, passing her son into the welcoming arms of Harriet.

'Not at all!'

'And 'iz 'port and quinine? Is that 'iz?' she quizzed, knowing full well that it was not.

'Course!' exclaimed Harriet. 'John took a while to settle, iz orl.'

Daisy shrugged and changed her tack.

'Iz eet like Bessie Brownbag's potion?' she suggested, with a giggle.

'What yo' sayin'?' Harriet peered at her sister.

'You remember, the Jolly boys at pace eggin'?'

Daisy moved across the parlour and clapped her hands before announcing in a dramatically low voice:

> *I've a likkle bottle in me pock'ole. Dat'll cure the itch,*
> *the stitch, an' mek'ole dead lamb's tail twitch.*

Harriet laughed, glad that the tenor of conversation had switched. Undermining her brother's fragile confidence would serve nobody. She turned her nephew around on her knee.

'I know owz t' mek a tail twitch,' she cried, tickling him. As she did she was reminded of her part in the resurrection play that Rampside celebrated every Easter.

> *We're three jolly toss pots, all uv one mind.*
> *We coom a pace-eggin' an' 'ope yo prove kind.*

She pulled a face which her nephew tried to copy. This exchange continued until they were joined by the rest of the family. After lunch, with her nephew back on her knee, Harriet dipped in and out of nursery rhymes. Her favourite never failed to make him cry with laughter:

> *This is the way the lady rides, niminy, niminy nim.*
> *This is the way the gentleman rides, trottity, trottity, trot.*
> *This is the way the farmer rides, bumpity bumpity bump.*
> *This is the way the huntsman rides, gallopy, GALLOPY GOOO!*

Daisy clapped along, and glowed with approval at the bond growing before her eyes. From under the wainscot like mist from the marsh an invisible balm enclosed the family, a swoon of bonhomie and unity. She thought of the 'God is love,' cry that had interrupted her brother's sermon. 'Love,' she tacitly acknowledged, 'the best medicine of all.'

That evening, with her son fast asleep, Daisy put down her book and leant towards her sister.
'Next summer, if I bring 'im oop, can 'ee stay 'ere wi' you?'
Harriet looked up from her darning. 'And you back in Smoke?'
'Aye.'
'It'd be no bother.'
And so, just like Harriet's arrangement with her brother, another family custom was established. Daisy's son from the age of four spent all his summers at Rampside under the care and guidance of Aunt Harriet. Only a day into his first visit he re-christened her 'Nanty', a

combination of 'nan' and 'auntie'. The name stuck and was soon adopted by the rest of the family, who had never much cared for 'Harriet'.

Not to be outdone, Nanty had many nicknames for her nephew. They were all terms of respect and fondness, his favourites being 'm'big mon' or 'big John' which made him feel grown up and accepted in his 'home from home'. When he was about eight or nine he began to unfavourably compare his real home in London with Nanty's due to its associations with the drudgery of school, exams and formality. Rampside wasn't like this; it came with no conceits. Provided he behaved as he was treated, he could be himself and do as he liked. Quite naturally he soon grew to love this place more than any other; it became his heaven on Earth. Nanty too started to count the days after April. She welcomed the summer migrants that always came, the golden plover and the arctic tern, but it was her 'wee mon' she longed for most.

'Nanty?' he enquired, when he was ten years old.

'Aye,' she replied.

'When can we walk to Fooley Island?' There was a suggestive note in his voice.

'Depends, pet,' she replied, looking into his open, blue eyes.

'And when we're out there will we see your island?'

'Y' mean "Seldom Seen"?'

'Yes.'

'Ah dunno.'

'Why?'

'It cooms an' goos, that's why.'

'What do you mean, "cooms an' goos"?' he mimicked her flat vowels.

'You'll see.'

'So when can we go?'

'D'pens.'

'On what?'

'Thar knows. Oop 'ere, one eye on t'weather an' t'uther on tide, 'owt else.' She made a rough calculation on her fingers. 'Mebbe Thursday... mebbe Friday... we'll see.'

He accepted the explanation. There were forces greater than even Nanty could control. That night he lay in bed thinking about where these forces lay... and what moved them. Of course, he'd heard talk of the terrible Rampside earthquake in 1865. Everybody nodded ruefully about that.

He got out of bed and crept across the floorboards to the window ledge and watched as the day drained away to the west. A gleaming light on the coast blinked twice and was gone. Soon, even the half-light would be spirited away. A breeze rustled the brittle leaves of an old apple tree; he shivered and climbed back into bed. A squall was coming.

As he grew drowsy he saw the world as a gull might – flying over salt marsh and miles of sinking mud with holes that could bury a ship. He glided on over dark waters rolling with the ebb, over the shallows where waves broke over black-blistered bladderwrack up to the high water mark; the soft sand and moon-white shells. This was the remote coast of 'Seldom Seen', a soft mist melting into one diaphanous deception after another; mountainous dunes, a storm tossed forest and waterfalls turned to spray and fog. Then, finally, his destination; a crenelated castle built of nothing but dark air. A granite-grey shadow holding a square of primrose light, a latticed casement of misshapen glass. He peered through... and fell asleep in seconds...

Downstairs Nanty simmered the first ripenings of summer fruit for jam. These were the best of times, when the garden repaid for the graft put in. As she labelled a dozen jars her concentration wavered to her 'big yoong mon' upstairs and the fun they'd have on their day's trek into Foulney's wilderness. She recalled his first or second visit to Rampside, when he'd crawled to the end of the garden beyond the gooseberry. She liked this and called it 'venturin'. It was something she would indulge because she liked it too; to go to the end of things. It didn't matter what or where; paths, roads, piers, even islands. With pleasure she noticed that he often gazed wistfully towards Roa and

Piel Island. Little did she know that almost a century earlier while summerin' in Rampside the poet William Wordsworth had been similarly drawn:

Four summer weeks I dwelt in sight of thee:
I saw thee every day, and all the while
Thy form was sleeping on a glassy sea.

Nanty's 'big mon', however, was becoming more interested in what he could *not* see, particularly after reading a local geology guide given to him by his father. After some consideration he wrote about it in his holiday journal before sharing his conclusions with his aunt. He thought he should perform it like one of his uncle's homilies. He stood up and cleared his throat before announcing:

'"Fooley" Island is very low,' he started, falteringly. 'This is why you cannot see it from the village. It comes from Cumbrian mountain rocks left by glaciers on the seaside. They got worn into billions of smooth pebbles and for centuries have been carried south by the tide to make a very long finger out to sea.'

'If tha ses so, me yoong mon,' Nanty commented in an impartial tone. He looked up and their eyes met. She accepted that 'Fooley Island' was as she found it but he, she realised, needed to know why.

Thursday arrived with the threat of another squall so there would be no excursion. Nanty took the opportunity to drop off some provisions at one of her sister's but returned in a flustered state.

'I moost know, OOH!' she held her hands in the air and spun round. 'Them playcards at the station says:
                    "COLLAPSE OF LANCASHIRE"!'

Her nephew watched helplessly as she grabbed her purse and disappeared. Five minutes later she was back with the penny sheet paper. She thrust it at her 'wee mon'.

''Ere, tell me. Oi knows it soomat reet bad.' Trembling she sat down, head in hands. 'Reet bad,' she repeated.

He quickly scanned the paper until it dawned on him what was wrong.

'Haha! No, Nanty, not an earthquake.'

'Tell me, tell me,' she begged.

'It's just cricket. Yorkshire beat Lancashire by an innings,' he crowed.

'Ooo! Silly game, frightenin' me. An' don't you zound so cocky. Tha' wuz an earthquake, before yoo wuz thought uv.'

'Yes, Nanty, I know.'

'I'm tellin' yo' t' trooth. Thas why 'ouses 'av cement on t'walls, coovers oop cracks.'

On Friday the weather and tide combination was agreeable so the duo set out past the strange depression called 'Conk 'ole' where the village ends and the mile-long causeway to Roa begins. Halfway along the banked road they turned left to follow a serpentine trail between salt marsh and open sea. Miles of mud glistened below the blue hum of the day. Ahead lines of bleached pebbles and sediment curved into the shimmering distance.

'Mind where yer walkin', them stones could be eggs.' Nanty breathed heavily.

'But,' he complained, 'my book says the nesting is over by early-summer, and it's already July.'

Nanty pondered the point as she passed her picnic basket to her other hand.

'Agh books, what do they know?'

'They're written by experts, or-ni-thologists,' informed her nephew as if that were the end of the matter.

She advanced a few steps then stopped, abruptly. With a vigorous gesture she indicated that her nephew should do likewise. She crouched until their heads were level. She pointed along the winding shore.

'Well, m' big mon,' she wheezed, 'He's nivva rid a book, haz'ee?'

He followed the line of Nanty's arthritic finger to the skulking silhouette of a fox. The boy's eyes widened. He was awestruck by a simple discovery. He held his aunt's neck and squeezed her in excitement. For the first time he'd replaced a belief with something much more valuable: knowledge.

'Do you think he's seen us?' he whispered as the fox continued its meandering search for food.

'Oh aye,' she smiled, '"eez bin watchin' uz all day long.'

Her 'big mon', suddenly enthused, ran round his aunt in a circle. Books were good but this was better… far better.

'The spring tides must've washed away the nests,' she added in a matter-of-fact way. 'Birds keep doin' what birds duz.'

'And what's that?' he asked, laughing.

'Yow knows well enough. Now, come along, mebe we'll see "Seldom Seen".'

'Where Nanty?'

'Reet oot tha' if we're looky, id'll be thur.'

An hour later they stood at the end of the spit where the dark mud rippled as hard as tree bark.

'It hurts my feet,' he said dancing around looking for crabs to put in a bucket.

Quietly she laid out the picnic; tayter cakes, apples, cheese with fig chutney and other treats.

'What d'yer mean, don't like pickle onion!' she exclaimed later. 'Like yer feet, yer need breakin' in.'

'But it's vinegary.'

'Ain't owt wrong with it, soom fellers don't knows when thez well hoff.'

'If I eat it can I shoot the airgun tomorrow, please?'

'Yo' rapscallion! Goo on then, orl of it mind.'

He forced it into his contorting mouth, pretending it was far worse than it was. She loved the performance but their conspiratorial leanings even more. For these few weeks he was her responsibility and she'd introduce him to things that his parents in London could only guess at.

He grew quiet and looked towards the sea until his eyes hurt.

'Nanty?'

'Yes.'
'Why can't I see "Seldom Seen"?'
'Praps yer lookin' wrong.'
'Nanty! How can you "look" wrong?' he teased.
'Hast yo a book that could tell uz?' she teased back.
'Funny, haha. How about you tell me what it's like, *your secret island?*'

She struggled to pick details from a sketchy memory.

'It wer real, aye…' she started hesitantly, '…ova' thur…in mist when I sin it, wi' grass…sond, er…shells an' pieces a' wood…' Her unspectacular words faded into the white noise of space…

'A shipwreck?'
'Oh aye, if yer wont.'
'Well, it's all gone.'

Nanty reflected on the shared disappointment. She had hoped for 'Seldom Seen' because it represented the 'prize' at the end of a long walk. She kicked herself for even mentioning it. It wasn't called 'Seldom Seen' for nothing. She felt responsible and wracked her brain for an answer.

'Mebbe when oi seed it,' she muttered slowly, 'oi wuz somewhere else.' The beguiling suggestion hung in the air before provoking a shriek of delight from her nephew.

'A whole island disappeared,' he cried, 'but how?'
'Same way as nests, I spose.'
'But a whole island, Nanty? With a castle, a king and queen.'

Nanty laughed.

'Oh m' big man', she marvelled, clapping her hands together, 'you're a one!'

He looked along the shingle edge that no map would define.

He imagined the squiggle on vellum and 'saw' it fade and reappear as the tides came and went. He walked up and down the shore and for the second time that day tingled with an exquisite excitement.

'Nanty.'
'Aye?'
'Don't worry, I believe you. There's no icebergs on maps either.'

* * *

The next morning Nanty holding a basket of washing turned the corner at the moment the pellet left the air gun. Three hundredths of a second later the robin's breast was punctured and its heart ruptured. Blood was forced into the bird's gullet as it tumbled onto freshly dug earth among raspberry canes.

'John Yerbury Dent!' she cried.

Dropping the basket she rushed past her stunned nephew. Her face puckered in anguish as she picked up every 'gardener's friend', her friend.

Nanty did not admonish. This was not her way. She took life as it came. This would be treated like every other slight, there'd be no histrionics. Nature is cruel, ships go down but nobody blames the waves. She had said the gun could only be fired in the garden and accepted with a shrug that her 'big mon' simply had another curiosity that would be satisfied. She did not share his interest but she'd never stand in the way of his nature. If her 'yoong man 'ad a mind t'do summat' he'd be helped.

Nanty left him without saying another word. She knew when to let him 'stew in 'iz own juice.'

Her 'big mon' sat motionless trying to unscramble his mind. She had never called him even 'John Dent' before, but his whole name? This shook him. He adored this place, its straightforward simplicity, but now tears of frustration blurred everything he'd betrayed. He'd lost his compass, his orientation with the familiar, the foundations which made him who he was. He tried to play with an old bike but the distraction lasted only minutes. If only the day could start again. The hours dragged, terrible hours, gloomy black hours. Why had he been so foolish? The shadows on the grass ceased to lengthen. Even if he ran away he knew he'd still be tethered to the frightful sight of Nanty's white-knuckled fingers cradling her loyal companion. He pictured the tinge of delicate blue around the flame of its breast, its perfect honey brown wings. In death the robin had revealed its pristine beauty… but with a bead of blood bursting at its beak.

There would and could be no relief. Thoughtlessness had pushed him from the simplicity of childhood into the adult world of complexity, doubt and consequences.

The sun eventually dipped behind a sentinel pear tree. Underneath stood a sandstone wall strangled by ivy and brambles. The air, as sometimes happens, even by the coast, stood still. And with the stillness, a silence broken occasionally by the ascendant withering of curlews. He listened intently for the next but heard only his gasping breath.

Inside her parlour Nanty stopped stirring the hot pot and checked the time. She tucked a corn-coloured curl behind her ear and peered through the back window at the bowed shape of her disconsolate nephew. She decided that he had suffered enough and pushed at the old back door. It scraped on the worn step; he looked up.

'M'big mon, wash yer 'onds, yer tea's nearly ready.' There was no change in her singsong voice, he was her 'big mon' again… Nanty never mentioned the incident again. It was as if she'd already forgotten about it. He, on the other hand, never would.

Early that night a soft breeze whispered in from nowhere to gather up the secrets of the day. Thereafter, the silent deeps of the western sky arched through towering columns of stars and waited. Then from the raven north flashed the first aurora flicker. Its emerald phosphorescence shimmering and blending within the waking dreams of Man.

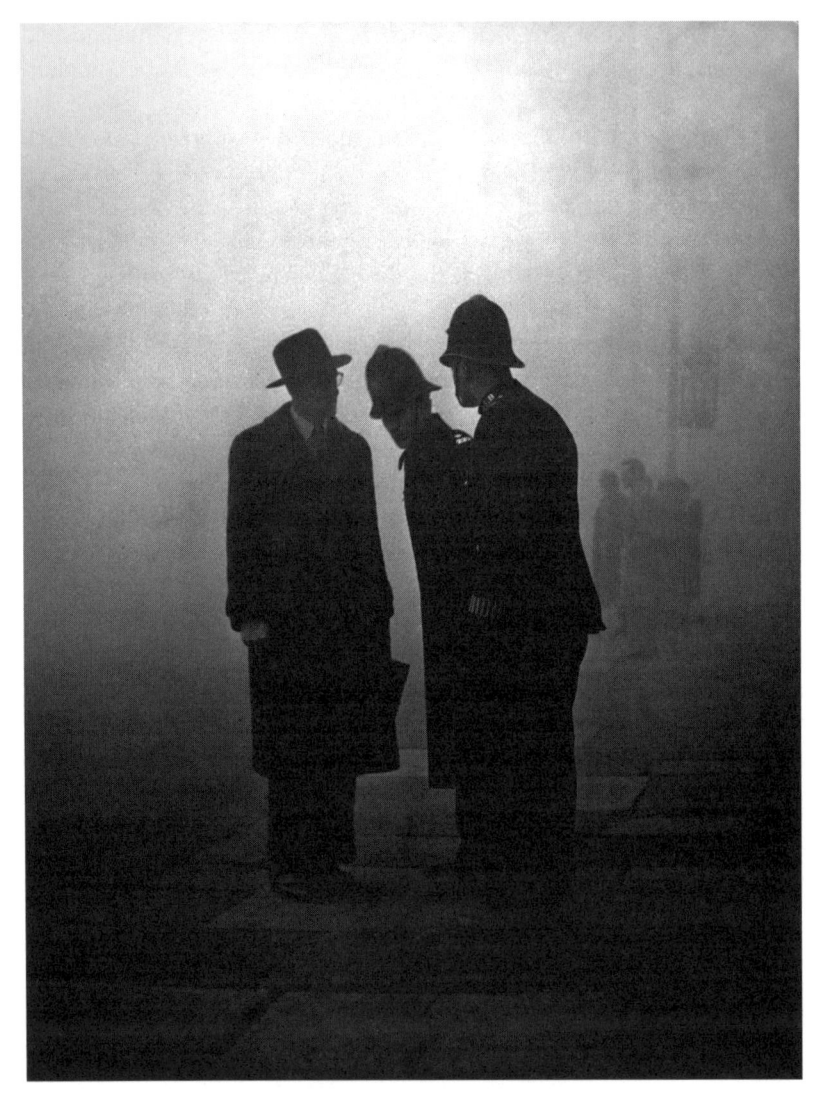

London and the smog smeared streets of the 1950s.
[©Alamy, photographer unknown]

2

London, April 1956

In the mid-1950s geo-political forces seeped into the fabric of society like damp in a rotting wall. With charred grins and crumpled faces ordinary men and women funnelled themselves down smog-smeared streets and headlong into the glare of post-war propaganda: 'peace, progress and prosperity'. Some wondered how faith in slogans would be rewarded.

A gaunt traveller from an antique land lurched backwards onto the pavement.

'Look where yer goin' mate!' bawled the cabbie through a swirl of exhaust.

He fell in with the stream of plodding pedestrians until a spasm of gut-wrenching pain forced him to stop. He clutched a lamppost. As the agonies withdrew he faced the hopelessness of his task. 'Easier to drift with the bobbing herd,' he told himself. 'Driftwood has no roots, I'll drown downstream... nobody'll notice.'

After floundering for several hundred yards he re-surfaced against a telephone box, a blatant piece of pomp and kitsch. Gagging for air he pushed his face up to the glass and read a card by the receiver:

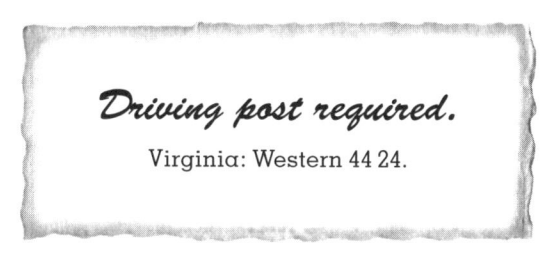

Driving post required.
Virginia: Western 44 24.

Overhead pigeons spiralled in an up-draught. He shivered; his toes hurt and would hurt more if he rejoined the moon-faced crowd. Back came the whine of his dilemma, 'Get buffeted by flatfeet or lie down and freeze to death?' He tried to distract himself with the words of a poem but couldn't remember them... or even the poet. Another blast of air twisted the trees overhead. He glanced up and vaguely registered the arthritically limbed grotesques hectic against a wild sky. 'One day it'll all be mush in a sinking swamp.' He imagined a constricting vine shooting from the drains and lassoing his ankles. 'Yeah, yeah, yeah... I know,' he warned, 'it's gonna drag me under too... into the wasteland pulled by the sucking sickness of junk.'

The traveller fidgeted inside his crumpled suit as waves of pain and panic swept from his body throughout what was left of his mind. He must confirm the address but had forgotten which pocket it was in. His shirt, dark with sweat, stuck to his ribs. 'Oh, yeah,' he recognised, 'those old incompatibles are back: neurotic urgency and inertia.' This was familiar but alongside the cloyed purpose, the twitches and demoralising brainfog, not even he could miss one huge, troubling irony: London.

'London, for Chris'sake, its sheer unutterable drabness,' he muttered. 'Torpor over clay. Layer upon layer of creamed shit turning mud into nest for the great democratic bitchmother. Cradle and bed for all those white Anglo Saxon small-minded Protestant whore whelpings hounding me forever... yet here I am, forced curlike to sup on my own vomit... to cobble a future out of the ruins of degeneracy; mine from theirs.'

A black spirit-voice cast a further net of entanglement over his torment:

'Your misanthropy is stoked by self-disgust,' it reminded him.

'But London, of all the bubbling cenotes,' came his indignant rebuttal. 'London, the rotten rancid tit of the old world, the progenitor of every vile form of corruption spawned by Homo sap's curdled ballsack of fear, discharged as if it were the elixir of life.... America's the poxy mongrel, but London the congenitally inbred monster, doubly infected by myth and hypocrisy.'

LONDON, APRIL 1956

Another blast of air threatened to tug the address from his fingers.

"'Ere! You lost?'

The sharpness of a real voice shocked him. A misshapen, bulbous woman with lipstick more hideous than the phone box pushed her face into his.

'You look lost, mister. Can I 'elp?'

She was a flower out of season, a bashed dahlia. He felt too sick to respond.

'Please yerself, darlin', I was only asking,' she huffed before sinking back into the human swell.

Emptily he looked after her, down again at the scrap of paper and up at the nearest front door. 'Come on, you asshole!'

The house numbers made no sense but he had an aversion to asking for help; the familiar's gloomy voice was telling him he didn't need it: 'You're above asking.'

After another buffeting he entered a plush hallway with several brass plates and a large poinsettia as vulgar as phone-box lips. He rang a bell and an interior glass door was opened by an efficient-looking woman. He took off his hat.

'Yes? Can we be of assistance?'

'I was told to come here ... to see the doctor.'

'Oh?' She eyed beads of sweat on the man's brow.

'Yes, I have a letter of introduction.'

'I'd know if we had a consultation.' Her voice snapped like scissors.

The knot in his intestines twisted. She noticed his grimace; her lips pursed.

'This *is* the address,' he tried to suppress the mounting torment, 'I was told t-to come ...... I rang, surely ...'

'Yes, you said. But there's nothing down ...'

'I am sure this is right ....' He fumbled inside his jacket and shakily held out an envelope with a US stamp.

Taking the letter she closed the door, checking it was locked. He watched as she disappeared. Two minutes later she was back.

'Dr Maclay will see you. Please, this way.'

She escorted him through an oak-panelled but deserted waiting room into a plush office with blinds and a consultation desk angled towards the door. A man in his mid-fifties, in a dark three-piece suit and sober bow tie, got up and extended his hand over the desk.

'Hello, I'm Dr *William* Maclay. So you're Mr Burroughs?'

'Yes, and I'm, er, Mr *William* Burroughs.' said the visitor. They shook hands limply.

'There's been a misunderstanding,' said the doctor, 'but, please, now you're here, sit down.'

'Oh?' Burroughs looked around, hesitating. This place didn't look right. It felt like a lawyer's office. And his secretary hanging around like a bad smell.

'Please, sir, do make yourself comfortable,' repeated Maclay. 'This won't take long.'

Burroughs lowered himself onto a hard chair.

'We're referring you to another doctor,' informed Maclay in a detached voice.

The visitor jumped to his feet dropping his hat. 'What! Why?' he cried.

'Please, try not to worry. This is in your best interests, I assure you.'

Burroughs held the back of the chair.

'This doctor isn't far away,' continued Maclay. 'My secretary will give you his details.'

'But I thought that *you* were to treat me; I was assured, my fam—' Burroughs interrupted himself with a loud sneeze. Snot dribbled down his face and between his long fingers. He stifled another sneeze with his handkerchief pulled from his trousers.

The doctor made a face and recoiled. 'It is regrettable sir, but it would seem I am the *wrong* Maclay.'

'What!?'

'Yes, the *right* Maclay is a psychiatrist and has a worldwide reputation. He lives in Queens Gate too, you probably should be seeing him.'

'Two Maclays, two *Doctor* Maclays.' gasped Burroughs, disbelieving.

'Yes, that's right,' confirmed the wrong Maclay, laughing, 'we also have the same initial. Confounding isn't it?'

LONDON, APRIL 1956

Burroughs couldn't see the funny side.

'But please, don't worry. You're not the first to get this wrong... and won't be the last. We're even the same age.' Maclay giggled.

'I don't understand. I've come from Tangier... you....'

Maclay checked his amusement and interrupted his visitor. 'What I should also explain, this area of medicine isn't mine.' Maclay gave a little, self deprecating shrug trying to ignore Burroughs' dribbling face. 'Your... er, complaint... well, it requires a particular form of specialisation, as I am sure you can appreciate.'

'But I am in need. Please!' Burroughs shoved the sopping handkerchief back into his trousers. 'I'm in dire straights... you gotta help me...'

Dr Maclay edged himself further from the desk. 'Now listen to me. I would not know where to start. We are referring you to someone who is experienced in this matter... er, field. I assure you.'

'This other Maclay?'

'No, not him. He cannot see you either... but he's recommended another doctor.'

Burroughs started. He had confronted this bullshit before... heartless bastards who couldn't wait to see the back of you. 'But you gotta help me.' he pleaded.

'I can assure you, sir, it'll be better this way.'

'What about this English licensing system you have? I dunno, does it extend to US citizens?'

'That isn't at issue. This other doctor will treat you in his own way; if I interfere it might set you back.'

'But I am in terrible pain, surely—'

'I'm sorry, but you'll have to accept what I am saying.'

'But what if this doctor doesn't want to help either?'

'Oh he will,' Maclay forced a grin, 'you have our word.'

Burroughs' body shrank. Slowly he sat down again. He only had one card left to play. 'Surely you can write me a script?' he mumbled, 'I can pay.'

Maclay scoffed. 'Oh really Mr Burroughs! You're in London now, not Timbuktu. I shouldn't need to remind you that our codes of practice would not permit what you're suggesting. I repeat; this is the most appropriate course of action. Furthermore, the other Maclay, the *right* Maclay,' the doctor emphasised, '*he'll* check your progress. Now, if you wouldn't mind … the quicker we finish up here the sooner you'll be dealt with.' Maclay nodded to his secretary.

'Sir,' she tried to get the American's attention. 'If you could come with me.'

Burroughs gripped his pounding temples. His brain was scrambled; he couldn't find anything to say. He was being stitched up, it was obvious.

'Sir,' the secretary's voice insisted. She picked up his hat between finger and thumb and let it swing before the long and pallid face. 'This way … please.'

Burroughs stumbled into the waiting room. His ears started to ring. After a few minutes the bad smell re-appeared, offering a sheet of folded notepaper.

'Here you are, sir. I wasn't able to speak to the doctor himself but left a message. You can contact him yourself, these are his particulars.'

'Ugh?'

'To make a consultation. That's his number, Western: 6738.'

'What's this, his name?'

'No, that is the borough, Ken stands for Kensington.' she smirked.

Burroughs' misery clicked shut. This was it. There would be no escape, no cure. Now he'd die like his uncle. His mother had told him. She had known, everyone knew, just a matter of time …

* * *

An hour later and not far away John Yerbury Dent, a 66-year-old doctor, slammed shut his front door at 34, Addison Road, w.14. He pushed back his bushy white fringe with nicotine-stained fingers to get a better view of the sky. The wintry grey was giving way to a bright afternoon. Perfect weather to try out his new camera. He could hardly wait to get to the park.

LONDON, APRIL 1956

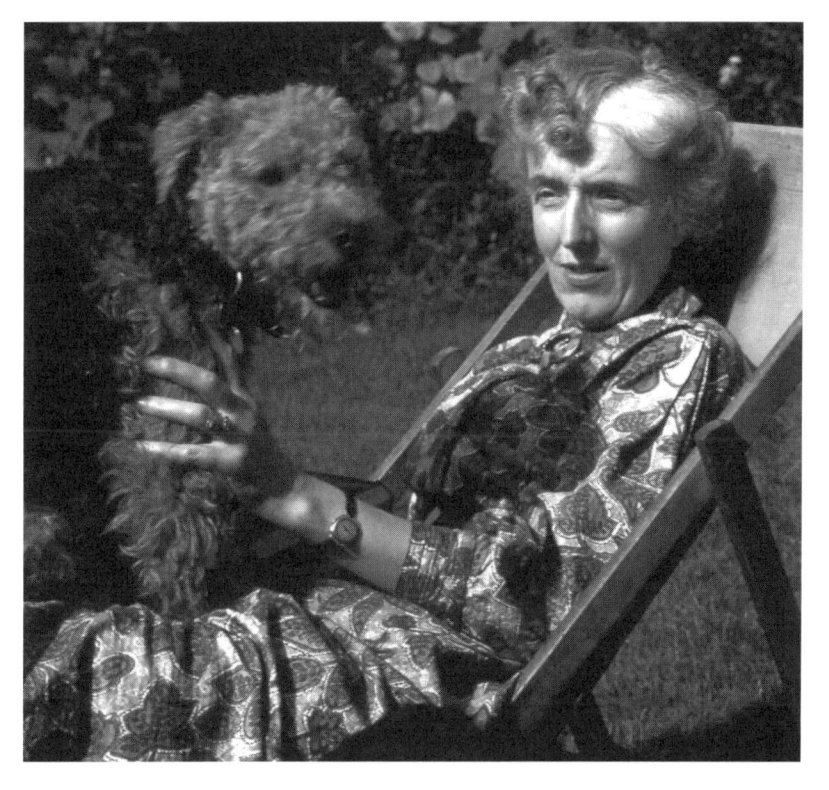

Rhoda Brenan with Peel, a black and tea coloured Welsh terrier, 1956.
Rhoda was married to Blair Brenan the brother of the Hispanic writer, Gerald.
[photo: John Yerbury Dent]

His partner, Rhoda Brenan, several years his junior, had already left for the daily constitutional with their curly haired terrier, Peel. Dent always left last as he liked to walk briskly. Rhoda preferred a slower pace. With any luck they'd arrive at The Orangery together and enjoy a relaxing hour away from the coal face.

Dent was trying to lose weight and a walk instead of lunch seemed logical. This was fine but he'd noticed that his dinners had got bigger. Was this yet another example of the absurd way good intentions are corrupted by any number of tiny deceits and compromises? He concluded that every one of life's challenges are beset with contradictions and maybe life was all the better for it. If existence were reduced to manageable episodes and happy endings how dull it'd be. In fact Dent was amused at the thought that any of the puzzles that dog mankind were solvable. Progress was illusory though he did notice that he was making good time on his way to the park. At this rate he'd overtake Rhoda long before she got there.

Apropos of nothing, he suddenly found himself imagining the world beneath his feet. He often liked thinking of the earth's crust in this way; he called it 'geologising' and thought it preferable to theologising. Well, that was what he had said last night at dinner with some churchgoing friends. 'At least geology can be scientific whereas Christianity,' he had argued, 'can only remain subjective, like *witchcraft*.' Stressing that last word may have been unnecessary but whenever he was bored he liked to stir the pot. Now, however, his mind fluttered over something quite different; a very peculiar subterranean vision. Some way off the rumble of an underground train could be imagined if not felt. This was immaterial to Dent since he knew it was there, just like the signalling between the hemispheres and lobes in the brain. Instantly and to his great delight the entire tube network; stations, tunnels, and platforms, transformed itself into a brain map of terminals, dendrites, axons and synapses. Atoms rushed this way and that like billions of time-lapsing commuters. They couldn't stop monitoring, checking and reminding. So many mediating currents of chemicals flowing deep throughout earth-brain and all in the blink of an eye: the royal-blue Piccadilly line, the blood-red Central line and the acid-green acetylcholine. He smiled to himself at his glorious conceit; its simplicity and complexity…

'A penny for them?' Rhoda enquired.

'Oh, my word, there you are!' Dent replied, ramming on the brakes.

Rhoda, her face reflecting the brightening sky, shone with pleasure. 'You were miles away!'

'I know,' Dent acknowledged, without any impulse to pretend otherwise.

'Little Johnny, head in the air,' she teased.

'Well, not in the air, exactly.'
'What?'
'Oh, never mind.'
They hugged and proceeded onwards hand in hand.
'So, what was so engrossing?' she asked.
'Oh nothing... really.'
'Mmm. You enjoy your thoughts, I can tell... but they'll never exist until they're shared.'

'But,' he protested, 'if I talk and walk, I'll get out of breath and collapse. Then you and Peel will have to carry me, then you'll collapse and that would be unfair on Peel, a poor terrier having to drag the two of us home.'

Peel seemed unaware of his responsibilities as he hurtled after a squirrel. Rhoda managed a breathless smile.

They emerged from a tall avenue of chestnut and lime and stopped to take in the spreading sky. She lit a Senior Service cigarette and handed it to Dent before lighting her own. They sat down on a bench. They enjoyed these moments, just themselves and their energetic terrier.

Several minutes passed as they welcomed the becalming sights and sounds of life. Dent was on the point of closing his eyes when Rhoda asked, portentously:

'Do you think mankind is on a road to nowhere, imprisoned as we are on this lonely planet?'

'Oh, I wouldn't say that. We're unable to accept our limitations, you know?'

'But surely we are likely to run out of space.'

'But not *in* space, how would that be possible?' Dent teased but Rhoda wasn't going to give way.

'I am not convinced that humanity will ever colonise space, if that's what you mean?'

'Why ever not?' he argued. 'Not so long ago we sailed into the unknown believing that we'd drop off the edge, but it hardly stopped us. We've never recognised any physical boundary, and our reaction to discovery only spurs us to go further.'

Rhoda's mind jumped to a painting of Renaissance Italy with richly robed inventors flinging their designs to an enthusiastic crowd of merchants. Simultaneously Dent's thoughts swept effortlessly from the past into a philosophical appraisal of the future:

'This never ends because ambition is unlimited, and feeds on itself. Now we have to deal with the universe as a whole; with each breakthrough we just extend the potential for further curiosity... and the possibility of more territories to inhabit... and exploit.'

Dent was dissatisfied with this summation, there seemed to be something missing.

'You see, that's what organisms do, not just humans; we're nothing if not entirely predictable.'

'Now you put it like that.' Rhoda smiled.

'Humanity seems unable to co-operate anyway,' he threw in. 'Outer space for a few powerful souls may be their only answer.'

'Oh, before I forget,' Rhoda interjected, 'back here, on Planet Earth, Macker the shrink's secretary rang this morning. He's referring a patient who'll be in touch.' She let the information sink in. '...I wonder who it'll be this time. Another "hopeless case"?' There was a hint of annoyance in her voice.

Dent waited for a second. 'Agh, Macker's not so bad, you know...'

'Why doesn't he treat them himself? He could, couldn't he?' said Rhoda, firmly.

'Why?' said Dent. 'He has always appealed for alternative approaches and would only refer a patient if he believed he'd be better off elsewhere.'

'Or that *he* might be better off with his *patient* elsewhere,' she snapped. 'Wasn't it Mackers who sent you that raving Mother Superior? You remember? The one kicked out of the Army?'

'I don't discuss my patients with anyone,' Dent responded in a flat voice. 'In any case, no, it was not and you're being unfair on Mackers. He's up to his ears with the yahoos at the Maudsley, poor man.'

Rhoda paused. She watched some small children in the distance rolling around on the grass. She wondered where this conversation was leading.

'I was just curious if you've ever thought of retiring?' She lit herself another cigarette.

'Oh! You've never asked me this before. Do you think I should?'

'No, I think it should be entirely up to you. It is just that you don't have a partner, somebody younger to carry on your work. I just wonder if you did you might find it easier to let go.'

'That is a good point, except I am still learning. My treatments are certainly not infallible, they can always be bettered.'

'But there has to be a limit to what one man can do. You run the Society virtually single-handedly; you look for sponsorship, fill and pay for its blessed journal, run a busy practice and a small nursing home and take on patients from doctors who cannot be bothered. What about us, your family?'

Rhoda hadn't realised she would throw in the last point, but there it was, the elephant... amok in the room.

'Ah, so that's the problem.' Dent raised his eyebrows. 'Have the girls said something?'

Rhoda looked away. Her waves of grey-blonde hair framed a thin, pale face. She knew as well as anyone that medical care was a responsibility John never shirked. After all, he couldn't choose his patients. They came to him in various stages of disrepair and at all hours. John just took it all in his stride. He even, she sensed, enjoyed the uncertainty. 'It keeps me on my toes,' he had said, 'forces me to evolve my thinking... prevents bad habits.' But Rhoda was also beginning to appreciate that this was far from the full story. John needed his patients as much as they needed him; it was a curious contract and provided him with a sense of benign fulfilment which she could never share. Recently it had occurred to her that the patient/doctor boundaries were being blurred but perhaps that was understandable as John was very much the 'hands on' sort of practitioner. With so many 'hopeless cases' being turned around why should he change? No, she would have to admit it, *she* was the problem, *she* had grown tired and wanted an easier life. It had been so very exciting fifteen years ago, despite the war. They had seemed on the threshold of something with endless possibilities, a new understanding between psychiatry and medicine, but suddenly there was no unity of purpose. Nothing had quite materialised, even their closest 'allies' seemed to be jumping ship. It depressed her to think about it and sooner or later her feelings would have to come out...

Rhoda stood up as a dark shadow swept across the park. She inhaled deeply from her cigarette and stood as tall as her elegant frame would allow. A blackbird chattered fretfully at some hidden danger. She waited for the commotion to die down.

'No, I confess, this is my problem. I just wonder when life might settle down.'

'Parenthood is probably something I've failed at,' sighed Dent. 'I do my best but must accept that my work has left me conflicted. A doctor has to put his patients first but a father must do the same for his children. Something has had to give.'

'Oh look, I hadn't meant that at all,' Rhoda asserted, unconvincingly. She looked away, struggling to understand what she did mean. 'You do your best, but you're a one-man band trying to sound like an orchestra. If I am angry it isn't with you, it's with your bloody silly colleagues. They're lazy. None of them put in as much as you do and many show a deliberate inability to appreciate why your ideas are important. They should be doing more, much more.'

Dent laughed. 'Well, they probably *are*, for their children!'

'Oh, no!' exclaimed Rhoda, 'That isn't it either, the children adore you. You respect them and treat them as equals.' She flicked away her cigarette stub. 'Though I do think we could try and include them a bit more?'

'Oh?'

'Yes, I think this is a negative side of your Quaker ancestry kicking in, that damnable contemplative bubble of quietism you all inhabit. It can be quite daunting, you know, for others to penetrate.'

'Such as?' asked Dent.

'Well, when the cousins spent all their Christmas money on toy soldiers. They couldn't understand why it upset you.'

'Couldn't they?'

'Well, of course not!'

'And did it show?'
'Did what show?'
'I mean; did it show that I was upset?'
'Oh for pity's sake! Of course it did! They know you. You could have explained yourself, nobody would have minded...'

Dent reflected for a moment on the incident and recalled his response. He felt he'd been petulant.

'Well, I was being ridiculous, all the tub-thumping by warmongers I have to listen to. Banging on about Russia now. It never ends, you know how I feel. And then the children go and buy a platoon of dragoons with bayonets and bagpipes. Now...,' Dent's voice switched from indignant to solemn, '...if there's one thing worse than being murdered by bayonet it's by bagpipes.'

Rhoda chuckled; her body shook. It took her a moment to regain her voice.

'I only hate one thing more than bagpipes,' she said, still giggling.
'What's that?'
'The bastards that play them.'

It was John's turn to laugh.

'And since this has come up,' Rhoda continued, 'I think this is a perfect example of what I mean. You should just explain yourself, it is understandable, we all have grave doubts about conflict, the endless sabre rattling.'

'You're right,' agreed Dent. 'I think the inevitability of human aggression has always upset me. Perhaps unduly.'

'Well, there's no need.' Rhoda's voice rose slightly as she dived in at the deep end. 'You're turning into your dad. He was the quietest man I've ever met. All that bustling humanity and endless smiles. You'll end up two peas from the same pod. I bet you never saw him explore his feelings, not profoundly. Do you ever stop to think how frustrating this can be?'

Rhoda walked away from the bench to examine the emerging lilac of a collapsed wisteria.

'How do you actually differ from your father, I mean *really*?' she asked.

Getting no answer she turned back and realised she'd lost John's attention. He was searching deep inside his hold-all. He reminded her of an old horse eating oats from a sack.

He emerged holding a smooth leather case. He opened it revealing the shiny chrome and glass sparkle of a new camera.

'It's a German model,' he announced. 'I was at the book fair last Saturday but nothing. Then, coming home, I saw this. "£12 pounds," he said so I said, "£9, and not a penny more," thinking we'd meet halfway. But he accepted! I've been worrying that something won't work, but so far everything appears shipshape. I want to try it out and give the film to Onions before the shops shut. How long have we got?'

'You're fine, it's only two-ish,' replied Rhoda. 'There's nothing apart from our promise to do some gardening together. The committee doesn't meet until eight.'

'Good. Now, let me see. Any volunteers to be my model? Peel's scarpered.'

'Oh, you know how to spoil a gal,' Rhoda replied, ignoring the invitation and feeling more than a little frustrated. She sat down to light another cigarette. Dent twiddled a dial without knowing what it was for. He peered through the viewfinder, trying to locate the distant chimney pots. Suddenly they snapped into focus, vivid terracotta edged in sunlight.

'Good, all seems clear. Lens too, no mildew.' He mumbled to himself while fiddling for the shutter release. 'Where is it?'

'Where's what?' asked Rhoda, irritation returning to her voice.

'The knob.' His thick index finger stretched over the top of the camera. 'Ah!' he cried, 'I think I have it.' He pressed the shutter release but nothing happened. 'What's wrong? It's not working.'

'Really, £9 is suddenly sounding expensive,' she crowed.

'Aha! No, I bet you can't take a photo unless there's a film in it. That'll be it.'

Rhoda looked skywards as Dent blindly fumbled in his bag once more, this time for the latest Ektachrome-x36.

Rhoda mumbled away, almost to herself, 'How many times are you going to find a willing friend prepared to sit in the freezing cold while you look for your knob? I've been here before, you know.'

Dent laughed. 'Once or twice,' he admitted.

The film was soon loaded. He stood to photograph everything and anything. He just needed to use up the roll.

'Now then,' feigning sternness, 'how can I get the job done if you don't take this seriously? Steady the ship, boys!'

Again he raised the camera to his right eye, this time trying to catch Rhoda unawares. Instinctively she looked away; she knew the drill. She was in her mid-fifties, attractively tall and smart. She wasn't Bloomsbury, not quite one of those that somebody wittily commented: *'live in Squares, but love in triangles'* – well, not the first part. She was shabbily bohemian, and proud of it. Dent, by comparison, could've been pulled from the hedge behind him. They appeared a slightly incongruous couple but their speech and shared glances revealed a relaxed intimacy. They'd lived tempestuous lives, adventurous and open. They knew many who lived in a twilight world of deceit but their *ménage*, shared with her husband Blair, was a relaxed, amicable affair. Her annoyance with John stemmed mainly from his apparent self-sufficiency. She loved the knockabout discussions and sparky meal times but then he'd disappear for hours sustained solely by his interests; his geology, hundreds of atlases, manuscripts and books. His engaging re-emergence full of bonhomie would melt the frustrations that were only truly dissolved by shared pursuits such as gardening and their days out. She treasured those fleeting moments more than she was prepared to admit, even to herself. How many more would there be? Perhaps this was what was eating her up.

Dent scanned the flowerbeds and skyline. As he did so he inexplicably found himself recalling the death of a young woman he had treated nearly forty years ago. He sat down and closed his eyes, but she was still there, stricken. Once more her flame was going out and like a battered old moth, Dent was being drawn in. He recalled the hospital swing doors and fumes of carbolic and chloroform. Up the back stairs and into the mixed ward past stretchers and hurrying nurses to a row of beds. Once more to the last bed on the left with a curtain round it, her bed. He remembered pulling the sheet back and looking down. Now he could smell her, feel the imprint of her death seep into him. It spread through his mind to the core of his trembling body until consumed by emotion he caved in.

'What's wrong?' Rhoda cried.

'I am sorry,' said Dent, holding his head.

'What's come over you, tell me,' insisted Rhoda, well-aware of how increasingly often John could become a hostage to thought.

'Ah, I'm all right,' he sighed, as if trying to recover his breath. 'Not my imaginings this time, more my memories. I'm fine, really, but just like that,' he snapped his fingers, 'I was back at St Pancras alongside that poor woman with meningitis. You remember; the one in my memoirs? It is quite extraordinary how abruptly the brain can unlock a memory… something about the camera perhaps, the smell of its leather case or the way the sunlight spread in the glass? I don't know. Anyway, it all came flooding back… everything… it gave me quite a start, won't happen again.' He smiled.

Rhoda was unconvinced. She knew how his feelings could suck him dry… turn him to a husk vulnerable to the forces of a pitiless universe. She shivered as she turned her face towards the horizon, to the clay roofs shining above the thrum of early afternoon traffic. 'Yes, I remember,' she murmured. She was staring into the distance but it was John's story that danced before her eyes. She sidled closer to draw comfort. These reveries were becoming common, but she didn't know why.

For a minute or two they sat in silent recognition of another anonymous victim of austere living conditions made worse by war. Rhoda knew that Dent's character sprang from both his experiences and an empathy outside her range. Much of his motivational strength lay in a sense of universal humanity bent towards healing. It wasn't difficult to appreciate. Abruptly, it occurred to her that this too might be fuelling her growing sense of disquiet. She'd laboriously typed up those memoirs years ago in an attempt to drum up feedback among their circle of literary friends. Dent had had some limited success with his first book and it had momentarily bothered him that he'd never succeeded as a writer. Perhaps though, if she were to be entirely honest, it had bothered her more. She should accept that he'd moved on. He'd let that fire go out because he'd been able to light another... it was she who had been left behind raking over the embers, chatting up insufferable publishers... those heady evenings with the Gollanczes at the book club.

'Politics,' said Dent, firmly.

'What?' said Rhoda, more than a little confused.

'You asked me in what way do I differ from my father.'

'Oh, yes,' said Rhoda, remembering.

'When I gave up on religion I needed something else. That's when I developed an awareness surrounding social injustice and a dislike for authority. I became a right little so-and-so.' He grinned while taking another photograph before continuing.

'That's why I've failed. Paradise on Earth is as illusory as the one in heaven. I think I fooled myself there.'

'But you haven't failed, John, not at all.'

'Oh, if only that were true. I entered into correspondence last year with America. This morning I received another letter that in their opinion apomorphine is addictive and dangerous. Progress even amongst my peers is impossible. In fifty years they'll still be saying that Dent owed his success to "aversion or his magnetic personality". I am absolutely hamstrung, surrounded by the cloth-eared or worse.'

Rhoda was suddenly struck by the darkening in John's face. His eyes tightened. His voice squeezed out from under his sandy moustache.

'The worst thing, though, is that medicine is not being informed by good practice. We're going in a wrong-headed direction and just when doctors should have more say in policy we're being dictated to by bureaucrats who wouldn't know one end of a syringe from another, a hernia from a haemorrhoid.'

He slung his camera over his shoulder.

'What would your dad say?' wondered Rhoda out loud.

'Well, to take your point, he'd smile and read a book on mountaineering. Maybe he was right. I've overreached myself,' Dent observed, ruefully.

'You're still very like him.'

'I don't think sons or daughters like to hear that. They like to hear that they've learned from previous generations and moved things along.'

'And you have, but progress isn't linear is it?'

'Well, it's rarely straightforward. I think in medicine most doctors are reliant on old procedures, and even when science provides answers there is resistance. But of all human activities medicine should be an understanding of how to make things better. That is not happening, not uniformly anyway. And doctors who absent themselves from any political sensibility are among the worst offenders, the most unethical.'

Rhoda sat back, struck by the forthrightly critical voice in her friend, confidante and lover.

She knew he despised bad practice but this was new. This message echoed in the sunless parts of her mind. It frightened her.

'Explain yourself,' she demanded.

'Oh dear, we haven't got all day; but these letters from America confirm it, I'm afraid. You see, what they are saying is categorically untrue. It is unscientific and science is objective; I cannot falsify my observations. I'd have more success pushing water uphill. But here, in respect of apomorphine, how I use it and what for, there is a wilful effort to falsify its properties and discount my findings. It is only through analysis that science has value. The suspicion is that commercial imperatives are both driving and distorting research. If it is happening to me where else is it happening and to what end?'

Peel joined them and jumped onto the bench. Dent stroked him while continuing to run the rule over medicine's improper tendencies. 'How many other initiatives are ditched because they won't make somebody rich – or worse, how many damaging approaches are adopted because they will? Sadly, this is becoming endemic with doctors taking lessons from salesman, I ask you! Our health ministry should set an example and remain independent from political favour and only take its cues from best evidence. The government cannot be impartial; therefore, research and medical policy have to remain the preserve of an ethically based and cooperative scientific community. Everything which is currently happening points in the opposite direction; the erosion of medical autonomy.'

'I see.' Rhoda nodded and pulled her cigarettes from her handbag. 'One for the road?'

'One more, and then home,' said Dent, unwinding his slide film and putting it in his jacket pocket.

Rhoda offered two packets: Gold Leaf and Senior Service.

'Name your poison,' she said.

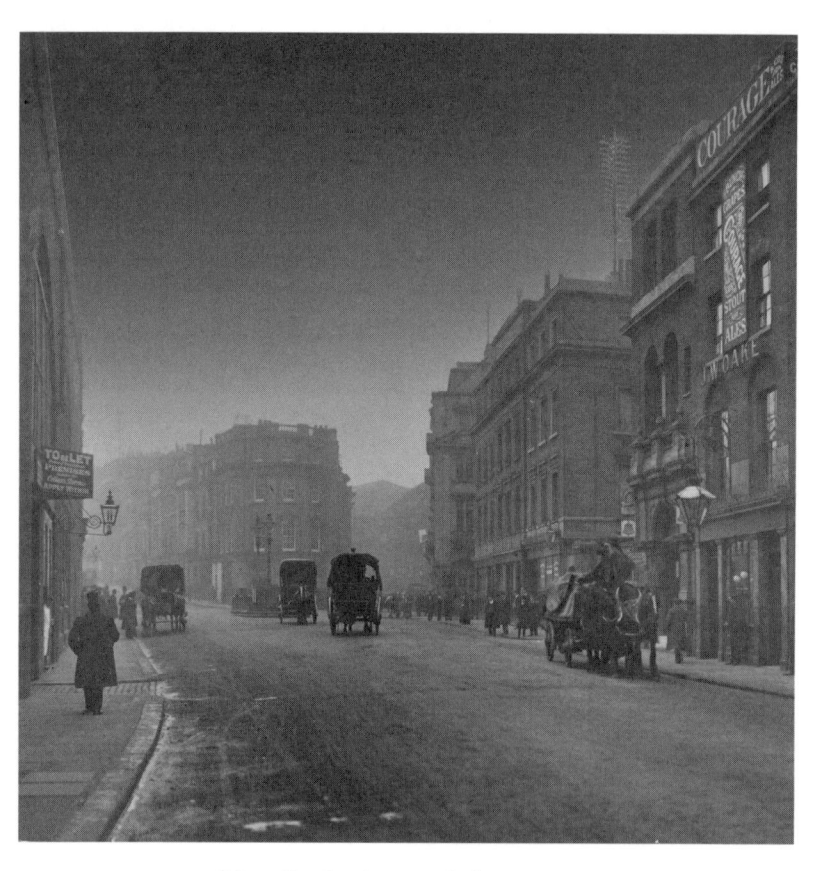

Edwardian London, a typical street scene.
[©Collage, London Picture Archive 2018]

3

From Science to Séance

On his eighteenth birthday John Yerbury Dent took in the scene around Temple Tube Station. He was a few minutes early for a rendezvous with his uncle and watched intently as a thick river mist gradually shrouded the Embankment. A blonde girl in a long coat arranged piles of books and periodicals on shaky trestles. Nobody seemed interested in her wares. Droves of office workers, their footfall muffled in the fog, shuffled down the steps, all too eager to get home for the weekend, their well-earned prize tagged on to the working week. Perhaps in a hundred years with most jobs done by machines, mused Dent, it'll be two days on and five off. That would be better for all concerned. He imagined a time when people would stop, browse and learn... you can never know too much.

 He'd raise the matter tomorrow at dinner, an occasion to celebrate his birthday. It'd be interesting to see what his dad and two uncles thought about this idea of more leisure time. They were brothers, all doctors, trained nearby at King's College Hospital and married to three sisters; the Parks from Rampside, that unassuming village on the edge of Morecambe Bay. This marital harmony between families wasn't that remarkable and was assumed in part to be attributable to their shared religious convictions: the Dents with their Quakerism, the Parks their Methodism. Nevertheless, John wondered, how much pressure had his Uncle Louis and Aunt Emma been under to tread the same matrimonial path as their siblings? It was understood, if never openly discussed, that Uncle Louis was not entirely at ease with himself or with the world he couldn't escape from. Maybe this disquiet was why John had always felt drawn to him as compared to the rest of his relations. For instance he was secretly proud of the fact that Louis did not suffer saints gladly, preferring the company of publicans and sinners. This subversive streak was also characterised by his convictions surrounding education. 'Yes, knowledge is useful,' he had said, 'but only because it permits criticism. Understanding must be Man's ultimate aspiration, remember that.' Perhaps because Uncle Louis was childless he had taken much more than a passing interest in John's education. 'You can learn as much knee-deep in an Epping pond catching newts as in the British Library,' he asserted. And this was not just empty rhetoric for he often joined in and didn't mind when some of John's amphibians escaped from the bathroom and ended up among his dress shirts. John ran these thoughts through his mind like a blind man might run a chain through his fingers ... feeling for the weak link, the explanation to the enigma that was Uncle Louis.

'Ah, JACK! There you are. Come on or we'll be late.' Uncle Louis bawled John's nickname in his usual manner, with a gusto that made passers-by stop and look.

They walked briskly up Arundel Street towards the shiny new and austere statue of William Gladstone. Uncle Louis, as his nephew knew, harboured an intense dislike for all politicians but Gladstone was in a class of his own.

'Spit for your country, Jack,' he demanded. Uncle Louis spat and was displeased when his nephew didn't follow suit. He stopped. 'Spit, come on, SPIT!'

'But Uncle Louis, it says on the corners of the plinth, "Brotherhood, Aspiration, Courage" and, er, "Education" – surely worthy ambitions?'

'But not upheld by that windbag. A typical politician, Jack. He'd've eaten his grandmother for a vote. So come on, damn you, SPIT!'

'Or the day's over?'

'Yes.' Louis was in no mood to climb down.

'You'd send me home on my birthday?'

'Yes.'

His nephew thought for a moment before catching his Uncle's eye. Fixing it he spat into both his hands, rubbed them together and raised them as fists; the pugilist's pose.

Uncle Louis roared his head off before grabbing his nephew round the neck. 'You little rascal. I'll get you for that.'

Reacquainted with their knockabout camaraderie they marched towards Lincoln's Inn and entered the lecture hall on the dot of 5 p.m.

They found a couple of seats near the back of a steeply banked auditorium. It was packed and filling with tobacco smoke. Eventually the hubbub of voices died as a thin bespectacled man approached the lectern. His voice was both whispery and disdainful.

'Ladies and Gentlemen, I shan't keep you as I know you'll be eager to hear from our main speaker but afterwards there'll be the usual questions and then a brief explanation of our plans for next year. Yes, that's right, Christmas will soon be upon us and to fit in with the academic year we have just three more talks after today. The subjects covered, dates and times of these are on the noticeboard near the entrance.'

He paused to hold up a thin pamphlet. 'These details are also in today's newsletter which costs one penny, representing excellent value. It is supported by donations from business and this price helps us to reach as many as possible. By buying it today you will be helping to keep the price as it is. Thank you.'

His voice shifted; a darker, less whispery tone emerged. 'Now, there's just one further matter. Last Friday afternoon the guest speaker was set upon by a group of ruffians as he left the hall. I understand that no real harm befell the Bishop of Gloucester who nevertheless took offence, as he put it, to this, er, "outrage". We humanists may wish to usher in a more secular age but giving the bumps to our Christian leaders does us no favours, even if it was his birthday. I should not have to remind anyone that the Rationalist brotherhood seeks to emphasise the values of cooperation even with those it profoundly disagrees. It is with amity uppermost in our minds that we will win new friends. I have written to the unfortunate bishop in the hope that he bears us no lasting enmity. It is hoped that this will be the end of the matter.'

Dent noticed that Uncle Louis was finding it hard to contain himself. Tears were beginning to stream down his face.

'Are you all right, Uncle Louis?'

'Don't, Jack.' He stifled a snigger.

The man at the lectern frowned as he peered towards the back of the hall. He shuffled his papers.

'Ahem. So, now, without further ado, it gives me great pleasure to introduce the learned and widely respected physicist, holder of the Romford Medal, Sir Oliver Lodge.'

A portly, white-bearded gentleman ambled towards the lectern to modest applause.

'Good afternoon, I trust that what befell the Bishop of Gloucester won't be my fate.'

'Better mind your Ps and Qs,' announced a heckler to a few cheers.

'I hope I can do more than that,' replied Lodge. He stood away from the lectern. 'Throughout my career I have been spurred by my ardent pursuit of discovery. The stimulus of standing on the threshold of new understanding is like nothing else, I can assure you.'

'Better than conjugal bliss?' somebody called out.

'Oh yes, though admittedly that may come a close second. I can still recall the giddy thrill I got when, for the very first time, I watched particles of atoms respond to electrical charge. It is with me still but regrettably I frequently forget the name of my wife.'

This disclosure was met with a ripple of solidarity.

'I jest,' he continued, 'but recently at a séance in Cambridge the clairvoyant suggested that my wife, Mary, wanted to get in touch with me. I had to inform her that she must be mistaken as I was not yet a widower.' Lodge laughed behind his hand. 'She'd probably mixed up her mesmerism with my magnetism.'

The audience rumbled in arcane appreciation.

'Anyway, as you may or may not know, my reason for addressing you today is to reiterate my renunciation of the monistic view of the universe as pronounced by Haeckel in favour of my own appreciation of a dualism including the metaphysical which, just as real as the atoms I have referred to, is quite observable. Please, do not misunderstand me; I like much of what Haeckel says. I am sure his view on Darwinism is perfectly sensible. However, as you will see, I differ sharply over his one-world view...'

Lodge's lecture was conducted in a respectful but humorous atmosphere maintained by an attentive audience. In the bar afterwards John Dent felt a bit let down that he hadn't been asked to the previous week's entertainment with the Bishop of Gloucester but it wasn't long before Uncle Louis revealed his full hand. He led his nephew over to a smartly dressed gentleman with clean features and slicked-back hair.

'Jack, meet Edwards; he's introducing us to Madam Scarlett tonight.'

'Hello, Jack,' said Edwards in a smarmy voice. 'Will this be your first séance?'

'Yes,' said John, uncomfortable that he'd had to declare his virtue so soon.

'Well, we all have to take the plunge sometime. How old are you?'

'It's my birthday today, I'm eighteen.'

'Oh, many happy returns! And Sagittarius,' added Edwards, raising his eyebrows. 'You probably have special powers being born on the cusp.'

'What's that?' asked John.

'You don't know?' scoffed Edwards.

'Why would he?' said Uncle Louis, chipping in.

'Well, with your deep interest in psychical research, Dent, I would've thought you'd've educated your nephew by now.'

'I do not believe, Edwards, in indoctrination. Education is better self-inflicted, when it springs from within. If, after tonight, Jack wants to learn more then he will find his own path.'

'How sensible.' Edwards backed up his compliment with a recital:

The wise old owl who lived in an oak,
  the more he heard the less he spoke.
The less he spoke the more he heard,
  why can't we all be like that old bird.

Neither Dent seemed impressed.

'Yes,' said Uncle Louis drily, 'something like that. But Edwards, if I can ask for your discretion. You see, there's family politics to consider. My brother, Jack's father, doesn't exactly see eye to eye with me on this and so we, Jack and I, have to be tactful.'

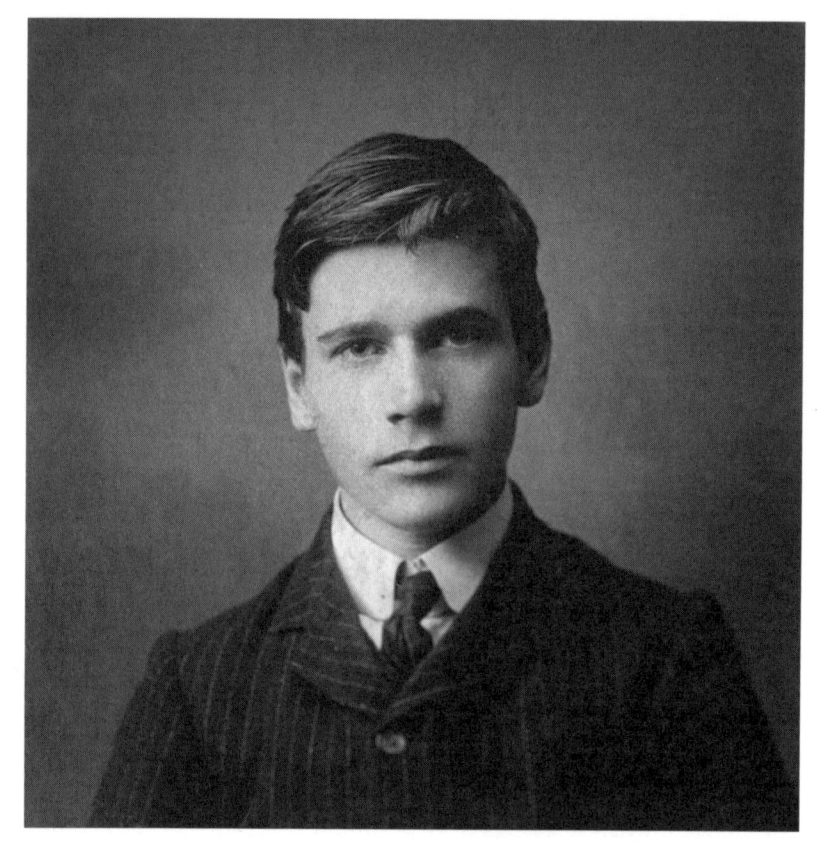

John Yerbury Dent on his eighteenth birthday, 23rd November 1906.
[photographer unknown]

'Oh, yes, fear not. From now on I'll be very sensitive. Mea culpa,' said Edwards, sounding anything but sorry. 'What do you think of spiritualism, Jack? I'd really like to know.'

'Well, I haven't read much about it,' John volunteered, 'but there's clearly a link between it and scientific breakthrough.'

'Do you really think so?' asked Edwards, smoothly. 'You see, though I am involved, I cannot bring myself to believe in any of it. Perhaps it's because of my religious upbringing.'

'I have bullied myself there, too,' said John, 'but it won't do anymore. In our search for an earthly paradise every discovery shows us another place where it isn't. Materially religion and spiritualism are baseless but those that have tried to communicate with the dead have developed tremendous ideas which are both verifiable and useful; telegraphy, the wireless, radiography and so on.'

'My word,' said Edwards, 'are you saying I won't be able to pull the wool over your eyes?'

Louis clapped his hands. 'Ah! Excellent. So, you see Edwards, mind how you go.'

'Agh, right,' calculated Edwards, looking at his watch. 'We could *go now* if you're ready.'

'Where is it?' asked John.

'The Lamb 'n' Flag, a Charrington House. About a ten-minute walk,' replied Edwards, moving towards the door. 'The séance is held upstairs.'

A little while later the three men stood at the front of the pub. It was crowded. The young Dent played with the intoxicating taste of pale ale and tobacco smoke... and with it the flavour of anticipation. He sensed that Uncle Louis was opening his eyes to more than just Oliver Lodge and a séance. But what? He was nervous. Suddenly, red and sapphire sequins flashed by the back stairs. It was difficult to see the cause until a lithe girl leapt from a chair onto the bar. She embraced the sudden shouts and quickly turned them into orchestrated cheers by punching the air. Alerted by the din more people from the street squeezed towards the bar. The premises began to shake as the girl started a storming dance and to roars of approval her negligee disappeared. Delighted she urged greater effort from the crowd. The cheer that followed the removal of the rest of her clothing was heard in the next borough. The pub was bouncing.

The young Dent was transfixed by the girl's power. With a wave of her hand, the thumping beat was silenced. Her attention had been taken by a tall bowler-hatted gentleman who sat motionless at the end of the bar reading a newspaper. Fatefully he looked up as the apparition approached. Upset by his indifference she removed his bowler hat, revealing a bald head. She looked surprised and the pub guffawed. He looked around, suddenly aware of his predicament. Wedged in by a mob and without his hat he was trapped. He blushed, his crimson pate shining in the gaslight. She gyrated and coyly used his hat to mock him and protect her modesty. Teasingly, she offered to return his hat. He stretched out his hand but this was cat and mouse. She waltzed to the other end of the bar and gestured that she was tired and would like to sit down. She tried to use the hat but, of course, it gave way. She shook her head and tried again until a wag yelled, 'Sit on his head!'

She thought this a brilliant idea and edged back towards the shiny bonce. With her back to the pub she lowered herself towards it. As skin met skin the pub exploded. She wiggled to find a comfortable position and brought the house down. After more wiggling she stood up to her full height, earning many 'ooos' and 'aghs'. Turning round she signalled to the hatless victim that this was hot work and she could do with a drink. 'Help the poor thirsty lady,' came the cry. Expressing signs of frustration at the gent's coolness she tapped him on the shoulder. She would return his hat in exchange for some beer. 'Gooo on, give her a drink, why don't yer?' urged the wag to ironic cries of sympathy. The gentleman finally relented and offered her his tall glass. She took a deep draught until the glass was half empty. With a half a pint in one hand and the hat in the other she leant against a wooden pillar as if it were a lamp post. Inexplicably she hit on the idea of putting her left breast in the glass. She leant forward and discovered to her delight that it fitted perfectly! She then realised that even if she leant backwards the beer couldn't spill. The crowd cried tears of joy as she formed an inverted C shape until the glass was upside-down. Further cheers accompanied the same trick with her other breast until the back of her head touched the bar. She curtsied and returned the glass to her victim, indicating that he could have his hat back if he drank his beer. When he hesitated, she wagged her finger. The pub joined in: 'Go on! What's wrong with yer, drink up!'

Cowed by the unrelenting pressure, he raised the glass to his lips and took a sip. The girl shook her head. She insisted; he must drink it all. Following jeers questioning his manhood the demoralised gentleman emptied the glass. At last the girl returned the hat and with a final flourish, vanished.

The crowd thinned and the three men were able to find a small table.

'Well, from Oliver Lodge to dear little Lily, quite a leap there, Jack?' said Edwards, grinning.

'Lily? You know her?' asked Jack.

'Yes, she also works for Madam Scarlett upstairs. Extraordinarily versatile, wouldn't you agree Dent?'

Louis was quiet.

'When will it start, the séance?' asked John.

'In about thirty minutes or so. Would you like to meet Lily?' Edwards looked at the young Dent waiting for an answer.

It was John's turn to blush.

Edwards stood up. 'It'd be better if you came upstairs. Why don't we all go up?' He suggested. 'I've got to talk to Madam Scarlett anyway.'

'Yes, all right,' agreed Louis, 'lead on.'

They climbed two flights of stairs and were shown into a small sitting room with sparse furniture: a pile of wooden boxes and a suitcase stood against the far wall. A single light hung from a central rose.

As they sat down Edwards left. A minute later a fully clothed Lily entered. She had removed her wig, revealing short-cropped hair. 'Hello, I'm Lily, and you are?'

'John Dent, hello, and this is my Uncle Louis.'

'Oh, we know each other, but it's Lou-ee,' assured Lily.

'You're nearly right,' said the young Dent, trying to be helpful, 'it is spelled the French way, but pronounced Lou-iss, like the town.'

'Oh,' said Lily, doubtfully. 'You mean all your family know him as Lou-iss?'

'Yes, that's right.'

'And his parents always called him Lou-iss?'

'Yes, of course. Is that a problem?' The young Dent was confused.

'Don't worry about it, Lily,' said Uncle Louis, firmly.

'But,' she protested, 'this means that all those spirits that have been talking to you, calling you Lou-ee all these years? This means you've known all along it's nonsense.' Lily was upset.

'It doesn't matter,' said Louis. 'Please! I really don't mind. I never have.'

Lily recoiled slightly before sitting down. There was an uncomfortable silence. Louis finally spoke up.

'You see, Jack, Lily has often been your grandmother's ghost or spirit, calling me Lou-ee, the French way. I don't mind, I really don't, not at all. We all have different personas, why not names? I think it is one of the things that spiritualism permits. An opportunity to be someone else, nothing wrong with that, is there?'

'Hang on a minute,' said Lily, visibly annoyed, 'before we go any further, who is he, John or Jack?'

Louis looked at his nephew, 'Shall I explain?'

'I will. My birth name is John, but my family always called me Jack.'

Lily made a gesture of incomprehension.

'Jack doesn't want to tell you why,' smiled Louis. 'The truth is he's shy... about his height... or lack of it.'

'I don't *see* at all,' said Lily.

John tried to look indifferent.

'Tell her, Jack, or I will,' his uncle goaded.

John sighed, 'When I was young,' he started, 'very young,' he emphasised, 'we used to play hide-and-seek. There was a small ice box under a side table that I hid in. Nobody could believe anyone could fit in so nobody looked. Of course, I could hear everything and when they all gave up I jumped out!'

'That's right,' said Uncle Louis, 'so we called him "Jack-in-the-box". Then just "Jack".'

'Not a very interesting story,' said John, clearly bored.

'Oh, no!' enthused Lily, her eyes sparkling. 'I love it!' She got up and kissed John on the lips. 'Wonderful,' she gushed.

'Er, really, w-why?' he stammered.

'Because that's how I got into this lark. I used to hide in boxes and throw my voice; got me started.'

'But that's because you're double-jointed, not a shrimp, like him,' said Louis, mockingly.

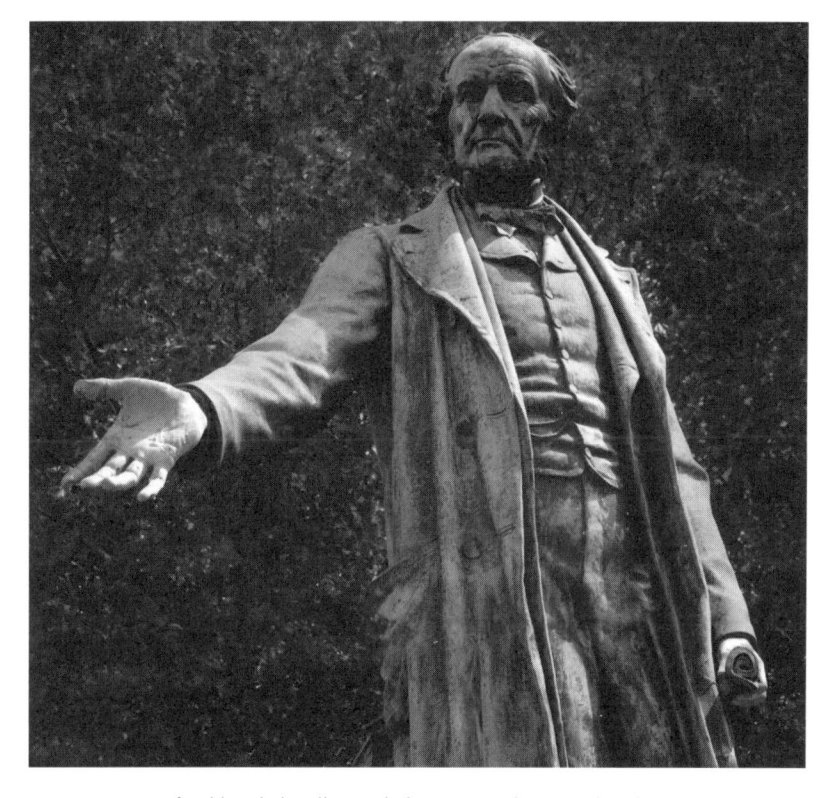

Statue of red handed William Gladstone outside Bow Church, London.
[photo: JWS]

'That's not fair,' said Lily. 'Young John is far from short now, a fine fellow.'

'Mmmm,' said Louis, 'maybe.'

'What would you have done, Lily,' asked John, trying to remain cool. 'I mean, if you hadn't been able to hide in boxes?'

'I'd've ended up a match girl like my mother, with a phossy face. And that's no life, believe me. Died in agony she did.'

'Phossy face?' asked John.

'Yes,' said Louis. 'More accurately "phossy jaw". Most of the workers got it at Bryant & May due to the phosphorous they handled. It caused a reaction when it came into contact with saliva and rotted the jaw. We came across a lot of it in Bethnal during training. Quite terrible; the mouth and jawbone collapse. And Jack, another thing *you* should know,' Louis' voice grew teeth, 'those poor women, afflicted with that terrible condition had their wages stolen to pay for another statue to that bastard Gladstone.'

'Oh yes!' recalled Lily, 'we still paint 'is hands red every year on account o' that.'

'Quite right, too, the buggering blowhard,' swore Louis making no effort to conceal his outrage.

'I didn't know,' said John, reflecting that he might spit next time. 'I am sorry.'

Lily looked at him kindly. 'Not your fault, love, but not a word of a lie; I still get the 'orrors thinkin' about what Mam went through. She had to soak her mouth in gin to kill the pain. There was nuffin' else …'

A long pause followed. John twisted uncomfortably at the thought of a face rotting from within. Eventually he was distracted by some sounds from outside. The bar below was emptying and shouts echoed along the street. From somewhere further away a muffled scream …

'Who was the man at the bar?' he asked, 'the man with the bowler hat?'

'Ah!' exclaimed Louis, 'you see Lily; he's cottoning on.'

Lily got to her feet and stood behind Louis, her form melting into the shadows. She hung her arms over his shoulders before running her fingers up his neck and cheeks, ruffling his hair and humming. Gradually a soft melody emerged, its wistful delicacy quite at odds with the lyric:

> *My name is Lily, I'm a whore in Piccadilly*
> *My sis does the same along the Strand.*
> *Daddy sells 'is arse'ole*
> *Daan the Elephant an' Cars'ole*
> *An' on the 'ole the family's doing real grand!*

A loud knock on the door and Edwards returned.

'Right, come on. The circle is called. Madam awaits.'

They trooped out, climbed another flight of stairs and entered a carpeted room with ceiling-to-floor black velvet curtains. A circular table was set in a dingy pool of yellow light. Edwards pointed to everybody's prearranged places. Lily, John noticed, had disappeared.

Edwards opened the curtain and helped a tall woman in a scarlet dress and black shawl to the only high-backed chair at the table. Even in the dim light John was able to make out that her eyes were blank, like pots of curdled milk. She was probably blind.

Behind her appeared two more women who sat opposite each other and finally a middle-aged man with a round red face. Edwards helped him to his seat next to John.

'Thank you, circle, for coming tonight and giving us the opportunity to combine our energies. Please,' she spoke imperiously, like a governess charged with authority over unruly children, 'if we could join hands, letting our arms rest on the table, thank you.' The circle obediently adjusted to this arrangement. 'Welcome everyone, on this side and in the next. My name is Madam Scarlett and without further ado I would like to introduce you. We have with us two Dents, Dr Louie and his nephew John. Welcome, John; your first séance, I believe.' John nodded. 'He may be a conduit in his own right,' Madam Scarlett continued, 'and we will certainly try to discover if he has special powers. Dr Louie, of course, we know and will certainly be keen to converse again with his parents…. We are also delighted to entertain our esteemed and occasional visitors from the Hampstead circle; Miss Fortescue and Miss Selfridge, welcome. Of course, Mr Edwards, to whom we are deeply indebted for organising this circle and last but not least, another first time visitor, from Kensington, the distinguished scientist and highly acclaimed academic, Professor Gove.' There followed a brief moment for exchanged glances and strained smiles.

'And now,' Madam Scarlett's voice wandered into a highly affected register, 'I wish to share with you a little story which confirms the special powers of spiritualism available to our gifted and highly attuned followers.' She drew herself up against her ornately carved and high-backed chair. John Dent was reminded of *Alice in Wonderland*'s Queen of Hearts, another ridiculous figure.

'Many years ago I became aware that my carriage clock,' her voice wavered, 'my precious gran sonnerie, made by the esteemed Parisian, Jacot, had stopped working. I mentioned this to my beloved aunt at a garden party who had exactly the same model. She divulged that hers had developed an identical fault and, being familiar with its delicate mechanism, knew how to fix it. She promised to visit to conduct the repair. A week or two later and in the middle of the night I was suddenly awoken by a sweet chime. My precious Jacot had struck the hour, 3 a.m! I got up and sure enough it was once again working perfectly. I believed it had fixed itself and thinking nothing more about it went straight back to sleep.'

Madam Scarlett paused and gave a small sob. 'Well imagine my shock when on the morrow, exactly seven years ago tonight, I learnt that my dear aunt had in the early hours passed that night from this world to the next. Clearly, though, she had kept her promise with regard to the repair and since that day I haven't even had to wind the clock. It still works, perfectly.'

The medium's story, John Dent noticed, had been delivered in an increasingly haunting voice while almost imperceptibly the gas-lighting had dimmed. He wondered if these circumstances were designed to conceal rather than reveal what might happen next. After a few seconds she added:

'We in touch with the afterlife have no trouble in accepting the veracity of these events. It is evidence of the power of our spirit brethren to intercede on our behalf. I am grateful to my dearest aunt who was herself a very open-minded lady and it is my fervent wish that one day she will permit a materialisation.' Madam Scarlett paused. 'Who knows, perhaps tonight?'

'Oooo yes,' said one of the Hampstead ladies.

The other tittered nervously and brought her hands to her face.

'A heart-warming tale,' said Uncle Louis, arching his eyebrows. He had heard the yarn before.

'A beautiful story beautifully told. Thank you,' said Edwards, anxious that Louis' faithless manner should not be dwelled upon.

'Ooh! What was that?' asked Madam Scarlett suddenly.

'What?' said Edwards.

'I didn't see anything,' said Uncle Louis.

'Neither did I,' said Madam Scarlett, loftily, 'I *felt* something.'

'Oh dear!' one of the Hampstead ladies gasped.

'Yes. A faint brush of my hair, when I was thinking of the Professor. Oh yes! There it is again!'

As the circle looked around apprehensively the table started to vibrate. It suddenly rose several inches before crashing to the floor. Both Hampstead ladies squealed.

'Ah HA!' exclaimed Madam Scarlett. 'It seems we're in for a lively evening.'

She turned her face to the ceiling and raised her voice to a quivering falsetto. 'Is there anybody there?'

There was silence; nothing except for the sound of breathing.

'Is there anybody there?' she repeated. 'Knock once for yes.'

'And two for no?' ventured Gove.

'That wouldn't make sense, would it?' asserted Edwards.

'Oh, yes,' said Gove, 'silly me.'

'Quiet please,' commanded Madam Scarlett, 'I *shall* be allowed to concentrate. Please, circle, summon our energies to the matter at hand... to the presence of our friends and loved ones in the spirit world.'

Cowed by the strident words the circle bowed their heads. Outside a peel from a distant church bell and the sharp clicks of a passing drayman's horse penetrated the thickening atmosphere. Soon every sound faded from consciousness as the group began to relax.........

BANG! The circle jumped.

There was a flurry and approaching footsteps, very loud footsteps. One of the Hampstead ladies shrieked.

'WHO IS THERE?' Madam Scarlett demanded. 'Declare yourself. Do you want to speak to someone here? One knock for yes, two knocks for no.'

The silence returned but steeped in terror. Finally, after mounting tension, there was a single emphatic knock followed by gasps.

'Agh! Our spirit friend who touched me earlier,' said Madam Scarlett. 'I feel certain someone is trying to reach one of us. Are you trying to speak to Professor Gove? One knock for yes, two for no.'

After another long pause came a single knock.

'I thought so,' said Madam Scarlett, leaning forward, permitting more of the yellow light to fall on her wax-like face, her mauve lips and stagnant eyes.

'Please, we must know who you are. Are you a relative?' her voice a baleful wail.

There was another single knock, the sound you might expect to hear if you banged a broom handle on a floorboard. Young Dent imagined that Lily was yawning as she did it.

'A parent?'

There were two loud knocks.

'A brother?'

Two more loud knocks.

'A sister?'

Another pause, then a single knock.

'Ridiculous,' said Gove. 'I never had a sister, how preposterous!'

'Wait!' insisted Madam Scarlett. 'We will reserve judgement.'

The circle bent its collective ear to the darkness. The hush fell like snow in still air.

'Did you, kind spirit, know your brother?' the medium asked haughtily.

There was another strained pause, then two very loud knocks followed by a congested puff from Gove. One of the Hampstead ladies held her cheeks in a look of horror. All eyes turned to the professor.

'Are you sure you didn't have a sister?' asked Madam Scarlett, sounding like a shopkeeper catching a thief red-handed.

Gove removed his hands from the circle and shielded his eyes.

'I tell you, I don't know,' he pleaded. Gove's earlier poise had all but evaporated. He wriggled.

Madam Scarlett ignored his protestations and returned her attentions to the spirit world. 'Are you, kind soul, trying to reach your brother?'

There was a single knock.

'Did you, wandering spirit, expire in childbirth or shortly after?'

There was another quick knock.

'Then you shared the womb with your dear twin brother?'

A very quick knock followed, slightly louder than all the rest.

Madam Scarlett breathed out and raised her hands as if in prayer.

'And are you, kind spirit, well? Happy in the afterlife?'

There was a brief pause before the knock.

'And your brother has nothing to worry about, because one day you will be together again?'

There was a final emphatic knock. The curtains billowed and muffled footsteps receded into silence.

'Well!' said Edwards, 'How wonderful. You have someone who loves and admires you.'

The professor held his cheeks in horror. He slumped forward onto the table and started to blub. 'My poor sister, my poor, poor sister.'

'Please, Professor, pull yourself together.' Madam Scarlett straightened her back. 'Your dear sister simply wanted you to know that she has always been watching over you and is quite well, she's happy, in no pain.'

This news drew a further wail from Gove who finally sat up, his face streaked with tears.

One of the ladies got up and put her arm around him. 'There, there,' she said, 'I lost an infant sister, too. She was only three and I don't remember her. I'd love to hold her hand one day.'

'And you surely will,' said Madam Scarlett, getting up. 'I am certain of it.'

John Dent caught Uncle Louis' eye, but Louis wasn't giving anything away. After a few minutes of small talk he signalled towards the door. It was time to go.

They caught the last Tube. John read his cheap Rationalist Press reprint, Haeckel's *The Riddle of the Universe*; Uncle Louis the newsletter and a review of *The Doctor's Dilemma* by George Bernard Shaw.

When they got home John's parents were already asleep. He thanked Uncle Louis for an eventful evening and went upstairs himself. His uncle wished him a good night and said something about an exciting day tomorrow. But it was the day he was leaving that filled his thoughts. The Lodge lecture seemed weeks ago as John's mind spun with the sights and sounds of The Lamb 'n' Flag; the mysterious Lily and Madam Scarlett able to orchestrate emotion so easily. But the clearest pictures were the imagined. A broken down slum, dimly lit. In the front room sat a woman. With one hand she cradled a bottle of gin, with the other, her rotting jaw. In the shadows stood a young and helpless Lily, crying. Later they crept outside and defiantly painted Gladstone's hands... bright red... like match-heads. This pitiful scene dissolved into the gloriously clandestine painting of Gladstone's hands ... like match heads. Of all the day's events it was this clear expression of solidarity that had impressed him most.

The next day Aunt Emma arrived at 6 p.m. and stood her nephew's wrapped present to one side of the fireplace. She then went upstairs to see her sister Daisy, who was unwell and wouldn't be down for dinner. John's father Harry came into the drawing room and asked Louis and John whether they'd had a good time yesterday.

'Any Fabians at the Oliver Lodge Lecture?' he asked.

'Oh yes, lots,' enthused John. 'Afterwards we went to a séance,' he volunteered.

'Oh!' said Harry, 'you didn't tell me you were going to do that, Louis?'

'And if I had your beloved son may have missed the experience of a lifetime.'

Harry sat up. 'A séance is nothing more than a disappointing evening spent with charlatans. There's nothing in it, so why do it?'

Louis looked from his nephew to his brother.

'I think you will find, Old H, that despite your misgivings Jack and I had a terrific evening. He met some unusual people and as long as he lives he'll never regret it.'

The door opened and Aunt Emma's head appeared.

'Your mother would like to see you, Jack; not for long.'

John got up and left.

Harry felt he had to speak out; he was glad his son wouldn't hear what he had to say. 'The trouble is, Louis, séances are dominated by cheap manipulators of fear. People want a thrill; it's vaudeville, nothing more. And even if there is something in it, it is too dangerous. Life is hard enough as it is without complicating it by reintroducing those that have left it.'

'Maybe,' said Louis, 'but isn't it interesting that those who object most are those that go to church on Sunday. And what is the resurrection if it isn't the same game; incantations to the dead only with grander attachments of compliance and ritual?'

'Well, religion has its purpose,' pointed out Harry.

'What?' cried Uncle Louis. 'Religion demands obedience in this world by terrifying people with fear of punishment in the next. That's tyranny, nothing less.'

Harry hesitated before speaking. 'You know full well,' he started, 'religion serves society in other ways. If there was no moral guidance, no instruction by which to shape our lives there'd be chaos … anarchy. You wouldn't want that. None of us would.'

Louis scoffed as he lit his pipe. 'Nonsense. Think of the other ways in which society is kept in check. Universal education for one and fear of penury for another. Consider the Fabians; some of the most civilised people we know, motivated by simple feelings of altruism. They aren't in need of some genuflecting, sexually constipated cock in a frock to tell them what's what. The sooner we can rid ourselves of all that, the better. I don't know why you're so resistant.'

'I'm not. In fact I agree with you that religion is cheapened by professionalism. Why, for instance, would I go to a cathedral for guidance on Sunday when I can just as easily find it at the bottom of the garden on Wednesday? A spiritual life is highly individual and no less important for that. No, what I am really objecting to is interference with the dead.'

'Well, I want to know about it.'

'You mean, despite everything you've said, you think there is an afterlife?'

'Yes, most definitely.'

Harry turned and looked into the fire. He was not often pressed to lay down the law.

'Well, if that's the case then I forbid you to involve Jack. He's got some decisions to make about what he wants to do with his life and this cannot be allowed to distract him. Is that clear?'

Louis wandered over to the mantelpiece and leant against the black marble. 'Well, I suppose I have always involved Jack in my interests. And I never thought this should be any different.'

'Does Emma know you feel like this?'

'Of course; you know she does. It was she that introduced me. Me! The biggest sceptic alive. Yes, many of those involved in so-called psychical exploration are rogues, worse than bookmakers, but I'm hardly alone. Some of the greatest minds of our generation are hooked on it.'

John entered and returned to his seat. There was an uneasy silence; the fire glowed like a smelter's cauldron.

'How's your mother?' asked Louis.

'I don't know, she seems quite distressed to me. I would have thought with so many doctors in the house you should be telling me.' The atmosphere grew thin; the heat seemed to have sucked the air from the room. Louis broke the silence:

'Your father has been telling me that you've been thinking about what you might like to do next year. Any ideas? Cambridge?'

'I've decided,' said John.

'Oh!' said Louis, eyeing his brother.

Harry shrugged. 'Don't look at me, this is the first I've heard of it.'

'Yes, I'm going to be a doctor, but one who makes people better, not worse.'

'What do you mean, "worse"?' asked Harry.

'Mother tells me you've been giving her morphine, not for months, but years!' John's voice rose sharply. 'Now she can't leave it. This is outrageous – you, a doctor! I just don't understand. So yes, not architecture, or engineering but medicine. I'll go to King's.'

John stood up; he was shaking visibly.

'Please, Jack, sit down,' said his father. 'We can explain.'

Louis walked over and put his arm around his nephew. 'It isn't your father's fault. I also thought it best; Uncle Herbert too. We all discussed it. Your mother has terrible arthritis; we thought we could monitor the situation. It is only in the last few months that it's become ... er, difficult.'

John disentangled himself from his uncle. He was not going to be mollified. 'But there must be a better way?'

'There isn't; she says so herself. It's the only medication that works.'

'Works!?' questioned the young Dent. 'She's worse now. So "works" is not a word I accept, sorry.'

John sat down and the room returned to a strained silence relieved by a knock on the door. It was the cook. 'Dinner is served.'

'Thank you, Abba, we'll come through,' said Harry.

As Abba left Aunt Emma returned. She tried to catch Louis' eye but he was lost in thought. She picked up her present for John. 'Before we go through, Jack, I'd love to see you open your present.'

'Yes, all right.' John ripped off the wrapping before Uncle Louis could intervene. He held up a shiny ouija board.

'Ah ha!' Aunt Emma exclaimed, her face beaming. 'We hope you get as much fun out of this as Louis and I have out of ours.'

'Thank you, Aunt Em, Uncle Louis. I'll put it in the shed and try it out next full moon.' He made a ghostly hooting noise.

'Excellent!' exclaimed Aunt Emma, clapping her hands. She briefly admired the board with her nephew, its inlaid pattern of light and dark wood before propping it against the sofa. 'Come, dinner's getting cold.' She linked arms with her nephew and they walked out.

Harry jumped up and closed the door, rounding on his brother;

'This is too much, Louis. Do you hear me? Too much and it has to stop now. I won't say it again and I leave it to you to tell Emma. Is that clear?'

Louis was taken aback by the resolute tone of his brother's voice. He hesitated.

'Damn it, Louis! If you won't obey me I will forbid you to have anything more to do with Jack; anything. I mean it.'

Louis felt sick. He prided himself in seeing the funny side in every situation but the smouldering rage in his brother gave him no leeway.

'I understand, Old H, I won't mention it again.'

'Ever?' insisted his brother.

'Never. You have my word.'

* * *

A month later and a couple of days before Christmas John was seated by his mother's bed. For some time she had had trouble sleeping but found that being read to helped. John had grown accustomed to the role.

'What would you like to hear?' he asked.

'You choose.'

'A novel or poetry?'

'Oh, a novel.'

'Dickens, Wells or Brontë?'

'Brontë every time.'

'Charlotte, Emily or Anne?'

'Ah, that's hard. Well, how about Anne, there's only two.'

'You're right.' He opened the glass-fronted bookcase. '*Wildfell Hall* or *Agnes Grey*?'

'Let's try *Wildfell Hall*; it's a long time since I read that.'

'I've only read her sisters.'

'Oh *Wildfell* is the best of the lot, and particularly challenging.'

'Really? I thought they all sang the same tune.'

'But Anne goes further, her character jumps ship, which women just didn't. Anyway, I'm not about t' tell you, you'll have to find out...'

John closed the bookcase and turned towards the bed... there was a sudden cry from downstairs, followed by approaching steps on the stairs. The door opened. It was Harry.

'Louis,' he said. 'He's dead.' He crossed the room and half fell against the bed, sobbing.

'No!' cried John, 'I don't believe it.'

Daisy sat up and reached out to her husband. 'How?'

Harry mumbled something into the eiderdown.

'Suicide?' repeated Daisy, incredulous.

'Yes!' Harry cried.

John sat down on the bed next to his father, extending a hand to his heaving shoulder. 'I don't understand.'

Daisy sat back with her hand gripping the bedstead.

'Oh no!' she said two or three times, rocking back and forth. 'To think that you two never made up.'

Unsteadily Harry stood up. 'Well, now he knows I'm right!' He looked at his wife as if expecting a response. With none forthcoming he turned and went back downstairs.

John moved towards his mother and they held hands. 'I just can't believe it,' he said. 'I'm numb, quite numb.'

'Yes, me too,' was all his mother could say. They hugged each other.

'I'd better go and see your father,' she said eventually. 'He shouldn't be alone.'

'No, you're right. I'll wait here.'

John moved back to the bookcase and returned *The Tenant of Wildfell Hall* alongside the volumes by Anne's sisters. As he closed the bookcase he looked into the distorting Georgian glass reflecting the shadows from across the room. He peered into them and imagined Louis therein, watching him. 'Well, are you?' he found himself asking the empty room. There was no answer; nor did he expect one. He knocked the frame of the bookcase with his knuckle...twice, and bowed his head.

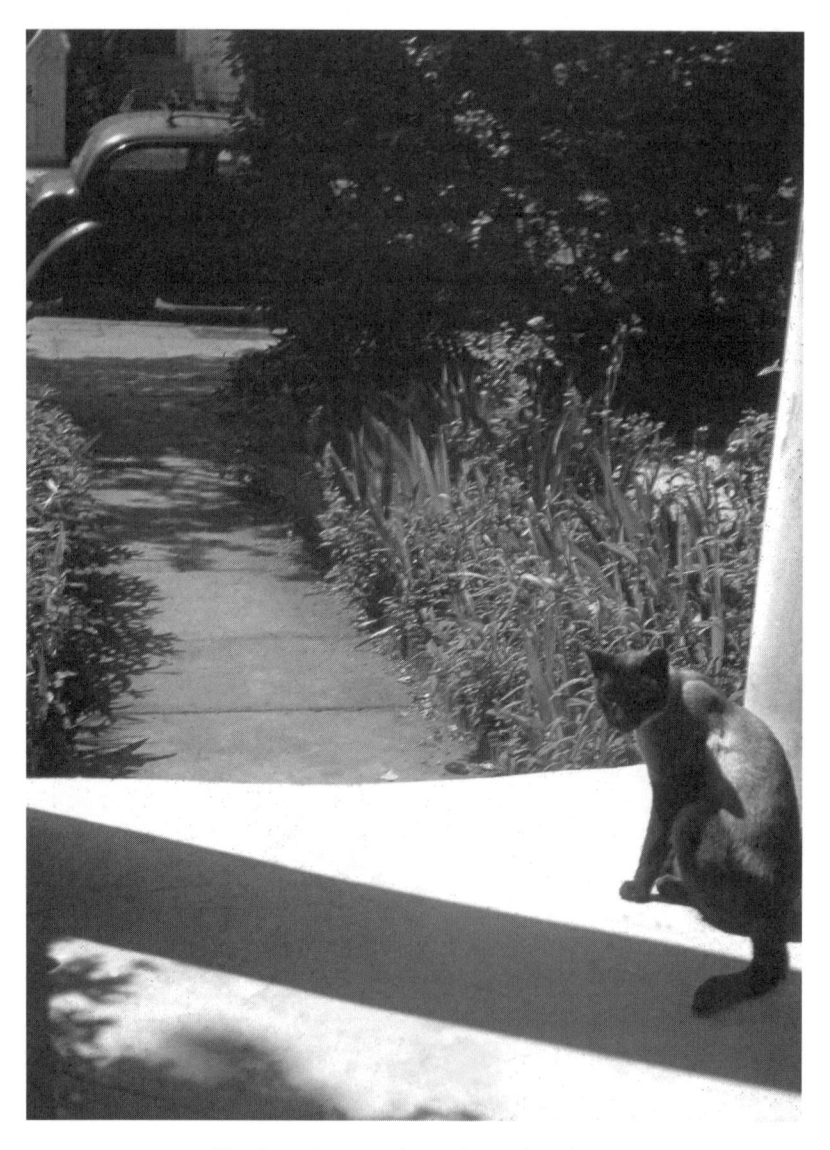

The doctor's car, garden path, porch and cat.
[photo: J.Y. Dent]

4

Siamese Fighting Fish and Ulysses

> The quality of mercy is not strain'd
> It droppeth as the gentle rain from heaven
> Upon the place beneath; it is twice blest;
> It blesseth him that gives and him that takes...
> – Old Bill Shakespeare
> Portia, *Merchant of Venice*

By mid-afternoon, William Seward Burroughs, a leaden-eyed and compulsive opiate addict, paranoid and down on his luck, entered Addison Road, W.14. Every cell in his shivering body screamed at him to leave. They knew what they craved and this was hopeless.

'A waste of time, you motherfucker.'

'Shut up.'

'Shoulda gone to Piccadilly.'

Addison Road was a wide, almost deserted street filled with shabby villas. The grey traveller hesitated outside No. 34, a detached corner house. He checked the address and looked down the short path leading to a stuccoed portico sheltering a large black door. In its centre a brass devil door knocker glinted. He advanced a few steps and, unsure what to do, stopped. Yes, it was hopeless... the 'Dilly boys' would know. Fatefully, Peel jumped out of his kennel. He stretched and shook; a typical canine welcome. His long chain rattled... loudly.

Burroughs stepped back and sneezed as the front door swung open. A stocky man in red socks and braces and an unbuttoned white shirt appeared.

'Hello, I'm Dent.'

'Ugh, hello, I'm Burroughs,' the traveller said, wiping his face. 'I am er, sorry, ah, I, er... saw a Dr Maclay. I haven't an appointment but it's urgent, you see. I was worried, er...'

'Agh worry,' interrupted Dent. 'Such a curse, isn't it? Never mind, please come in... sorry about the dog... there's worse inside: cats! You don't mind cats do you?'

Fumbling with his handkerchief Burroughs edged into a large hallway filled with sunlight and the mustiness of old books and wood polish. Dent reached out and felt a limp handshake but failed to meet his visitor's gaze buried under the brim of a wide hat and thick-framed glasses.

Undeterred, the older man continued to talk, almost to himself. 'I am delighted, Mr Burroughs, you came when you did, in the nick of time as it happens. You see, I was about to pull on my gardening boots but you've saved the day, thank you.' Dent's gratitude merged into a warm rumble of laughter while he put on a jacket without tucking in or buttoning up his shirt. 'And this, Mr Burroughs, is Onions. Please, let him have your coat.'

A youngish, smiling man appeared and helped Burroughs with his mac.

'And your hat, sir?' he suggested, in a fey voice.

'Oh yeah, my hat, sure.'

'Ooh, before I forget, Onions,' said Dent, 'here's my photographs of the park. When you get a chance perhaps you could drop them off. Could be a breakthrough, change the course of photography.'

'I thought you'd already done that,' said Onions, tittering.

Dent joined in with more throaty laughter.

'...And perhaps, Onions, if you'd be so kind and help Rhoda with the roses. We'd be most grateful. *I'll* make the tea. Mr Burroughs, do you like tea?'

Burroughs steadied himself against a mahogany newel post.

'Perhaps you'd prefer something stronger?' said Dent, not waiting for an answer. 'Well, I'll make the tea anyhow. Please, follow me.'

Dent disappeared down a wide corridor leading to a warm parlour.

SIAMESE FIGHTING FISH AND ULYSSES

A large kettle half on and half off the Aga's hot plate steamed gently. Burroughs struggled to keep up.

'This won't take long, Mr Burroughs. I'm parched and sweet tea greases the wheels.'

Dent lifted a pile of books from a throne-like chair he'd hand carved out of oak many years before. 'Please, Mr Burroughs, sit down while I sort this out.'

Burroughs vaguely noticed two eel-like creatures on the chair's broad back. Were these the fish who swim to the Sargasso? He sat down gingerly squinting at the titles of the books the doctor had thrown on the table. The doctor warmed a large earthenware teapot while casually observing his visitor.

'If you like libraries you've come to the right house,' he chuckled while measuring three teaspoonfuls of loose-leaved tea. 'Please, if there's anything there you like, take it.'

Dent poured in the boiling water. 'Perhaps you don't like reading?' he asked, clattering some mugs and utensils onto a tray.

'I read this as a kid.' Burroughs held up a golden-brown book so Dent could read the spine.

'Ah, yes, *Lives of the Hunted,* great stories.' Dent stirred the pot with a long silver spoon. 'Too late for my childhood but we found our girls loved them, couldn't get enough.'

'Yeah, I dug them,' said Burroughs, his voice scratched like a dry twig outside a window.

Dent picked up the tray and slid it into a dumb waiter.

'RIGHT, let's go upstairs.'

Dent's solid frame moved back across the hall and up the wide staircase that doubled as a depository for more books. Every step supported mixed piles of every age and genre. Burroughs stumbled and steadied himself against the bannister. Dent noticed and slowed down.

'Sorry about all this.' He waved towards the stacks of books. 'I'm trying to sort it out, but if you break a leg, I'll fix it, no fee.'

Dent listened for a reaction but none came … this was noted.

The two men crossed a gallery landing and entered a large room at the back of the house. Two full-height Georgian windows overlooked a deep rambling garden. Between the windows a rococo framed oil hung above a marble Buddha, pure white. With his serene face and hanging eyelids the enlightened one gazed meditatively over a cluttered coffee table towards a brightly illuminated aquarium stocked with tropical fish. A sapphire and crimson shoal glinted amongst bubble-pearled reeds. Against the far wall stood a matching pair of huge Georgian glass-fronted bookcases crammed with volumes arranged in tight formations. On the lower shelves there appeared to be some ancient manuscripts, atlases perhaps.

'Please, Mr Burroughs, sit down, make yourself comfortable while I get the tea.'

The visitor dropped heavily into an upholstered chair beside a consultation desk pushed tightly against the wall. His right hand immediately pinched his temple. Leaning over the desk the doctor pulled on a blue cord. There was a hollow roll that grew until the mechanism clattered to a halt like a milk cart in a tunnel. He lifted out the tea tray and plonked it on the desk with a crash. Out of nowhere a Siamese cat leapt onto the visitor's lap.

'Agh, Ulysses!' said Dent. 'He's banned. I do apologise. He likes fish, you see...wheedles his way in.'

The doctor picked up Ulysses and carried him to where he could get a perfect view of the flickering aquatic display.

'Ulysses?' wheezed a startled Burroughs, trying to calm himself down and ignore the contradiction between Dent's words and action.

'Yes, we name our dogs after British prime ministers and our cats after your presidents. Not a great president, but what a name!' Dent laughed alone.

'Is it obvious; I mean, that I'm American?' croaked the traveller, trying to engage.

'Well, it just so happens I had a crash course on American accents last week. There was a medical delegation from the States interested in our drug laws and I showed them around. What part are you from?'

'St Louis.'

Dent looked up. An airy image of Uncle Louis loomed in the

distorted glass of the bookcase. His memory still tugged him, still threw his voice down the decades. *'Spit, damn you. Spit!'*

'Ah, T.S. Eliot's hometown,' said Dent, regaining his poise, 'and New York, have you lived there?'

'Sure,' said Burroughs, wrapping his left arm around his stomach.

'I only ask because one of those visiting doctors mentioned their drug problem. He said it's tough in New York, an epidemic. You wouldn't know anything about that, would you?'

Burroughs spluttered before sneezing. Dent handed over a large box of tissues. Their eyes met for the first time. 'It isn't good, is it?' asked the doctor, gently probing. 'What is essential is to stop the same thing happening here.'

'Can you do that?' grunted Burroughs, wiping his long, dripping nose.

'We must try,' responded Dent, sitting down a few feet in front of his visitor. 'Actually, we can do better than that. We must force the World Health Organisation to recognise that criminalisation is not the answer. It creates a black market with more people becoming slaves to criminal gangs. Your country's example proves it.'

Dent stopped talking to concentrate on the American. He registered a shabbily suited gentleman. Forty-ish, bloodless face, thin hair, emaciated, jumpy. He placed this information alongside every case he'd ever encountered, portraits stretching back forever. Their faces came with all their baggage; their defining characteristics, backgrounds, and circumstances. Dent's casebook was bursting at the seams but he'd never tire of adding another because everyone is unique. This visitor's preliminary sketch was already in the sub-section marked 'compulsive'. The doctor noticed he brooded like a sick animal. He hadn't let go of his stomach since his arrival and he twitched... almost continuously.

'I haven't spoken to Walter Maclay, but is this why you're here?' Dent asked, not wanting to waste time.

Burroughs brushed some imagined dust off his grey trousers. He didn't want to talk about the Maclays... it was too confusing.

'Yeah, I have an opiate habit. Twelve years … can't shake it …'

'I know Maclay well, and if he sent you then it is with good reason. Please, when you're ready, tell me your story.'

At first there was nothing until a hesitant wheeze emerged. It sounded far off like the distant rattle of a night train, but lonelier … more desolate …. It chilled the doctor to hear it.

'Someone back home … in the States, recommended London, said I should come … I dunno …' his body squirmed. 'I was in Tangiers … I've done my best to kick … it's no use … futile. An' each time harder, I burn … give in … I've tried, I dunno … so many times …. This killed my uncle, it's gonna get me too … my back's to the wall, I need help, a cure … anything ….' The bleakness of his report wiped away what remained of his physical resistance. He bent forward to stifle a moan … to stem another belt of contorting agonies … 'Aaagh …'

And that was it. A few fragile words. Dreadful, down in the mouth words destined to fade into the void … to disappear immediately … until the doctor, unseen, stretched out and retrieved them. He'd never forget them. They'd outline his preliminary sketch; to be used later to flesh out his portrait, his diagnosis and treatment. They'd provide shape … form … depth; help fill in the clues both psychological and physiological. Each dimension as critical as the other. As a practising doctor he knew that most scientific books are written by those who 'never go to sea in small boats' and in any case 'books are a poor substitute for people'. Once more at sea he would lean overboard and grab the drowning man. Later, when he'd dealt with the biological crisis, he'd plot a recovery. The drained features were not unusual … nor were the pinched, hollowed cheeks, the candle-grey skin smeared with sweat, the persistent neurasthenic twitches, birdlike. His drear, joyless bearing indicated shame … the words he used … and those he didn't … or couldn't. The doctor knew what had to be done. For the time being there was no point in discussion; if he didn't intervene soon this fellow might sink without trace. Here was a man running on empty, at the end of his resources: physical, chemical and emotional. The terminus was up ahead, the end of the line.

The doctor moved from his chair, slowly and deliberately. He crouched and placed a hand on Burroughs' shoulder. When their heads were level the visitor felt his shoulder being squeezed...firmly. At first he heard nothing until as if from childhood there came an owl wing's voice, half-whisper, half-supplication.

'It is a good thing that you are here...I have everything we need. Please try not to worry.' The soft voice faded into the gentle hiss of the air filter from the fish tank, like the twilight murmur rising out of the rain forest. 'I assure you,' he felt the nape of his neck being rubbed, 'no matter what you may believe, or what you've been told...we can beat this.' Vaguely he felt his forehead being touched...his fringe being pushed back with a strange intimacy...not unwelcome. 'Of all man's ills,' the voice continued, 'this thing you complain of comes with the best hope of health, the strongest likelihood of complete recovery. I assure you.'

Burroughs' drawn features didn't change but underneath his inhabitant depressed spirit had been served an eviction notice. 'A good guy,' he thought. 'I have come to this cavernous shit-hole and stumbled upon a good guy.'

His croak etched the air, 'Thank you, doc.'

'Are you sure about everything you've said?' Dent asked.

'Yeah. I'm ten years in, easy.'

'How old are you?' Dent shifted his attention to Burroughs' wrist.

'Forty-two.'

'Are you sleeping?'

'No, impossible.'

'And how much of these drugs have you been taking each day?'

'Sometimes twenty, thirty grains a day, recently more.'

Dent watched the second hand on his watch as he took Burroughs' pulse but continued to talk. 'And have you been taking other drugs?'

'Just opiates: paregoric, eukodol, demerol.'

'Alcohol?' Dent could smell it on his visitor's breath.

'Well yeah, but that's not the problem.'

'You drink but believe it's under control?'

'No, er, I mean yes.' Burroughs took off his glasses and screwed up his eyes.

Dent was quiet for a moment. 'Do you remember when you last took opiates?' He briefly felt the nape of Burroughs' neck before sliding his hand down to just below the shoulder blade.

Burroughs tried to think. What day was it? Wednesday. He had landed in London on Monday, no, Sunday. He had taken a hit to get on the plane and another before his London transfer, in Paris. Sweat stung his eye, the light smeared, he couldn't concentrate.

'Take your time, there's no rush,' affirmed Dent, listening to Burroughs breathing. 'You're safe here, quite safe.'

Burroughs moved his free hand back to his brow. He must answer.

'Yesterday morning, doc. Early, dolophine.'

'Agh, methadone,' said Dent, moving his hand back to Burroughs' jutting shoulder. 'You probably know this but heroin has a faster action and less unpleasant side effects.' He paused. 'Would you like some?'

The doctor felt the jolt.

'Where?' The American's tone shifted. 'You'll write a script?'

'A prescription?'

'Yeah.'

'No, I won't do that.'

'Well, how, man, how?' Burroughs' voice was racing.

'I give it to you!'

'When?'

'Right now. Would you like that?'

'Man, what d'you think?'

Dent smiled. He let go of the American and stood up. As he did so Burroughs unwound his arm from his gut...the tightness receded. Junk time, his scuttled mind told him, could readjust, realign itself behind the shifting intersections of chance and opportunity.

'Excuse me a moment,' said Dent. He left the room, closing the door.

The grey wolf scanned the terrain.

'He's probably ringing that shit Maclay,' the bleak spirit whined. The wolf jerked.

What was that? A noise from the street? He sniffed.

'Course I'll wait.' His words escaped like a curse. 'I can't escape, I'm trapped. Iron teeth scrape my bones, rip my guts.' He stood and looked down into the garden at a thick bank of swaying trees fringed with April green. It could be the entrance to a forest, perhaps a jungle. That's why the natives take yagé he realised, there's no horizon... an expanding consciousness is their only escape... he didn't hear the door open...

'Please, Uli.'

The grey wolf jumped. He swung round. The doc was holding the door open for the cat! He was talking to the cat!

'Oh!' Burroughs fell back into the chair. 'I thought you said summat else.'

Dent said nothing. Carrying a case under his arm and drying his hands, he returned to the desk under the dumb waiter. He draped the towel over the arm of a chair, pushed the tea tray back against the wall and got to work.... The cornered beast craned his neck, glimpsing a needle... the hairs along his back rose to the chink of glass on glass, nostrils flared... his skin shivered, ears cocked... guts churned. All his hopes and fears colliding through every single one of his 35 trillion cells... Come on, old brujo, I'm dying back here, dying.

At last the doc stood to one side. A sparkling syringe, surgical tourniquet and several small bottles were laid out on a spotless white towel. The wolf's back straightened... this was it; gloria in excelsis. The father, son and holy ghost of sacred sacrament... exquisite corporeal salvation, alle-fuckin'looyah.

'Right,' Dent said, firmly. 'Injectable diacetylmorphine otherwise known as heroin. I prepared it myself. Now, you have no objection to heroin?'

Burroughs squeezed out a frantic laugh.

'Just one thing, Mr Burroughs. Offering you this,' Dent gestured towards the desk, 'is not an undertaking on my part that I will treat you. This simply enables us to establish where we're going. There are house rules we need to go through, is that clear?'

'Yes, yes... I get it,' he snarled; rabidly prehistoric.

'Well then, please, when you're ready. I assume you know what to do. The syringe is appropriately filled, a single grain. When you've finished, we'll chat. I must pump ship.'

Dent promptly left the room. Burroughs pulled his chair up to the desk and found himself the reluctant participant of another maddening argument.

'Hey, look at you. A drop of God's own with full medical consent,' his dark spirit taunted.

'So what?' Burroughs replied. 'He's a Johnson, a good guy, there's a level of trust here.'

'You know all relationships are predicated on exchange.'

'But no hypocrisy.'

'How can you tell?'

'I can tell.'

'You're kidding yourself.'

'This croaker's straight, on the level.'

'You'll pay, you always pay.'

'But no script, nothing to trade, no forgeries.'

'You wait…'

'…and no questions to make me feel like dirt.'

'They'll come, they always come.'

'Shut it!'

'Just a friendly warning, kid…'

'Look you asshole, beat it!'

The junky rolled up his sleeve. He was glad the croaker wouldn't see his pitifully thin arm, its desiccated, pockmarked skin. Part of the same shrivelled WASP body he'd poisoned for so many years… in all those places and now London, the mother ship with its sonovabitch conservatism, cloying reserve and patrician snobbery; as turgid as shit in a hose pipe.

The colliding ironies, real and tenuous, gripped him as tightly as the tourniquet. The vein bulged; that same ole blue-grey, simpering body, yearning for love or the next best thing. He steadied himself and slid in the needle. A hit. Cardinal red plumed in the glass. He pushed the stopper... within moments the agonies withdrew. Furious waves collapsed down jagged rocks and melted into the muted monotony of a flat calm. The monster was fed. For an hour or two it would do no more than lick its lips along the shoreline...

Slowly the junky's attention was drawn to a languid movement. Fluorescent colours merging one into another. How is that possible? The hues shimmied beside a lump of feldspar quartz, giving it everything... that ole 'come and fuck me sideways' scenario... a fin dance more flouncy than flamenco... a witchy dream of purples, turquoise and poppy petal reds. Dammit! Everything was incongruous; the thickness of that oak chair, a domestic library, a fish that makes peyote redundant and a cat called Ulysses. The Siamese heard his thoughts, tuned in and stared like cats do. Burroughs blinked first. His attention shifted, he floated under a cliff of books. He scanned the strata; dark blues, reds and browns. Rich seams of scientific and literary pedigree; Swift, Wells, Huxley, Newton, Darwin, Havelock Ellis. The saintly scribes, their names embossed in gold, stretching in every dimension... forever... one volume stood out, as vivid as malachite: '*Ulysses* – James Joyce.' He looked at it blankly; he thought of the magic of chaos. He sat down.

More dreamy minutes passed before the old doc returned and poured out a very dark mug of tea.

'Bit stewed, never mind. Help yourself, there's milk, sugar and biscuits.' He turned towards the middle of the room seemingly in no hurry to do anything... measuring the silence.

'What sort of fish is that?' asked the traveller, struggling with the heavy teapot.

'Siamese fighting fish.'

The doctor looked away from his visitor's clumsiness. All confirmed addicts are specialists of their particular condition. Their beliefs lie deeper than a xenolith encased in granite. The doctor knew he could break through, not with lessons of morality or decency but with ideas and possibilities. He considered the shaking hand unable to prevent the tea from spilling. There was a digit missing... a sign of an industrial accident or some childhood trauma? People want answers, but this was only useful if they ask the right questions... usually when the spark of curiosity is fired from within, of the patient's own volition. Beliefs preserved by an addict's unique brand of denial rarely shift unless there's fundamental change... There must be no rules, this is no watertight compartment... everyone has his story, tale of valediction. The doctor would reach out slowly... a game of give and take. One false move and it'd unravel. Dent imagined what might lie within his isolated visitor... behind that stuttering paranoia... the clue that might offer the pathway to recovery and beyond. He could ask questions but that was never the way. First disclosure, empathy and understanding. He cleared his throat.

'This is just one of *my* many addictions,' he started, waving his hand at the fish. 'I used to write, but I'm in remission. I've umpteen habits but the few I admit to: well, there's collecting atlases; smoking of course. Some say I am addicted to silence. Then there's my awful driving and hoarding. I cannot stop collecting geological specimens and recently, tropical fish. You see, I never let a week go by without adding a new fish or two... When one tank gets crowded I *permit* myself a new one.' He smiled and shrugged at his own helplessness. 'I have three more tanks in the basement and they are all bigger than this one. It is a constant demand on my time when I should be doing other things...

'Anyway, apart from everyone's favourite, the Siamese fighting fish,' he gestured towards the submerged version of a peacock, 'there are "community" fish, the little ones in shoals. I find they impart a restful mood, probably due to their patterns of movement, a murmuration of aquatic suspension which helps all sorts... even the most self-absorbed *cats*...'

Dent stroked Ulysses as his voice tailed off. Burroughs watched harlequin and tetra mingle as if flocks of kingfishers. His fidgeting had stopped. He leant back and listened like a child to a bedtime story. Dent coughed quietly and continued.

'I do not know exactly when my weakness for a watery environment became a compulsion but there can be no doubt that that is what it is. From an early age I was fascinated by the understanding that our surroundings control us. With the help of my uncle I used to play tricks on tadpoles, preventing them from reaching the surface. Consequently they remained tadpoles. They need air, you see, to ignite the next stage of their development and we're all a bit like that. All change is movement and *all* movement is the result of a previous movement. It does *not* matter what it is, love in your heart, balls on a billiard table, atoms in the brain. It's all subject to the push and pull of environment and our reactions to it.'

Dent's words fell simply, like leaves from a tree. Burroughs thought again of the eels on that chair downstairs, those strange fish.

'And this is why you are here. Your environment contained drugs which have changed you and are now poisonous to you. Your experience of them was probably inevitable and now your exposure to them habitual, canalised. This is because your brain chemistry has been changed by cellular events and is now loaded against you. It will not allow you to stop using drugs despite bad things that keep happening. That is what we call addiction. It is not due to a lack of willpower. Asking a compulsive addict to be a teetotaller? I might as well ask Ulysses to take up the banjo. Your chemistry, like the tadpole's, must change for you to change. Free will has nothing to do with it and nor have morals, superstition, Freud's id, the imagined soul, or anything else. We can only react to our environment as our biology permits and our organism demands. I am a chemist not a moralist.'

Dent's visitor uncrossed his legs. He wanted to say that he'd spent half his life coming to the same conclusion but this old doc wasn't looking for plaudits.

'And so, you will be wondering, what can I do for you? Well, I can do a great deal, I can change your chemistry, a metabolic change that will combat your sickness and allow your physiological need for drugs to disappear. I can do this but I will need your help because this will not be easy. We have been lucky up to now, you have got this far, but you are no different from anything else in the universe. Every living thing reacts to its environment and when those reactions cease we die. Opiates do not discriminate. You're running out of time, and we both know it.'

The peripatetic doctor had driven his points home with the precision of a mechanical hammer. Every strike on centre. He'd gone round the room twice, drunk his tea and poured another cup, indulged the cat, put away some books, helped himself to others and fed the fish. He was back beside Burroughs and looking into the garden. He pushed back his wild mop of hair which seemed to be bushier than half an hour ago and turned again to face his visitor.

'So, Mr Burroughs, without further ado, tell me, why are you here?'

Burroughs was suddenly wide awake. The bedtime story was over. He panicked. If you're gonna screw up better to screw up quickly.

'Er, well, doc, er, Dr Dent, to be cured.'

'I cannot do that,' said Dent.

'But I thought you said you could er, change … I mean …'

'What I can do is help you. I can heal you with a treatment we go through … together. This is not a cure. You will always be an addict. You have an allergy to drugs for which there is no inoculation. If you do not crave drugs anymore that does not mean your allergy isn't there … it will be.'

Dent looked intently at his patient; he saw someone who needed information. He decided to press on.

'You see, the word "cure" is unhelpful. Strictly speaking there is currently no such thing. You have a susceptibility, a predisposition perhaps. This is quite possibly *both* heritable *and* environmental … not necessarily "either, or", as some like to say, but "both, and". In other words this is due to *both* your inherited traits *and* your environment in the widest possible sense. And this includes society's impact upon us with all its systemic structures; its language, laws and culture, its prejudices, taboos and fears. I am not surprised by you mentioning your uncle but I do wonder if these stories aren't simply the father to the fear. This story may have got the better of you and became a trouble you dispelled with drugs. In time you developed an extreme physiological need and now you're here. This chemical imbalance I can address, but cure? No, that is a matter between you and yourself. You'll always carry this with you; you'll be an addict until you die.'

The grey man covered his face with long thin fingers and swallowed hard. The clear way Dent had spelled out what deep down he already knew meant this was no time for argument. He trawled his confused mind for something to add but there was nothing... only echoes.

'So?' asked Dent, without a hint of impatience. 'That is why I need to know why you are here; I cannot help you until I know.'

The grey man shifted uncomfortably. He must answer.

'Well, doctor, I have been trying to work.'

'And what work is that?'

'I am a writer... who cannot.'

'Ah,' acknowledged Dent, 'that can certainly be difficult. So?'

Burroughs thought of all those people willing him on, his parents, brother, friends, Ginsberg, the others. But, this wasn't what the old croaker was after. He leant forward in a silent plea for the doctor to flesh out what he could not.

'What do you like about yourself?' the grey man heard; more soft words.

'I dunno, not much,' he drawled, more than a little resignation in his voice.

'Well, I cannot suggest what may bring contentment. This again is a matter for you. Most say they want "to be happy" but asked to define happiness no two people can agree.' The doctor paused, glimpsing a flicker behind the American's pallor. He pressed on.

'Some of us think we know what we want. But that belief can sometimes make us very inefficient and a man who is trying never succeeds. Aware of this inefficiency our frustration becomes unbearable... we become paralysed. Tell me, Mr Burroughs, do you think this problem is necessary to you as a writer?'

'No, definitely not.'

'So, is this problem the reason why you cannot write or an excuse for not writing?'

'Oh?' Burroughs looked up from his fingernails. He'd thought about this... but he'd never had it levelled at him. He was nonplussed. 'I don't know,' he mumbled.

'Would you like to work because that would be who you are?'

'I guess...'

'Well then...?'

'Yeah,' said Burroughs, 'I get it now. I wanna do what I really am, not this.' He pushed out his arm and poked at it with his fingers. 'At the moment I cannot do anything. I cannot wash, eat, get out of bed. What chance do I have... the remorse... it's killing me.'

Dent waited until he'd found his visitor's gaze. 'So, you're here for entirely selfish reasons. Not for your mother, the Pope, the Wizard of Oz. *You* have to want this for yourself... that part of you which is indivisible from your ambition, your *true* self.'

Burroughs found himself drawn to something beyond the croaker's steel-eyed intensity. His promising words offered a glimpse of a land he could imagine if not reach. If only...

'This task of overcoming drugs,' Dent continued, 'may be the last barrier to achieving who you'd like to be.... But, one step at a time. My treatment may provide you with the means to overcome the physiological problems of withdrawal and craving. I repeat...we can do that...together.' Dent paused and waited again until their eyes met. 'But the rest of it, this business of writing, you will still have to do all of that. Clear?'

Burroughs looked away. He fidgeted, re-crossing his legs while scratching his chin and neck.

'Well, Dr Dent, I think I get it. I've already some experience of writing, though success doesn't come easy.'

Dent looked over the top of his half-moon specs. 'What have you written?'

'Only one published book but I think you'd be interested...'

'What's it about?'

'The title is self-explanatory: *Junkie: Confessions of an Unredeemed Drug Addict*.' Burroughs coughed.

'Oh.' The doctor paused, 'What's it like?'

'Well, it's more than a confessional; I wanted it to be accurate, to give people a flavour of what's going down, really going down. As you might guess, some said I should skirt round the issues, but that's not my thing.'

Dent stood up and turned to look out of the window. He saw Rhoda and Onions on their hands and knees, digging. He liked roses, loved the garden... but really! They couldn't sustain him like the promise held in his visitor's last few words. He imagined him healed, with a clear ambition to write about his struggle with addiction. He wouldn't mention this now but what a benefit this could bring to so many.... He recalled Marty Mann's *Primer on Alcoholism* and the value her book had for changing perception in the US about this growing public health problem; and how one of his ex-patients, Patrick Riddell, had attempted to do the same in Great Britain with a book of his own; *I Was An Alcoholic*. He compared his thin, grey visitor's ambition to write and placed it alongside his sense of resignation at the medical and political indifference towards this growing health problem. The inevitability of more and more sufferers... people just like his visitor. Dent felt a rueful ache on top of his deep sense of frustration. He rubbed his cheeks vigorously... this was no time to get maudlin.

Behind him the grey man peered at his fingernails. He had been spoken to directly, in plain words. They'd cut him to the quick. He reviewed his predicament... but in a new light. Saw how acceptance by a discerning society could provide the stepping-stone to redemption. It wasn't difficult to understand... just impossible to do. Maybe he did want success because of the status but it had to be on his own terms... and maybe he'd run out of things to say... or was it the way to say it? He looked up at the croaker's silhouette framed by the window. A stocky figure, neither tall nor short. What mischief is it, he wondered, that in less than an hour the futility and desperation surrounding his problem could be challenged so radically? He played the sound of the name in his mind, Doc Dent, Dr John *Yerbury* Dent, as if searching for a clue. He envied him his position, an old time Londoner clutched to the bosom of the medical establishment. Doesn't need to travel because the world comes to him, that's cool. Burroughs' mind switched to all the other doctors he had known and met.... How they preyed on his sickness, how their cynicism had provided the justification for rejecting any thought of a medical career. Prestige ain't worth a damn without integrity. Burroughs picked at his skin as a mounting sense of loss consumed him. A nostalgia for a life he'd never own. His frustration threatened to tip him into a rage. But this was not the time. He'd have to stick with this crazy old croaker... his cure like every cure would fail. He'd end up just as sick, without funds and sink deeper into the mire... but he had no choice, this was his last chance saloon.

'How does your method work, is it this "British system"?' Burroughs asked.

Dent turned round. 'You've had other treatments?'

'Yes; slow reduction, cold turkey, Benzedrine, barbiturates, antihistamines... er, prolonged sleep...'

'Prolonged sleep? How does that work?'

'It doesn't. They knock you out with enough tranquillisers to sedate an elephant. You never sleep properly. Then, when you come round, you're still tired, still addicted to heroin but also to sedatives on top. An awful idea.'

'You'd never go through that again.'

'Never. It nearly killed me.'

'My treatment is qualitatively different.'

'Oh?'

Again Dent realised his visitor would need information but of the detailed variety. He returned to his chair. 'My treatment uses a drug called apomorphine. It is a back-brain stimulant.' He grabbed a sheet of paper from the desk and sketched out a profile of the human skull and brain. 'It works in this area here... the hypothalamus and beyond. You can call it the "back brain".' He indicated with a quick scribble. 'Think of the brain as two halves. The front and back parts represented by different ends of a see-saw.' He drew a line through the middle of the brain. 'Man gets anxious in here, the thinking cortex or front brain and it springs up.' He drew a slanted line through the middle of the see-saw. 'So we depress it with drugs; alcohol, barbiturates or opiates.... This brings the anxiety down but when the drug wears off it springs back up... so we take more drugs but in increased quantity...'

'Because of the increased tolerance...?' enquired the visitor.

'Exactly!' exclaimed the doctor, pleased by the American's ability to keep up. 'Anyway, I have found that this drug, apomorphine, stimulates this area, the other end of the see-saw,' he ringed the hypothalamus, 'and as it rises it pushes the cortex down but without the need for drugs. In other words, apomorphine re-regulates the brain until the front and back parts are balanced.' Dent scored several horizontal lines through the fulcrum of the seesaw. 'The main advantage of apomorphine is that when the apomorphine wears off the front and back brains *remain* balanced. You will have no compulsion to re-adjust it with drugs. You'll be a changed man.'

'I see,' said Burroughs, doing his best to concentrate and suppress his incredulity. 'Is it like morphine, this APO-morphine?'

'No, definitely not. It is derived from morphine but possesses none of its properties. It is certainly not addictive. It is psychoactive but not psychedelic ... nobody takes it for fun.'

Burroughs scratched his head. 'You know this, I mean for sure?'

'Oh yes. I saw this as a student. You see apomorphine has one main side effect; it is an emetic, it makes the patient vomit. However, when the vessels are tied to prevent the drug reaching the stomach, emesis still happens. It therefore acts indirectly by stimulating the vomiting centres of the brain.'

The doctor let the information sink in. He got up, walked across the room and picked up Ulysses, rubbing him playfully behind the ears.

'And how would you treat me?' asked the American.

'I have a small two-bed clinic where we administer an injection of apomorphine every two hours over a period of several days. This is important because this is what turns your brain chemistry back to that level see-saw I described.' Dent hesitated. He thought about what he should say next. He waited until he knew he had Burroughs' attention. 'I also promise to give you morphine whenever you ask for it providing you do your level best to avoid taking any.'

Burroughs digested the information. He needed to be sure he'd heard that right. 'You'll give me junk when I want?'

'Yes,' the doctor confirmed. 'To help regulate your withdrawal. We understand that this treatment can be daunting, gruelling even. But you will have round-the-clock care and I'll visit as often as I can.

The main side effect of apomorphine, as I mentioned, is this vomiting reflex. But, and I want you to be clear on this, this is not an aversion treatment. Any morphine we provide is simply to manage your withdrawal from heroin. We will help you directly with your cramps, hives, whatever else you encounter. The other side effect of apomorphine is that it is a somnambulant. You will probably have bouts of yawning, a prelude to sleep, but a natural sleep not the drugged consciousness you described earlier... with tranquillisers. Gradually your outlook will begin to change. You'll realise you can exist without opiates, look forward to a time when you won't even think about them.'

Burroughs checked a squeal of derision. He could not imagine such an existence.

'I'll also employ other approaches as and when they are useful but for the time being any further discussion is a waste of time. Indeed, Mr Burroughs, I'll be frank; any positives gained in the last hour will be driven out once you leave here and your craving returns.... But, please, try not to worry about this as it does not worry me... not in the slightest.'

Dent gave Ulysses two firm strokes along his back and put him down. His visitor had heard enough.

'So, Mr Burroughs, I am convinced you do want to be well and therefore I am happy to help. So, have you made up your mind... or would you like more time?'

'No, I've decided,' intoned the grey man. 'I need help, like you said, so I can survive to work... to write. It's why I'm here. I have no other reason to be in London. Your treatment, how much will it cost, and your fee?'

'Oh, I am not sure, what can you afford? On top of my fee there's the nurses who'll care for you, day and night. They're five pounds a day each and you'll be there for over a week, possibly ten days. Is that manageable?'

'Yes,' said Burroughs. 'And where is this clinic?'

'99 Cromwell Road, it isn't far. I'll write the address down for you.' Dent opened a drawer in the desk and lifted out a small light-green exercise book. 'You enter through an abortion clinic, next door. There's a receptionist, seven days a week. It suits everybody as both sets of clientele wish for discretion. Now then, where are you staying?'

Burroughs pulled a slip of paper from his inside pocket. 'An apartment: 44 Edgerton Gardens, SW3,' he said.

Dent wrote it down on the cover of the book. 'Telephone number?'

'2017.'

'Not far off,' Dent remarked, raising his eyebrows.

'Edgerton?'

'No, 2017, just 61 years from now…'

'Oh, yes…'

'Hopefully with ethical drug policies nobody should be suffering in 2017 like you are today.' Dent handed Burroughs the exercise book, a card and a small bottle. 'On the card are my contact details here and the address of the clinic. You can contact me or the clinic at any time day or night. The bottle contains two grains of morphine, not enough to kill you but enough to tide you over till Friday when we can take you. Please, try not to take any other drug. But, if you do, please let us know. Come on Friday at 11 a.m. and hand the exercise book to Sister Gibson. She'll be there to help you settle in and I'll be along later. Your treatment will consist of the apomorphine injections I mentioned and constant monitoring…'

'This Friday?'

'Yes, Sister Gibson, we call her Kate or Gibbie, will go through this when you arrive at the clinic, but there's an explanation in here,' Dent pulled open the bottom drawer of the desk, 'in my book. Here, take it with you.'

Dent gave Burroughs a small hard-backed book with black and white squiggly lines on the pink dust jacket. Burroughs thought of the zigzagging radio signals that Martians communicate with in comics. He read the title:

'*Anxiety and Its Treatment.* Anxiety?' he pondered.

'Well, yes,' answered Dent, getting up and moving towards the door. Burroughs stood to follow. 'Worry is biochemical, too,' continued the doctor. 'The use of drugs may often be traced to sudden trouble: maybe a bereavement, an unforeseen crisis, a terrible event. The number of ex-servicemen I end up treating is no coincidence…. As doctors we must be sensitive to these issues and the wider circumstances of the patient.' Dent carried on talking as he crossed the landing, 'Recently, at a symposium, an owner of a luxurious nursing home full of what he called "neurotics" said that all I am interested in is a material view of addiction. I responded by giving him that book, adding, "I do not know why you say that, the clue is in the title."' Dent boomed with laughter that faded to a long snigger lasting all the way down the stairs.

Burroughs felt gauche … inarticulate. There were so many things he wanted to say. His frustration was made worse by accepting the book. *He* was the writer … he reluctantly followed Dent back down into the hallway filled with the scent of freshly picked flowers and lower down, the aroma of cooking. Dent had to be getting on with his life.

'Now then, Mr Burroughs, you know what to do.' He handed Burroughs his coat. 'If there are any thoughts or questions you can always telephone here or the clinic. Remember, anytime day or night.'

Burroughs thanked Dent, pulling on his coat and lifting up the collar. 'I'm glad to be on the program,' he added.

'Treatment,' said Dent.

'Yes, treatment.'

'How will you return to your flat?' asked Dent, handing Burroughs his hat.

'I might get a cab.'

'Try walking. Always better to walk in a new city, helps to get your bearings.'

'Oh,' said Burroughs, shaking Dent's hand.

'Yes, it won't take long. And it's a beautiful evening. When you get lost ask for directions. Always useful, meeting people. Helps develop a sense of where we are in the world, a sense of belonging.' Dent smiled.

Burroughs couldn't tell if this was kooky bullshit or whether he was being laughed at.

'Till Friday,' said Dent.

'Yeah, sure,' said Burroughs, 'Friday, 11 a.m.'

He turned and felt the rush of air as the door slammed behind him.

The bemused traveller wandered onto Kensington High Street holding the tiny bottle of morphine in his pocket. He ran his fingers along its characteristic ridges. Its stopper was secure. He checked to make sure... for the time being he was safe. Junk compulsion, as the old croaker knew, had just erased everything that had been said and done. The junky transferred the bottle to an inside pocket; it'd be safer there.

'No one argues with the Chinaman,' whined his inner voice.

He pretended he hadn't heard it.

'You're a useless, no good junky,' it insisted. 'Don't think *you* can change.'

'Shut up,' Burroughs muttered, feeling for the bottle again.

'See, I told you,' crowed the dark spirit.

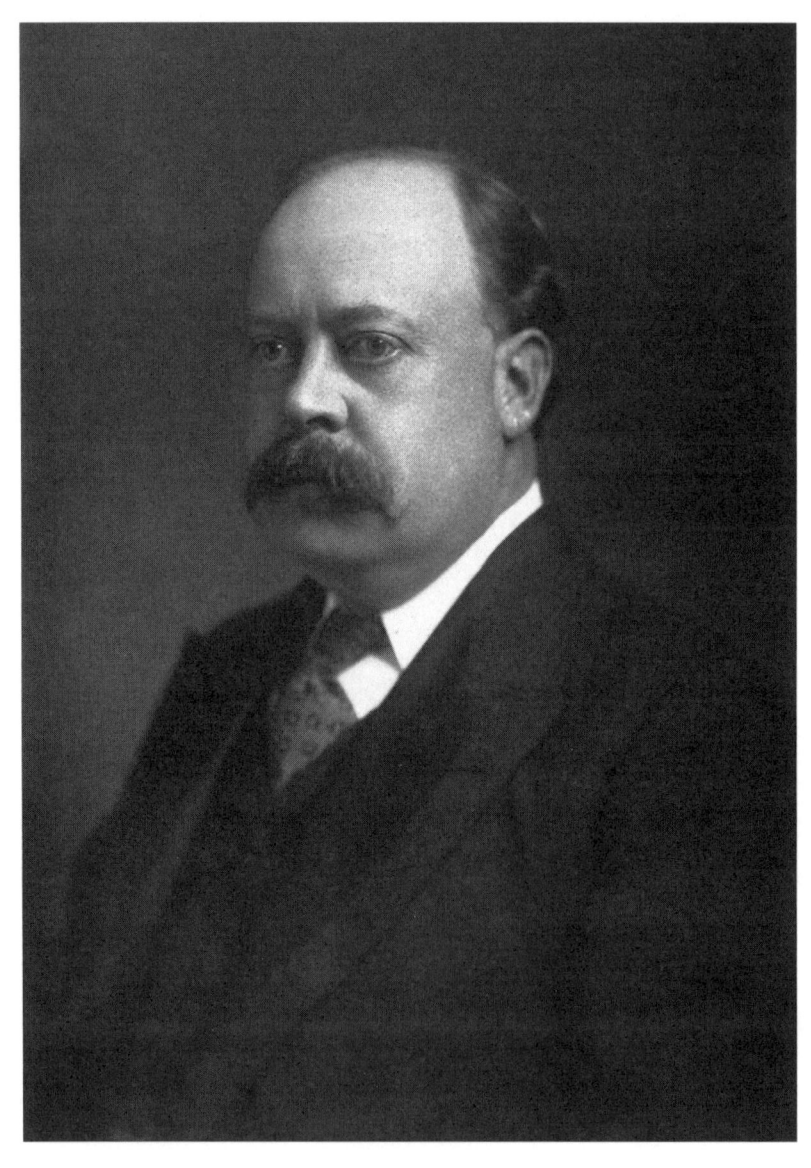

William D. Halliburton's (1860–1931) enjoyed a 34-year stint at King's College as Dean of the Faculty of Medical Science. [©Wellcome Collection]

5

Leave Well Alone

> Sitting quietly doing nothing Spring comes.
> The grass grows by itself.
> – Zen Proverb

Dent lay in bed, unable to sleep. Tomorrow he'd have to be on his mettle. He'd assisted in many births but only in the confines of the hospital under the watchful gaze of those who could intervene when things got hairy. But tomorrow was going to be different, very different. He would be on his own, working in the slums and encountering God knows what? Slum conditions were an extreme test. 'Stand on a newspaper and pour chloroform into your turn ups.' had been his senior lecturer's only advice. 'What?' he'd blurted, consternation and confusion drawing the blood from his face. The lecturer looked to the heavens.

'Oh dear, Dent. The newspaper is so you don't have to stand in filth and the chloroform will suffocate the bedbugs crawling up your legs. They'll eat you alive if you don't do as I say. Now, put away those books. Books are for librarians and for giving your examiners a lot of ruddy eye-wash. Doctoring? Well, you learn that off your patients. Best advice you'll ever get; now clear off. Go home and relax. And if you can't relax get drunk.'

Dent gulped at the memory. His lecturer had meant well but it wasn't helping him sleep. He tried to dissolve his anxiety by visualising his last visit to the country with Uncle Louis, the numerous butterflies they'd caught on Box Hill. This technique had worked in the past. He 'heard' the swish of the fine cotton mesh net as Louis danced through the long grass or under the broad span of oak trees. He 'heard' too Louis' triumphant giggles as he swept up specimen after specimen and as he called out an alphabetical list of his catches with enthusiastic asides:

'Admiral, *red, nice but common as muck.*
Admiral, *white, luvverly, a favourite.*
Blue, *chalk.*
Blue, *common. Rare this year, wonder why?*
Brimstone. *Lovely markings, look Jack, magical.*
Camberwell Beauty, *superb.*
Fritillary, *small, pearl-bordered, another beauty.*
Gatekeeper *or hedge brown.*
Hairstreaks, *white-letter and purple, such delicate markings, and different in Norfolk.*
Stag Beetle, male. *Look at its antlers,
  always remind me of forceps...*'

'FORCEPS!'

It was no use. The spell had been broken. Dent was sweating. He could never declare he hadn't been warned about doctoring. His father had spelled it out, and Uncle Herbert too. Only Uncle Louis had remained quiet. Naively he thought midwifery might be easier on the nerves... but no. There was eclampsia that could end in coma and foetal distress caused by any number of complications. Haemorrhages causing cerebral paralysis was all too common in the clumsy hands of a novice. He imagined fumbling with the forceps as the mother screamed in agony. What if it was a breech? He sat up, horror after horror grabbing his tortured mind. His mentor, Professor Halliburton would probably laugh and admonish him with those fat fingers poking out of his gown. 'I advised you from day one, Dent. Don't say I didn't.'

It was true. On that infamous introductory speech with the new intake at King's the esteemed and noble Halliburton had walked down the aisle in a flourish of crimson and black. A bullfinch among sparrows. He had climbed the steps onto the stage to peer down at the rows of fresh-faced youths.

Halliburton's well established form always rose sharply from the recesses of Dent's fledgling mind but his character had seared it like a branding iron. He was a tall man with a barrel-vaulted chest below a bulging, overripe face; one or other looked like it might explode at any moment. Conversely, his voice was not at all overblown. He spoke with the quiet assurance of someone reiterating a successful strategy. His oratory had been weighed and polished many times. His job was clear: he had to explain to the new year's intake that the road ahead was arduous and that many would drop out. 'We are here to learn, but many of you do not have what it takes…' he started, without intending to be unkind.

'First of all there is anatomy and this can be very malodorous,' he guaranteed. 'Yes boys, that's right, smelly. Rabbits and dogfish are commonly available for dissection but you won't like it unless you suffer from anosmia, the lack of any sense of smell.' He smiled. He had them on a string. 'Then there's human anatomy,' he continued. 'At this stage some more of you will be weeded out because while rabbits turn the air with their stench they won't turn your stomach quite so much as the body parts of your fellow man. I am not ashamed to admit that when a student I became facetious and jocose and even thoroughly vulgar in the company of our brethren's intimate bits and pieces. This allowed me to survive the disgust that it is now your turn to confront. For instance, I learnt to play French cricket with femur and spleen while our teaching professor had his back turned and it cured me of some of my apprehension about death and human fallibility. I fully expect many of you to resort to such coping strategies. You won't last a week if you don't.'

Dent, sitting three rows back, was surprised by this candid disclosure and found himself warming to Halliburton. Such openness in front of so many impressionable youths was as disarming as it was unexpected. Halliburton moved closer to the front of the platform to conclude and drive home his message. His stature swelled until it had seeped permanently under the skull of every student, helped, of course, by the sheer dreadfulness of his message.

'After dissection I fear some more of you will fall by the wayside in post-mortem study. The smell is no better but corruption of the human organism by disease requires a steely resolve. It is sobering work and will remind you how weak and corruptible the human body is. There will be obstructive, degenerative and inflammatory conditions that it will be your duty to understand and identify. At this stage the few of you left, will no doubt believe that the worst is over,' he paused momentarily as if affording himself a private joke. 'Well, think again because at this stage you must fulfil a stint in surgery. All manner of operations will be undertaken. Hopeless and explorative cases, you name it. And, make no mistake, at no time are our surgeons expected to shield you from any of the risks and complexities involved. Arteries will be cut, blood will spray the walls, even your faces if you're unlucky. Regrettably patients will die, sometimes quickly, sometimes slowly, often in agony. This whole process will take three terms and if at the end anything like a quarter of you remain I will be truly astonished. Good day, gentlemen.'

At the moment Halliburton exited the hall a hubbub of excited chatter arose from the students. Dent swallowed hard. Halliburton had told it straight. Why hadn't he listened to his father's advice? He could have done anything; engineering, architecture, industry, even politics. Well, no, not that; jail would be preferable to politics....

More restless than ever Dent rolled onto his side and tried to ward off the mounting anxiety with recollections of his first meeting with his friends: Dalton and Barnes. It happened that same September afternoon as the students, in need of fresh air, spilled into the quad. Self-consciously, small groups gravitated towards each other.

'Hello, I'm Dent,' he had said, approaching two freshers trying to look nonchalant.

'Delighted to meet you,' smiled one. 'I'm Dalton, from the Midlands.' His dark eyes flashed. 'It's disgusting, isn't it?' he added.

'What, the Midlands?' said the other laughing.

'Where are you from, then?' Dalton retorted.

'Liverpool. It'd be as smelly as Birmingham but we've sea breezes. Barnes, by the way.' They all shook hands.

'The boss doesn't want us to suffer any illusions about doctoring, does he?' asked Dent.

'We must have our eyes open,' said Dalton.

'... and pegs on our noses,' Barnes reminded them.

'Quite,' agreed Dalton. 'I suppose they need training to be gruesome.'

'How do you mean?' asked Barnes, pushing back his blond fringe.

'To get rid of the faint-hearted,' said Dalton. 'Out there we'll have to be prepared for any eventuality... things we can't imagine.'

'Ah, yes. You could be right,' acknowledged Dent, 'but medicine doesn't have to be so unremittingly grim, you know?' His voice brightening. 'There's fun to be had. Remember what he said about playing French cricket?'

'Any ideas?' asked Dalton, not expecting an answer.

'As a matter of fact, yes,' said Dent. 'There's a rite of passage every student has to go through. And I think we could all do with some light relief.'

'Care to let on?' asked Barnes, his tall muscular frame impressing itself on the others.

'Comrades,' announced Dent, 'follow me.'

He took his new colleagues to the very top of the east stairs. Giddily they looked down into the stairwell.

'This better be good, Dent,' said Dalton. 'I'm out of breath.'

'Strictly speaking, gentlemen, this laboratory is out of bounds but ideal for our purposes. Do you see that statue down there? That's Dr Todd, one of the highly esteemed founders of this noble institution.'

'What of it?' asked Barnes, peering at the bronze bust eight flights below.

'Well, every student with curiosity in his heart must also accept that every theory must be constantly reviewed... er, for it to remain within the realm of scientific fact. And gentlemen, if we are to remain true to this principle we must never accept the word of others; we must insist on our own observations.'

'Quite right,' said Barnes, giggling. 'We must remain sceptical.'

'Proper science,' added Dalton, rubbing his hands together.

'Yes, but don't we need a theory?' queried Barnes.

'I am coming to that.' Dent cleared his throat. 'Gravity,' he announced, 'is the force expended until and up to the point that a greater force is exerted. How are we to know that Todd down there has greater force than say... an egg?'

Cottoning on, Dalton's face lit up. 'Yes, I insist on confirmation.'

'Don't we need an egg?' asked Barnes.

Dent carefully produced a heavy linen cloth from his pocket and unwrapped a pure brown egg. 'Here, gentlemen, you will see an object I laid earlier. Gentlemen.' Dent offered the egg for examination. 'Please confirm my observation that this is an egg.'

Barnes took the egg and rolled it between his palms. 'It feels like an egg.' He passed it to Dalton.

'I agree,' said Dalton, returning the egg to Dent, 'but how do we know you're a hen?'

'That'll have to wait... today is all about whether Todd down there can tell us that Galileo and Newton got their sums right.'

'Yes, we cannot be sure,' said Dalton, giggling.

Dent moved to the balustrade and held the egg in exactly the same position that Uncle Louis had shown him. 'Nature is full of magic things that science has yet to grasp,' Louis had said, before dropping his egg many years before. Now it was his nephew's turn.

The egg took 2.3 seconds to fall eighty-four feet, reaching a speed of 48.9 miles per hour. It caught Dr Todd's bust just above the hairline, bursting into a thousand fragments; an instantaneous blend of albumen, yolk and shell.

Sitting a few yards from Todd's bust, the caretaker, an exhausted gentleman with drooping eyelids, recognised the sound. He had heard it hundreds of times. He sighed and turned over his tattered copy of

Marshall's Illustrated Almanac, as frayed and worn as he. Without looking he reached under his desk for the grey cloth, sponge and bucket.

An exhausted Dent finally distracted by pleasant memories drifted off.

* * *

When Dent awoke he was aware that he'd slept soundly. Half an hour later he reported for duty. There were no morning calls. Waiting nervously with the other apprentice clerks he peered into his surgical bag, at the leather box containing a shiny speculum and two pairs each of forceps and scissors. Secreted away in one of the side pockets was a small bottle of chloroform and in another compartment a pristine copy of *The Daily News*. He was ready.

At lunchtime Dent got the call, to attend and facilitate a birth along the borders of Gray's Inn and King's Cross. London sweltered under a humid sky. Sweating, he paused by a corner to work out his route. As he confirmed his whereabouts he spotted a quiet corner between two carts. Crouching between them he tipped the chloroform into his turn-ups. His hand shook as he spilled in all he had. 'Better to be sure,' he muttered returning the empty chloroform bottle to his bag. His heart racing he re-checked the address and proceeded into a narrow lane hemmed in by blackened walls. Piles of refuse almost blocked his way; a waft of putrid air made him gag.

The lane narrowed into a tight passage before opening into a yard with children of every age playing marbles or hopscotch. A boy of about ten ran up to him. 'Hey mister, what you 'ere for?'

'He's a doctor, en 'e, look at 'is bag,' shouted another. Soon he was ringed by clamouring children.

'Hey mister, you a doctah?' A sullen-eyed lad stood in front of him. 'If yer 'ere to see Gertie Clements, I know where.'

Dent stopped. 'Yes, thank you. Where?'

'Cost yer,' replied the boy.

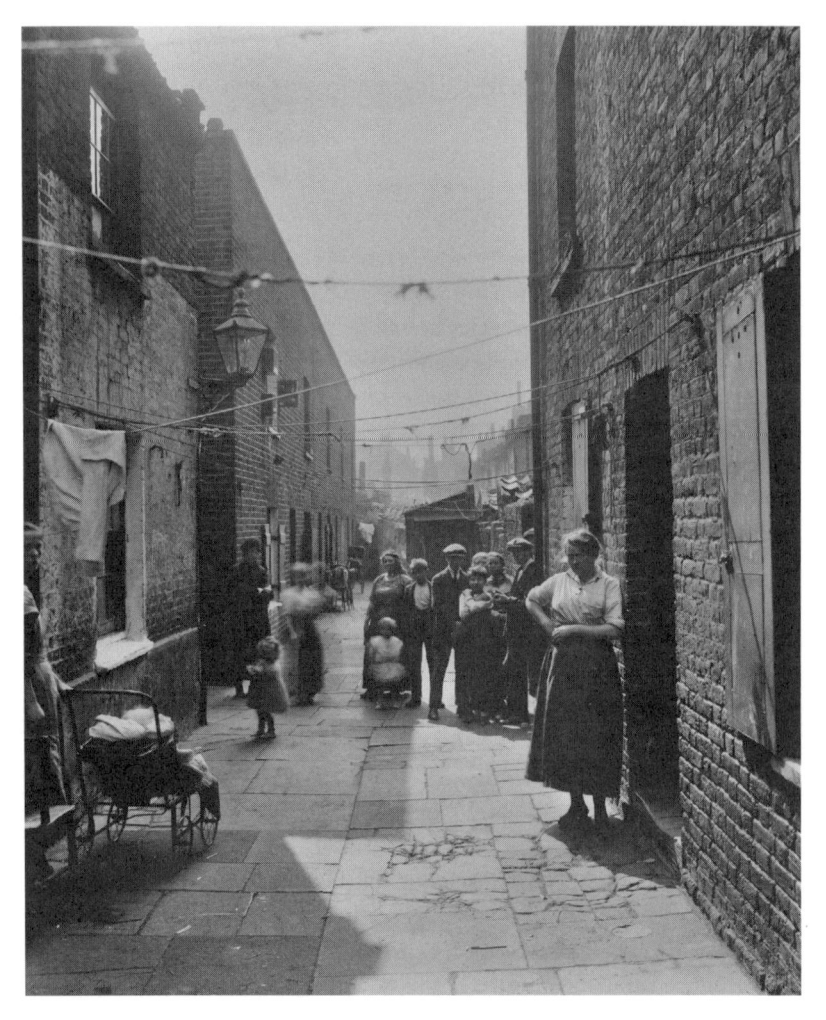

London slums around 1910 were awful. Small incomes were spent on the necessities but it was never enough. Disease and death were rampant.
[©Collage – London Metropolitan Archive]

'I've been called to help with a birth. I'm a midwife.'
Some of the children found this funny and ran ahead shouting. 'Itz the baby man, baby man.'

At the end of the yard an alley led to two rows of three-storey houses barely six yards apart. At the first house a number of children their faces streaked with tears and snot played in the dirt with pebbles. Dent picked his way through the group until he was stopped by a tall girl.

'In 'ere, mister,' she pointed towards the second house. 'She's upstairs.'

Dent heaved open a flaking front door and entered the hallway. As his eyes adjusted to the gloom a tremendous thud shook the house. 'Aggh!' someone cried and a snarling terrier shot across the hall and disappeared. Briefly there was silence followed by another terrifying thump directly under his feet. Fragments of plaster and blistered paint showered the floorboards.

'Hello!' called Dent. 'Anybody there?' Getting no answer he raised his voice: 'Is this the Clements' house, number 11?'

'No. This is twelve,' a woman's voice answered from the direction of the narrow staircase. Dent couldn't see her. He ventured onto the first step, craning his neck. 'But yer found 'er,' the voice continued, 'she's lyin' in up 'ere. Come up … an' pay no heed t' the bangin'.'

'What is it?'

'It's 'er 'usband and hiz ladz killin' time.'

'Killing time?'

'Yeah. Killin' time, killin' rats. There's loads of 'em. Dogs ain't bovvered, so he stamps on 'em, or bashes their brains out with what 'e can find.'

'Oh, is that all,' said Dent, trying to stay calm.

The woman's voice continued, 'Idiot uses farm dogs, flippin' 'opeless in town. Burrows dogs they are. I told 'im but 'eeza know all … are you from the 'ospital?'

As Dent climbed the stairs the owner of the voice loomed into view. She grinned, revealing long, lopsided teeth, like tombstones. He realised she was waiting for an answer.

[97]

'Sorry,' he blurted. 'I didn't hear what you said.'

'I asked if youz from the 'ospital.'

'Oh yes, y-yes, I am.'

'Ooo, fancy.' She pushed open a door off the landing. 'Sheeze in ere, and now you … a propah doctah iz'ere, I can scarpah.'

'Well, I'm not exactly a doctor, not yet.'

'Course you are, you come from the 'ospital.'

'Well, I …'

'Anyway, gotta scram. Be back laytah. There's buckets o' water an' a couple o' towels on the side. Shout t' one o' the boys if yer need anyfin'.'

The woman muttered away as she descended without looking back. 'Turrah.' She slammed shut the front door, leaving the slum to scurrying rodents, yelping dogs and a petrified junior midwife. Gripping his bag he tiptoed into the room. 'Hello?' he whispered. It was dark save for shafts of sunlight through shuttered windows.

'Agh, Doctah,' came a female voice. 'Thank the Lord.'

He walked into the middle of the room where a woman lay on a table draped with a blanket and sheet. It was too dingy to see clearly.

'I'm the midwife, and you're Mrs Clements?'

'Yeah, I ain't far off now.'

'Is this your first birth?'

'Second.'

'And did that go well?'

'That's a larf. Not bloomin' likely … 'ad a woman from the Mission. 'Opeless, she wuz. 'Ole fing took bad … an' ages, but I'm orlright now. You bein' a real doctah … wi klorryfum.'

'What was that?' said Dent, aghast.

'Klorryfum. All me mates 'av it. Yer dohn feel nuffin', they said, proper lovely, they said. So, I ses, that's what I'll 'av an orl, I ses. So I sent word t' the 'ospital, see … getta a doctah wiv klorryfum, they said.'

A dazed Dent stumbled towards the window and drew the thin curtains. It wasn't enough. He opened the shutter and lifted the sash.

'Hooray, it's baby man,' cried one of the children from the passage below.

'Show us the baby,' demanded another. The cries grew more insistent: 'Is it comin'?', 'Boy or gel?', 'Gissa look.'

He turned back towards the woman. The extra light revealed a horrifying level of squalor that stopped Dent in his tracks. He edged back to the woman and felt her belly. 'Have your contractions started?' he asked, feeling nauseous.

'Oooo yes ... quit hangin' abowt hey? Gi' us the klorryfum ...'

Dent ducked under the table to spread out *The Daily News*. The sheets of newspaper shook uncontrollably. He was stalling; the more he tried to think the worse his thinking became. A sudden wall of blackness descended. He was no longer in the room. He heard words, his words, but spoken as if by someone else.

'Err, Mrs Clements, have you had chloroform before?'

'Never!' she replied, 'but it's wonderful, ain't it?' She started to garble. 'I know them's thutz 'ad it, mind. Swear by it, they does ... makes yer 'appy, propah hapeee.'

Dent crouched lower until he was kneeling on the newspaper. He held his head while Mrs Clements continued to yabble at the ceiling. '"Getta proppa doctah," Myrtle said. She's got seven nippers, she should know, hey? Wi' klorryfum ... Am ready now, Doctah ... she sez it pongs.'

Dent looked up. 'Smells?' he asked.

'So what. I mean, getta whiff o' this place why don't yah?'

'Er, so you haven't smelled it before?' He scrabbled furiously in the bottom of his bag.

'Nivva.'

'Oh good, I mean, er, well, this certainly has a strong smell.' He grabbed a tiny bottle of sal volatile.

'Please, goo on, do me ova, why dhone yah.'

Dent sprinkled some of the smelling salts onto a handkerchief and applied it to Mrs Clement's face. To his horror she passed out ... instantly. Her eyes rolled to the back of her head. He slapped her cheek; nothing. Not even a deafening crash from the landing stirred her. She was dead to the world, perhaps she was dead? He checked her pulse; to his relief it was there ... and strong. What was happening?

Had she fainted? This was inexplicable. Everything usually done to bring someone out of a faint had just sent her into one! Dent, borderline hysterical, bit his finger... What could he do? And the baby... the baby!

'Hoi, mister!' came a persistent cry from outside. 'What's 'appnin'? Is it a dead un?'

Dent pushed down the sash to groans of protest and dashed back to the table. He would have to deliver the baby on his own! 'But how... how?' he wailed. He re-checked her pulse, then her breathing. Both were regular; his were not. He felt her abdomen and the surge of a contraction. She might be close. He measured her; he wouldn't bother with the speculum, probably three inches. No, it was four! It was difficult to see but he could just feel the emergence of the amniotic sac. He could break the waters but ...... no ... no, he wouldn't. He stopped. Something told him to hold fire, wait for the next contraction. He took a deep breath and slowly returned his palms to the woman's belly. He waited and listened. In those moments and unknown to anyone, unknown to any textbook swotted over or ignored, Nature's dispensary played its part. In evolutionary terms this exchange between baby and mother had been going on forever; cascades of oxytocin interspersed with pulses of adrenaline, waves of oestrogen, progesterone, beta endorphins, norepinephrine, hormonal floods and every other biochemical signal in favour of survival. The medical student simply took a back seat... Why interfere when there was no need... for several minutes he felt the rhythm of her steady breathing and at the moment that simply felt right pushed his finger into the sac. Fluid gushed over the table, his shoes and *The Daily News*. The baby's head dropped onto the cervix and the uterus pushed the baby free in a rush. The placenta followed, slipping off the table into a bucket. Plop! He tied off the umbilical cord, wiped the baby clean and wrapped her in one of the towels. She wriggled and miraculously changed colour... blackberry to strawberry. She was breathing! His first delivery and she would live! He temporarily used his bag as a Moses basket while he checked that the uterus was empty and cleaned up as best he could. Should he wake the mother and tell her the good news? Her face was motionless, she was still unconscious. He tentatively removed the hanky still reeking of sal volatile. To his amazement and relief she instantly awoke.

'Oh well done, Mrs Clements. Look, you have a beautiful baby girl,' he blurted. 'Six, maybe seven pounds. Look, isn't she wonderful? Well done!'

'That was luvverly, dint feel a fing,' she said. 'Klorryfum is magic, ennit?'

Dent changed the subject. 'Here she is,' he handed the newborn to her mother. 'Have you thought of a name?'

'We 'ad a boy's name but not a gelz.'

There was some frenzied barking from the rooms below. Dent wanted to share his elation with the father... the crowd outside the window... anybody. Dent pulled up the sash and leant out: 'Could you tell Mr Clements he has a beautiful daughter!'

There was some cheering.

'Show us, come on...'

'When her mother's ready...' He was distracted by the view. Back-to-back houses stretched in every direction, their backyards humming in the heat. Rotting waste, refuse, outdoor WCs, piles of discarded building materials, the odd dustbins and water butts filled with putrescence. Nothing was clean, not even the washing hanging out to dry. The air stank of infection and disease. It was horrific, something had to be done...

Dent's thoughts were interrupted by someone entering the room. He turned to face a man of about forty.

'Ah, Mr Clements,' greeted Dent, 'you'll be the proud father, congratulations.'

Mr Clements shielded his eyes from the harsh sunlight. He had a thin stubbly face. His dirty striped shirt hung over baggy trousers. The end of each trouser leg was secured to his ankles with baling string. Dent imagined adding string to his tutor's advice: 'Chloroform, newspaper *and* baling string. The essentials sir, for slum delivery.' He looked at the rat catcher's huge hob-nailed boots and thought of their recent purpose. Clements read his mind.

'Yeah, sorry abowt the bangin' but we 'ad a good day. Very profitable.'

'Oh good,' said Dent.

'Yeah, we musta catched thirty downstairs, an' half a sackful next door.' Mr Clements drew himself up to his full height and puffed out his chest. 'Tough work, knackered me out it has…' Dent moved to the right so that Clements wouldn't have to stare into the light. Their eyes met … momentarily.

There was an uncomfortable silence. 'Er, well done,' Dent's voice faltered.

'Ain't dun regular see … got t' stay on top of it … otherwise they take ova … vermin.'

'Yes, I can imagine.'

Clements flexed his arms like a wrestler. 'Are you done in 'ere?'

'Yes, it's all yours.'

Mr Clements returned to the door and whistled. Two Jack Russell terriers ran in, yapping, followed by a young boy with a long stick.

'Is this your son?'

'Mine not hers,' said Mr Clements, spitting and wiping his brow. ''Ere Mick, pull back the skirtin' and give it a poke …'

As the commotion of rat-catching resumed the junior doctor wished the family well, picked up his bag and walked onto the landing and down the stairs. He emerged into the bright sunshine, but his thoughts remained with the baby he'd just delivered. She'd been born into an environment that spelled nothing but struggle. The more he considered her plight the greater his sense of frustration. Any joy gained at a successful birth had evaporated along with the chloroform from his turn-ups.

* * *

'Were you called to the slums?' asked Dalton that evening.

'Yes, everything worked out in the end, a girl, seven pounds.'

'Then you won't have heard about Barnes?'

'What?'

'Smashed his leg on the rugby field yesterday. It's really bad, just above the knee. Word is that he might never play again…'

Dent was speechless. Dalton continued to fill in the details. 'They say… as far as breaks go… this could hardly be worse. Impossible to fix properly because of the knee…'

Dent looked vacant. 'Poor Barnes,' was all he could manage.

'Yes, awful. I am not sure if he's aware of much… he…'

'Who told you?' Dent interrupted.

'Abercrombie, Senior House. He advised against talking to him; said there's no point because he's off his head with morphine. He'd been screaming with pain and so they gave him extra…. They can't operate till the swelling's gone.'

'Poor Barnes,' Dent repeated. He felt empty.

'The pity is that half the field was waterlogged due to a burst water main,' continued Dalton. 'It was left to the players to cancel or not. It wasn't unanimous, but typically, Barnes insisted the game should go ahead.'

Dent tried to collect his thoughts. Visions of their friend injured and lying in hospital had robbed him of the opportunity to discuss the mysteries of sal volatile. Slumped in a chair he watched drearily as Dalton busied himself before leaving for a lecture. Alone, his thoughts remained with his stricken friend's miserable predicament. It seemed unimaginable. He looked out of the window and watched a cripple on crutches crossing the road. Slowly his thoughts returned to his dramatic day in the slums and Mrs Clements' faint… caused by what? Surely not by smelling salts? He also recalled the self-conscious look in her husband's eyes… the look of someone inhabited by shame… and sorrow… features of a life constrained by birthright and circumstance. The more fortunate members of society boast about equality as if it exists, Dent thought. But this is an arrogant conceit, a myth clung to by self-serving holders of power and control. Mr Clements battled all the discomforts, but also felt constrained by the falsehood that everything was his fault. He bragged about his rat-catching expertise but the hollow look in his eyes told a different story; his bravura was a sham. The reality was another mouth to feed that he had no use for.

His daughter would be lucky to reach adulthood. Something had to be done. He'd write a letter...to a local councillor. If nothing else it would dissolve his frustrations...and Barnes would approve. Yes, he'd do it for both of them. He reached for a compendium that bore the names of the local representatives. One name, a retired colonel, stood out.

30th June, 1913

Dear Sir,
    Today I have just returned from delivering a baby in the ward where you are a councillor. I was shocked by the insanitary conditions the inhabitants endure.
    I attended a dwelling with no running water, toilet of any description, or any lighting. It was infested with vermin and bedbugs and is by no means exceptional. People use the alleys and gardens for waste and water has to be brought from distant hand pumps. The neighbourhood is very overcrowded and runs the risk of epidemic.
    Doing nothing is not an option. Any sort of remedy which improves the living conditions of these neighbourhoods will bring benefit to us all.
    I look forward to your reply.
    Yours sincerely,
    J. Y. Dent.

A month later Dent bumped into the colonel at a civic function at King's teaching hospital, the Strand.

'Oh yes,' he had said gruffly, eyeing Dent through a shiny, gold-rimmed monocle, 'I remember your letter. No, I didn't reply. There's no point, you see?'

'What do you mean?' asked Dent, incredulous.

'Well, the more you do for such people the more you may do.'

A middle-aged couple joined them and struck up a discussion about spa towns in Switzerland.

Dent made his excuses and left early; he wasn't feeling well. He went out of his way and paused underneath the statue of Gladstone. He looked up at the austere features and saw all the lies at the heart of a controlling society. The hierarchies who purported community through education, health and philanthropy but were in reality more interested in shoring up their own authority measured in the accoutrements of petite-bourgeois kitsch: fancy clothes, window boxes and hiking hols on the Continent. Uncle Louis was right; politicians are the necessary but worst dimension of this farce. Local councillors were simply less conspicuous, a corrupting virus in its embryonic form. Dent coughed, a deep hacking cough. He felt terrible. He ached for Uncle Louis as he spat furiously into his handkerchief. He looked at the spreading crimson stain on the linen. Sure enough: blood, pulmonary blood.

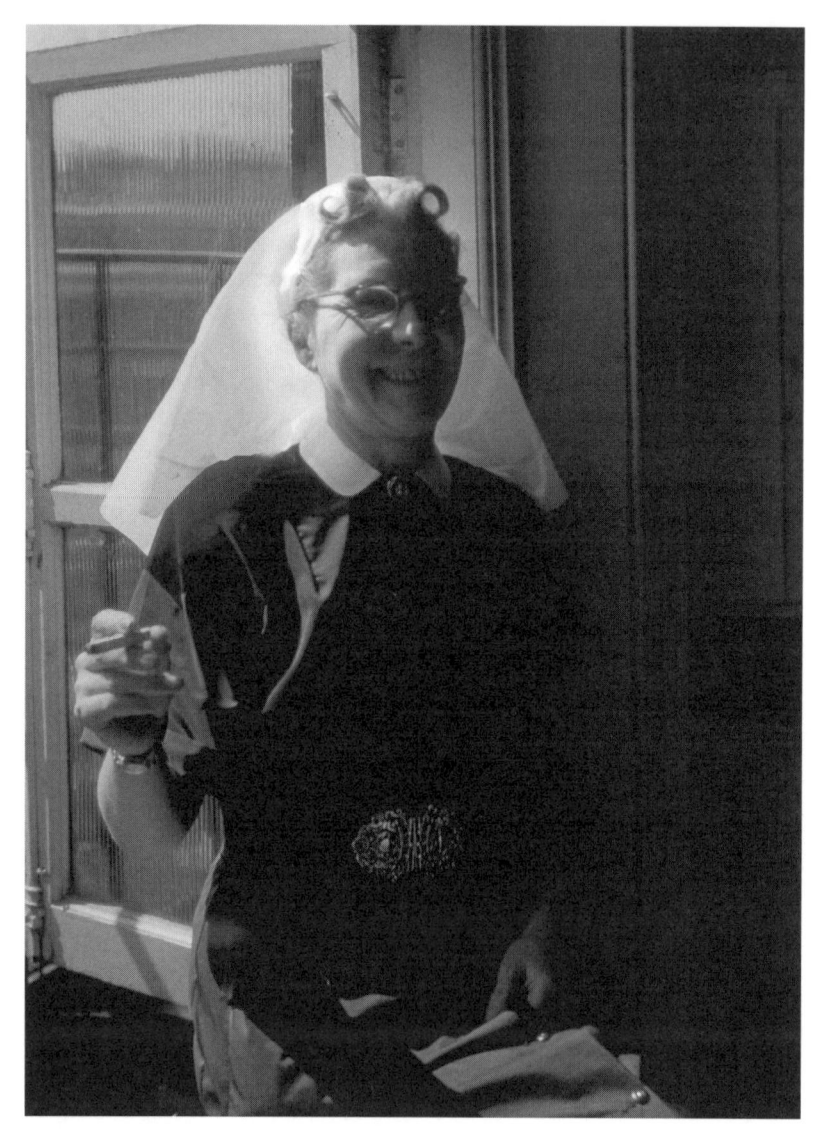

Sister Kate Gibson, or 'Gibbie', helped treat patients during the day shift. An example of her Notes appear on page 256. She is mentioned in Burroughs' *APO-33* (Fuck You Press, 1965). It seems everybody smoked, including the nurses. (photo: J. Y. Dent)

6

99 Cromwell Road

> An animal perfectly in harmony with its environment is a perfect mechanism. Nature never appeals to intelligence until habit and instinct are useless. There is no intelligence when there is no need of change.
> – H. G. Wells
>   *The Time Machine*

On Friday morning, the 20th April 1956, William Seward Burroughs took a left turn into Cromwell Road propelled by little more than a gust of wind. White cherry blossom shook above his drab hat; under it the last molecules of optimism were evaporating. He berated himself for believing there could be a cure for his problem. The sucking parasite of junk took its cue from every one of his viciously contorting cells: 'You dumb fuck. To imagine a cure could be dredged outta this filthy hole?'

He stumbled under a tall, mid-Victorian terrace sporting peeling paint and a 'No Wogs Dogs or Irish' sign. A crocodile of excited school children pinned him against black iron railings. He vaguely caught their excitement... something about dinosaurs?

'Sir,' one chubby boy whined.

'Yes, Johnson?'

'Fox called me brontosaurus.'

'Liar,' refuted Fox, 'I said diplodocus.'

Burroughs' face crumpled like wastepaper at another gut-wrenching spasm. At last the ribbon of schoolchildren crossed the road, leaving him free to blunder upon his destination, No. 99, shared with the clandestine abortion clinic. He dragged himself up tiled steps and through a pair of heavy swing doors into a gloomy lobby. A black marble floor stretched towards a formica desk and a receptionist wearing an ornate pair of horn-rimmed spectacles.

'So!' she announced, interrupting her manicure, 'you must be the eleven o'clock.' She put down her nail file. 'Just stay right where you are. *I'll* let 99 know.'

She moved backwards without relaxing her stare and opened a side door to reveal a steep flight of dimly lit stairs. Her neck twisted. 'Sister!' she screeched, 'HELLOOO, Sister. Yes, another live one.' The faint noise of a door opening and closing echoed in the stairwell.

'Two minutes and you'll be dealt with,' she said curtly, returning to her perch. He fell against the wall; its cold cut him to his marrow. The receptionist continued to stare; he felt as welcome as a cockroach.

Eventually, a middle-aged woman in a dark blue nursing uniform popped a smiling face round the door and beckoned that Burroughs should follow her up. Once on the stairs she briefly introduced herself,

'Hello, I am Sister Gibson. Dr Dent told me to expect you. So sorry about the reception. They're from an agency and quite unsuitable... and sorry too about these flights of stairs, five all told.'

They arrived breathless at a wide landing with several doors leading in different directions. Burroughs was shown into 'his' room, situated at the front of the building. It had a large bay window affording angled views up and down Cromwell Road. The high ceiling gave an airy feel. There was a steel-framed bed, turned down with crisp white sheets and a thick blue eiderdown. Busy floral wallpaper, pink and lilac, added to the potpourri of styles; living room, hospital and hotel. Everything was spotlessly clean and fresh, not that the downcast patient noticed. He dropped his bag on the floor and slowly undid his gabardine knee-length coat. Still breathing heavily he fell into a wicker chair by a small oak table. The coat he draped over trembling knees. Sister Gibson took her place opposite and started to take notes. She looked up and smiled.

'Now then, we never use patients' names here, we find it easier. We can give you a nickname, unless you have a preference?'

The patient looked through shivering fingers, trying to concentrate. 'Yeah, yeah, ok, I get it. Can I be "Chinaman"?' His voice trailed off.

'Yes, that's perfect, easy to remember. I'm Sister Mary Gibson, but some call me Kate, you're welcome to use either, whichever you prefer. We never refer to your name in the daily reports either. These will be yours. You may take them when you leave. Did Dr Dent give you a booklet?'

Burroughs grunted and pulled the exercise book from his holdall and dropped it onto the table. Kate looked at the cover.

'Is this your address, "Edgerton" Gardens? Just down from here?'

'Yeah,' drawled Chinaman.

Kate corrected the spelling.

'Now, you can ask me anything about…'

'My morphine,' interrupted Chinaman, 'when can I have it?' He let his head sink forward.

'Sorry?'

'Morphine,' he mumbled.

'Dr Dent will be along shortly, and we'll take it from there. Did he tell you that the treatment, the apomorphine, might make you vomit?'

'Sick? Oh, yeah.' He lifted his head and leant back, waving his hands impatiently. 'Like I'm flying.'

A faint shadow spread across Kate's face. She had worked with Dent for years. She could interpret sarcasm in any number of ways. The best strategy with a new patient was compassion laced with home truths… consistently held home truths.

'Well, you may vomit. If it happens take it as a sign that the apomorphine is getting through, but you'll do just as well if you don't.' She stopped talking and leaned towards Chinaman until she was sure she had his attention.

'The absolutely critical thing to understand is that this is *not* an aversion treatment.'

'Sure, yeah,' he croaked, 'Dr Dent explained. It's chemical.'

Sister Kate's eyes widened. 'Yes, that's right.' she smiled. 'Any sickness is just a side effect, nothing more. We use morphine and alcohol to stabilise your withdrawal symptoms. That's all there is to it.'

'Alcohol?' His face twitched.

'Yes,' she replied, 'we like to give it after the apomorphine. We find it helps.'

'Helps?' Chinaman sounded disdainful.

'Why, yes,' continued Kate, 'in the past it has helped relax the patient. All previous cases have shown this to be so.'

'But I'm not an alcoholic.'

'I did not say you were,' assured Kate, 'but alcohol is somehow linked to the metabolic change that happens; it helps to stabilise you … while apomorphine does its work.'

Chinaman shrugged. 'I been over that … in his book.'

'Oh, my goodness, you've read it!' Kate exclaimed, brightening. 'Well, you'll be the first that has. I tell Dr Dent nobody will bother.'

'I only …' Chinaman paused. 'I only read bits. What I wanna know is how many opiate addicts you've treated.'

'Me personally, not that many, about ten at the most. But Dr Dent has had experience of this for much longer than I have, more than twenty years or so. Usually our patients have developed a problem with alcohol and a few with prescription medicines; most morphine addicts come from a medical background.'

'Sure,' said Chinaman. His face lost some of its intensity as he looked vacantly at the floor, picking at his trousers. Kate was reminded of a mangy hen, pecking dirt.

'I suppose they're subject to temptation,' he mumbled, as if talking to himself.

Kate nodded.

'A liking for needles …'

'Oh, yes, they're certainly used to them,' said Kate, cheerily. 'But we also meet opiate addicts used to other routes: suppositories, smokers and pills.'

She put down her pen and sat back. 'You saw Dr Dent on Wednesday afternoon, is that right?'

Chinaman nodded.

'And he gave you some morphine to tide you over?'

Chinaman nodded again.

'... And you took it, and nothing else?'

'Yeah, goddamnit, just what he gave me, why do you think I'm dying here?'

Kate's met the flash of anger with a dead bat. 'Good, hopefully we won't have much need for morphine at all. There'll be charts for us to follow and you can see them whenever you like. You do understand, Chinaman, because every patient is different we have to be attentive. To that end we will be constantly running tests, particularly in the first few days, to see how you are. We cannot afford to base your treatment on any precedent.' She looked towards her patient to check he was listening.

'And please remember,' her voice a little firmer, 'we are always here and if there's anything you need, or need to know about the treatment, please ask. There's a chest of drawers and a wardrobe over there...' Kate pointed back towards the corner by the door. 'You can use those for your personal possessions. There's a linen basket in the bathroom for clothes that need washing. We could dry clean your suit if you'd like. There's a laundry in the next street. We change the bed linen every day. There's also some games, crossword puzzles, and playing cards. And a selection of books, some left by previous patients. If you cannot find anything interesting we can help. There's a wireless and a bell, there, by your bed. If you're having difficulties we sit with you...'

It was no use. Chinaman had long since stopped hearing anything. Panic possessed him as a new surge of agonies telegraphed their intent to twist him like a rope. He froze in an attempt to stem the contraction. It was futile. He winced, his torment released through a bullfrog croak. Kate responded. She extended her hand to his and slowly slid her warm fingers to his wrist. He felt her search for and find his pulse... that might surprise her he thought... the calm intervention had provided a distraction. She stood and helped him off with his jacket, took his blood pressure and temperature while asking some routine questions; when had he last eaten, was he drinking enough water, was he sleeping... constipated?

'I hardly sleep, and haven't been to the toilet in days.' He felt her reaction. 'Weeks,' he added, causing her eyebrows to arch.

'Yes, well that must be difficult... we can definitely help.' Kate's voice sounded solicitous.

'She just don't get it,' he complained. 'Look,' he grabbed her arm, 'I just need fixing. Morphine.'

'Well, can we wait until Dr Dent arrives? He won't be long.' Her poise intact.

'NO! Dr Dent said I can have it... any time. Dammit, he musta told you!' His voice wobbled between tears and hysteria. Kate watched and waited...

'I see how this must be difficult but let's wait until Dr Dent has seen you. He may want to ask you some further questions.' Kate took the hand gripping her arm and placed it back on the table.

'He promised!' The Chinaman ripped off his glasses and threw them across the table. 'The pain, it's a fucking vice, it ain't difficult to figure.'

'Look,' said Kate patiently, placing her hand on his shoulder, '... while we're waiting why don't you change? It'll help you settle in.'

'Settle in?' he squealed, throwing his arms in the air. Kate stood back as he fell violently against the back of the chair. 'Settle in,' he wailed over and over. 'This wasn't the deal... where's my fix? Give me what I'm paying for. Dent said I could have it, where is it?' He gripped his coat and stood up; things fell out of an inside pocket onto the floor. He kicked out at nothing, falling sideways against the wall. 'Where is it? Eukodol, paregoric, what do I care... Look, I'm not here for my health... what a bubbling sulphurous shithole this is. London!? Get with the program... COME ON!'

Chinaman slid down the wall into a heap. Kate picked up his coat, took his arm and dragged him up. She could feel his shoulder blades, probably less than ten stone. 'This way, Chinaman,' she said firmly.

Outmanoeuvred by Kate's calmness, Chinaman had nowhere to turn. Resembling a tamed animal he allowed himself to be shuffled across the landing to the bathroom.

He was weighed and given a basket with pyjamas, towel and a dressing gown.

'You can have a bath if you'd like,' Kate offered and noticed him flinch.

'Well, it's here if you want,' she smiled. 'Any time.'

'I know,' he murmured, scratching his neck vigorously. 'I'm a barn cat,' he mumbled, 'dirty and loathsome.'

The phone rang in another of the rooms off the landing. Kate went to answer it and returned immediately. 'That was Dr Dent,' she said, helping Chinaman back to his room. 'He'll be along presently. I'll leave you for a few minutes until he arrives. Why don't you change and try and rest?' Chinaman thought about the ordeal of getting undressed with aching joints. How long could he bear this?

'What time is it?' He sounded agitated again.

'Eleven twenty-five.'

'I've been here for hours.'

'No. You arrived slightly early. You've been here for half an hour, no more. Have you a watch?'

'Broken, like me.'

'Well, I assure you what I am saying is true. Would you like me to get you a clock?'

'Morphine. I want morphine, you're a nurse. Do your job.'

'Yes.'

'Look, stop agreeing with me. Just stick to the deal.'

'Wouldn't you rather wait for Dr Dent?'

'No! No! No! I'm in pain, terrible fucking cramps, my whole body aches, my head's about to explode and if you don't fix me now I'll die...'

'That's not likely, Chinaman, is it?' Kate's question did not require an answer. She left him alone, closing the door and any further discussion.

Painfully the American undressed and put on striped pyjamas. He placed both hands on the iron bed frame for support and closed his eyes. This was going to be his room for God knows how long. He climbed into the bed, trying to remember what the doc had said... it was impossible, his mind was shrinking, he was outta gas, finished .... Everything hinged on a crazy old croaker with a cat, books and a fish tank... and another evil bitch that hates me... in London for Chrissakes. Things could not be worse, his guts curled like barbed wire, his end was coming. What's that…whistling? His head jerked at the door. His body bowed, he shrank under the bedclothes. More voices…it's coming! He couldn't complain, he deserved to suffer. The bed creaked like his bones, his skull was splitting, his pyjamas already dark with sweat. He shrank, pulling his knees to his chin. Footsteps on the landing, the door swung open, he looked up.

'Hello, Chinaman,' said Dent, marching in, followed by Kate. 'So you found us all right. Well done.'

His patient covered his face with his palms.

'This is terrible, it is all hopeless,' he wheezed.

'Not sleeping?' asked Dent.

'No,' said Chinaman.

'And a battle getting here, I expect,' Dent added, feeling his brow. 'You've done well; the hardest steps are often the first.'

Dent sat down on the bed and took Chinaman's hand. He slid his fingers up onto Chinaman's wrist and found his pulse. A quiet descended as the old doc counted. His fingers were warm…strong.

'And how did you get on with what I gave you?' he said eventually.

'Took the last grain last night, I'm in terrible pain.'

'Yes, well, would you like some morphine now?'

'I begged the nurse but she refused, even after what we agreed.'

'Well, Sister Kate did the right thing.'

'Why? How?' Chinaman sounded crazed.

'Because of what we promised.'

'I *am* doing my best!' the Chinaman screamed.

'Yes, I believe you are,' said Dent. 'And Kate wanted me to see this for myself. You *are* doing extremely well, as well as any man could. I will prepare an injection of morphine now, a quarter of a grain.'

Dent left the room, closing the door. Kate moved to the end of the bed. 'Just do your best, Chinaman; for the time being that is all we can expect.'

He kicked at the bed cover at her pathetic, incomprehensible words. The eiderdown slid to the floor and Kate bent down and pulled it back over the Chinaman's feet. He kicked it off again.

'I'm hot!' he shouted.

'Would you like me to open the window?'

The Chinaman didn't answer. Kate eased the top sash down a few inches and waited.

Dent returned with a small case and box and set these down on the oak table in the bay. Turning to the Chinaman; 'Left or right arm?'

The Chinaman yanked at his pyjama top, breaking off a button. It fell to the floor and rattled across the boards. He pulled his arms from their sleeves and turned them over. 'Take your pick.'

Kate caught her breath at the signs of habitual narcotic use: black and red punctures like bee stings up to where you might expect to see biceps. Several holes looked vexed; almost septic. Dent sat down and massaged the Chinaman's right forearm for thirty seconds. His grip was assured. He applied the tourniquet above the elbow and wiped the injection site with an antiseptic swab. Kate handed Dent the syringe and he injected the morphine.

'What heavenly poison,' the Chinaman sighed.

'Venom,' said Dent smiling, applying a small plaster. 'Poison we swallow.'

'You're no snake,' said his patient in a terse comeback voice.

'And now the apomorphine.' As before Dent wiped another injection site and took a second syringe from Kate with a longer needle. He deftly pushed it deep into the muscle below the shoulder and delivered intramuscularly $C_{17}H_{17}NO_2$ but, unknown to both doctor and patient, the closest synthetic match to the brain's most beguiling messenger service, dopamine ($C_8H_{11}NO_2$). Chinaman didn't react.

'Now,' Dent stood up, 'in a few minutes you may vomit, you may not, it is immaterial. Kate or I will deal with it. You won't get much warning. If it happens it'll be in the next five minutes or so. Beforehand I'd like you to drink this whisky mixed half and half with water.'

'What time is it?' asked the Chinaman, beginning to feel calmer as the morphine kicked in.

'Eleven-forty,' said Kate.

'I never drink before midday,' said the Chinaman in a matter-of-fact voice.

'I would really rather you did,' said Dent.

'Yeah, I know,' said the Chinaman, 'but I have rules.'

'There are no rules here,' said Dent, 'only your voluntary submission to this treatment, one aimed at making you better. Now, it is up to you but if you wouldn't mind.' Dent placed the glass in Chinaman's thin hand and stood back.

The patient sighed and chucked back the whisky and water in one. Kate confirmed the time and entered some notes. She said something to herself, went out and returned with a bucket draped in a thick white towel. Dent sat down on the edge of the bed and felt Chinaman's brow once more. As he did so he thought about his patient. His loneliness, his jumpy paranoia. He didn't like the thought of this man in a strange place with no direct support. He'd ring Maclay, see if he could help.

'I feel tired, so tired,' said Chinaman, yawning and beginning to relax.

'Yes,' said Dent, his hand still covering the knitted brow, 'the apomorphine will help you sleep, you'll drift into it without noticing.' The doctor spoke steadily...calmly. 'By the way, would you mind if Dr Walter Maclay visits? He's very interested in alternative approaches to treatment. He's a well known psychiatrist, you'll have lots to talk about. Have you any objection to him dropping by?'

Chinaman didn't answer. He felt odd, his body hadn't been his own for years but this was new. What was it? He cocked his ear as if hearing music for the first time. Maybe a sonic warning, a danger signal? Perhaps the first tectonic shudder of a distant earthquake or Martian chatter using the buzz lines from the old croaker's book cover? He turned his head towards the remote signal as if it was aimed straight at him. He saw some majestic sandstone rocks vivid against a cobalt sky. Underneath some stones rocked. What was that? In their midst one pebble clicked and flew into the air, pushed there by spring water in its blind surge for the sea. The Chinaman lurched, his body jolted by every force left to him. Some he was reminded of...others he didn't know existed.

Spew hosed the bottom of Kate's bucket. She caught it all apart from the splashback which Dent wiped away. His insides erupted again, his diaphragm thumping the back of his throat. Enthralled by the novelty and winded by the exertion he fell back into his pillows gulping for air.

'Man,' he gasped, 'what was that?'

'Rest now, I'll be back tonight,' said Dent, wiping Chinaman's face clean with a damp flannel.

In a minute he was asleep.

* * *

An hour and twenty two minutes later the patient awoke. His legs ached; he didn't dare move as a cramp threatened to contort him. He slowly clasped his forehead.

Kate was at his bedside.

'What time is it?' he asked.

'One-eighteen.'

'I need more junk.'

'What?' she asked.

'Where's Dr Dent?'

'He's gone home. He'll be in later.'

'When?'

'After five o'clock.'

'How much morphine has he got?'

'What do you mean?'

'For me, of course!'

'Why, "of course"?'

Chinaman groaned. 'I need it. I've been on thirty, forty grains a day. You can't expect to fix me on that little sniff.'

Kate reached out to take his arm but he withdrew it.

'Chinaman, I need to take your pulse.'

'Why?'

'You know.'

'Know what?'

'We have to monitor you.'

'I know how I am. Stop checking on me. Time?'

'One-twenty.'

'Is that all! This is impossible. When's Doc Dent in?'

'I've just told you.'

'Isn't he supposed to be looking after me?'

'He is, and *we* are. Now come along, your wrist.'

Chinaman dropped his hand into Kate's. 'Have you got in extra?'

Kate ignored the question.

'You're gonna need it,' he warned.

'Now, Chinaman, would you like to pass water?'

'Water?' he shouted, 'you're deaf, aren't you? There's no way out, this isn't a cure. It's a failure.'

'We've just started,' said Kate. 'We have a long way to go, and, yes, there'll probably be setbacks.' She grasped his shoulders firmly. 'What I can assure you, Mr Chinaman, is that you will never be alone; we're going to go through this together. Sister Jones, Dr Dent and I; one of us will always be here until you've turned the corner. Clear?'

'Jones?' asked the Chinaman.

'Yes, she's your night nurse, I'm your day nurse. We'll get to know you very well, I'm sure.'

'p.m. Jones, a.m. Kate,' he reflected.

'Yes, like me, Sister Jones is committed to our work here. We switch at nine in the morning and nine at night, twelve hour shifts. Now, would you like to pass water?'

'As a matter of fact, I would.'

Kate bent down and retrieved a bed bottle. 'Can you manage?' she asked.

'No, I'm beat.' He sounded pitiful.

'Are you sure?'

'Deadly.' He drew his right hand to his forehead.

'Please yourself.' Kate lifted the bed clothes, grabbed his cock and placed it in the bottle. She could've been posting a letter. 'When you've finished just leave it here,' she continued, tapping the bedside table, 'for us to collect ... so we can run tests.'

'T-tests?' he blustered.

'Yes, the best way to discover when the metabolic change is

happening is to realise when your body has reacted. The sugar in your urine is the marker we use … the first indication.'

Chinaman's mind was blank. 'What have you done with my watch?' he mumbled as Kate referred to the notes.

'You told me it was broken.'

'No I didn't.'

Kate looked up as Chinaman looked away.

'Just tell me the time,' he urged.

'Two minutes later than what I told you two minutes ago.'

'I've forgotten.'

Kate returned to the bedside, undid her wristwatch and held it in front of him. When she saw that he had looked she placed it on the marble-topped comodino.

'Time for morphine,' he said, retrieving the half-filled bed bottle and handing it to Kate. 'It'd save me, come on.'

Kate took the bed bottle and went out. She reappeared with a tumbler of 50/50 water and whisky.

Chinaman continued to harangue. 'The morphine, where do you keep it, you gotta safe?'

She didn't answer.

'Are you allowed to keep it here?'

Kate returned to her note-taking.

'What would happen if the cops came?'

She looked up. 'Now then, Chinaman, are you ready for your injection of apomorphine plus two tablets?'

'What?'

'Tablets, yes. To be dissolved under the tongue.'

'Opium tablets?'

'No, apomorphine.'

Chinaman rubbed his face and sneezed. Snot ran down his face. Kate wiped it away.

'This is ridiculous,' he shouted, 'USELESS! First you make me wait for Dr Dent, then you hit me with whisky and now pills. I hope the cops come and bust you.'

Kate was a study of concentration. She left the whisky and water on the bedside table and silently injected her patient in the muscle under his left shoulder.

She fetched a clean bucket and towel and a small bottle of tablets, handing two to Chinaman. 'Under your tongue, please.'

'Under your tongue, please,' he mimicked taking the pills.

'One on either side of your mouth,' said Kate. 'They'll be gone in a minute or two.' She wiped his forehead and adjusted his bedclothes. 'As soon as the tablets have gone you can take the whisky.'

'No, I refuse.'

'That would be a shame. I thought you were going to be a model patient.'

'Well, now you know. My family's big in the States. They'll have cars here in no time. You won't know what's hit you.'

'Please, Chinaman, try not to talk. It is important the tablets aren't swallowed.'

'Why?'

'Because apomorphine does its work in the brain. I thought you understood this?' She hesitated while smoothing his hair. 'It enters the blood going into your brain ... here. That's what facilitates the change. We use nasal spray ... for the same reason.'

Chinaman sniggered. 'Nasal spray? More hokum. Anyhow, the pills have gone.'

'Good. Whisky, please.' Kate handed Chinaman the tumbler. He peered at the liquid and swirled it around.

'Health is wealth,' he said, and downed it.

'Thank you,' said Kate. 'I'll be back in a minute.'

'Don't go.'

'What's up?'

'Won't I need the bucket?'

'Not yet.'

'You expect me to be sick?'

'Possibly.'

'Why only possibly?'

'Some patients are never sick with apomorphine but as you already have been it is likely that you will be again … but there's still no guarantee.'

'I think I will be.'

'Ok, but it's still too early, take my word for it. Look, let me put this back,' she raised the empty tumbler, 'I'll be straight back … and then we'll talk.'

As Kate left Chinaman picked up the bucket and waited. He yawned. She returned and asked if he could expect any visitors.

'Nope,' he answered flatly. 'Nobody loves me.'

'I'm sure that's not true.'

'I'm a monster,' he assured, moving the bucket in front of him.

Kate stood close, placing her palm flat against the nape of his neck. She gently squeezed before sliding her hand down under his collar and onto the plateau between his shoulders. He grew aware of the spread of her fingers … the lightness of her touch …. Instinctively patient and nurse closed their eyes so they could tune in … to each other. She adjusted her breathing to his … and lowered her hand, her fingers stretching like dowsing rods … scanning the terrain for hidden forces … searching … searching. She reminded herself that when the tremor comes it's always faint … but unmistakeable … the prelude to the cascade … Her hand glided down further … hovering over ridges, over hairs … twitching … There! The first tell-tale pulse erupted into a convulsion. Kate wrapped her arm around his back as he purged himself. She gripped him; he heaved and rose before falling back against the pillows trembling and snatching for air. She smiled to herself, retrieved her arm, put down the bucket and wiped his face clean. Another obstacle breached on his journey to the sea.

He wanted to talk but his words were stifled by more yawning. He was too tired to think. He shivered as he began to relax … murmured something obscure … impenetrable.

In 3.1 seconds Bill Lee

HARDY TREE

Crashed
    Thru
        the
            Doors
                of   Bouncing
                      Deception ...   he reached out
... grabbed his subterfuge; surgical coat, lanyard,
stethoscope...he rolls over / coming to he's aware of the
incessant chatter of hustlers / pimps / salesmen / drugs 'r'
us / psychobabblers / LSD faddists / Friends of Apartheid ...
a creeps assembly at the end of his bed / bug repellant might
not be enough ...
Walrus arrives blowing nicotine through orange whiskers / his
distant oak and vellum voice commands the galleon, he tells it
straight ...
—Safe passage to port will require fortitude and a following
wind ... / here it comes boys whistling up the stairwell /
that ole drunk's standard / swirling around glass towers
—Human Congress? Ha! A nest of vipers, more like. Science?
You'll be lucky. A bureau concoct the evidence broadcast by a
complicit media. You're a gatecrasher, you'll see what we're
up against, watch and learn ...
Lee listens all right. Hears his rusty receptors opening / the
first grating push back on habituated patterning / a long lazy
wail echoes down river / the black ache of fog horns across
polluted water / out in the bay an old hulk's spine cracks ...
sinks deeper into mud / tough times ahead moans Bill / his
atoms jostle for attention / Suddenly a vile monster rises
outta the filth / curls a bat's wing around his shoulder /
—My name is Contessa Jewel, great name for toxicity, don't
you think? Now, come this way you radical little shit ....
Bill shrinks in terror ... and shame / buttons both his lips
an' overalls / the deceit an' self pity hurt
A steel and glass door slides open / the conference hall
expands as they advance ....

99 CROMWELL ROAD

An empty vessel's sense of entitlement approaches / offers massage in phony Welsh accent / oozes smarm / slag down a mountain ...
—Half price if you're a delegate from arseholes & abject / he grins / a right fuckin' chancer
—Hand relief my speciality he continues ...
Bill buries him in hot streak of projectile vomit ... Contessa throws her head back /
—Bullseye! she shouts. —A newbie, so much to learn ...
A head louse in Clarets scarf arrives in TV studio / exhibiting chronic traits of depression / hectoring, bullying, coercion, denial ...
Bilious Bill knows the signs / hoses him with puke; mandibles, thorax and tail / another cracking delivery.
More parasitism this way comes, advises walrus / Contessa climbs steps to lectern / nods to scheming cadaver in the shadows ...
—He's been dead for years / points out walrus —but few have noticed / propped up by close knit mob .... their blend of pietism'n'usury stains the air green .... like apomorepheeeen. Bill looks at his bed sheet and nods.
BigBiZ Convention fizzes / Contessa stumbles under weight of expectation / she wobbles / Bill recognises doubt / sees charade / ... world weary maybe but this was tip-top travesty / villainy on a pedestal / touch of the Harvard Tea Party, jeeeze.
—Wait! It gets better, grumbles walrus.
Contessa reads from auto cue
—Ladies and Gentleman, blessed delegates, offshore sponsors take heart / our mission is not over / yes there have been setbacks but we guarantee gerrymandering, half-truths, smears and let us not forget further lies and duplicity / we're still in control ....
<u>POWER POWER POWER POWER POWER POWER</u>! she punches the air ...
—Yes my cadre of cadets / the six P's / Power is ours and

[123]

we're not letting go
She opens her wingspan wide and pecks button with beak /
centre stage a fulsome red rose morphs into spinning roulette wheel /
—And THIS she screams —is algorithmically linked to our nerve terminals devastating the northern heartlands hahaha! .....
The delegates stand to cheer, wave betting slips, throw money like confetti at a whore's wedding.
Contessa, her poise regained, snarls:
—And your first bet is freeee / the harpy apes gangsterspeak / Lee sees class / decades of hypnopædic zealotry / ingrained inculcation / well-honed mannerisms / regular tax haven top ups / shags on a sofa / journalistic failure / the invisible biological bridges connecting antennae neck breasts and rib cage / this mouthpiece is almost the finished article with umpteen clones poised in the wings / sure a masquerade / but the war on the poor's a copper bottomed winner / nobody'll mind anyhow when everybody's TOXED to the MAX / the massive roulette wheel is now spinning so fast it becomes a blur / thugs from the building trade and Pharma hug like frogs in a ditch / Bill sprays a few until his stomach is empty / but the mindless never mind / fanatical stupefaction on steroids / Crazy drunk on adulation Contessa indicates everybody should unbutton their tunics
—Let it all go sisters! / everyone lathers themselves into peak hysteria / drugged cultists / Rule Britannia swells the stadium / Contessa bathed in pink sentimentality launches into CareinthecommoonityStFrancisofAssisibullshit#23 / tears of joy roll down the nation's face...bombast on plasma simultaneously stir ancient dreams; white cliffs, sunny uplands, a preference for make believe / the lights go down the conference is over / Lee stunned by the scheming orchestration watches everything immediately unravel / Contessa starts gibbering / her own posturing outta gas / she's finished / a vixen on heat no more ....

```
—Power for its own sake, she shrieks
—Agh, fuck it ... she kicks out at nothing ... falls on her
back ... arms and legs waving ... a dying cockroach
a loud bell rings ... someone drags her off stage .... throws
her in the trash ...
Outside the fireworks begin / Spidery pyrotechnics burst
against the sky as vacuous as the message / ordinary men and
women watch the display / elsewhere others look up wondering
if they'll be cluster-bombed / the bell rings again ...
```

The phone was answered in the rest room between the bedrooms. It was Dent. 'Hello Gibbie, how is Chinaman?'

'He's having a fitful sleep, very jumpy, unpredictable.'

'Anything unusual?'

'Not really, he's fearful, I'd say... not really compliant but at the same time doesn't want to be alone. He has no friends here, did you know that?'

'Yes, I spoke to Maclay, we're all he has. He's bound to be excitable.'

Gibbie laughed. 'He's certainly that.'

'Clinitest, blood pressure, breathing?'

'All normal.'

'Good. Could you tell him I'll be along later with Dr Maclay.'

'Yes, of course.'

'I think it important that he sees as many faces as possible. I do not want him to feel isolated.'

'Yes, I think that will help.'

'See you later.........'

* * *

At 6 p.m. Dent waited for Walter Maclay in La Dolce Vita, a small Italian restaurant on Cromwell Road. Guido, the proprietor, poured Dent his usual glass of Nebbiolo. 'Try some slices of vitello tonnato,' he offered. 'On the house,' he smiled. Guido had known Dent for years and one night divulged that he was homesick. Dent thought about it and asked him what his home was like. After one or two more animated 'chats' he suggested Guido should put up some pictures of the Langhe, Piedmont where he was born and raised. Guido warmed to the idea and threw out the Italian clichés: the Leaning Tower of Pisa, the gondolas of Venezia, the ruins of Roma, and replaced them with views of the Langhe: steep vineyards plunging under eiderdowns of fog that stretched to jagged snow-capped peaks fifty miles away. To the casual bystander it might have appeared odd that returning Guido to a familiar conversational environment could lift his mood. But the returning bounce in his step was noticed by all and hurt neither him nor his business. Those closest to Guido also saw that he became less reliant on caffè coretto to kick start his day though this was never mentioned.

Upon his arrival Maclay accepted Guido's offer of wine. He nodded towards a hilltop village surrounded by neat lines of viniculture lit by a setting sun. 'I'd like to go to Italy.'

'Me too,' responded Dent. 'Rhoda wants to do the classic tour: Siena, Florence and so on, but I'd prefer Guido's backyard. It looks far more intriguing, though he says it's quite poor.'

'Where is it?' asked Maclay, as Guido brought some more boccancini.

'Piedmont, an area around Turin.' said Dent.

'Probably wouldn't be very restful.'

'Well, I've already been to Venice and it was crowded and boring; every scene a Canaletto. A trip to Guido's hills and villages would be far more intriguing… full of rustic flavours just like his grandmother's recipes.' Dent slid the plate towards Maclay.

'You're too cavalier, what happens if you can't find a hotel?'

'Oh Mackers! I don't travel to read the *Daily Telegraph*.'

Maclay laughed; he was a pillar of the psychiatric profession. His organisational flair and reputation meant that he had been charged with managing mental health care policy under the spreading umbrella of the National Health Service. Part of this responsibility would

99 CROMWELL ROAD

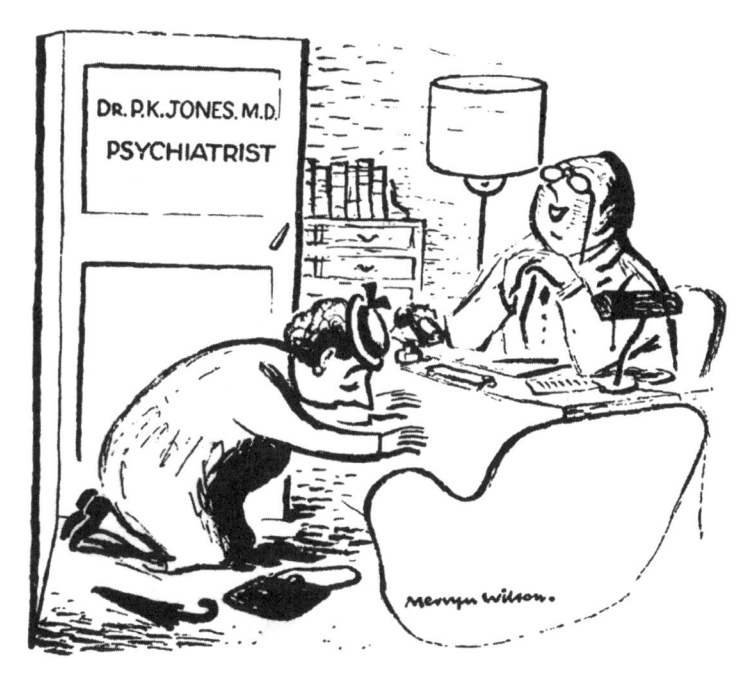

"*Good morning, Mrs. Todhunter. How's the inferiority complex?*"

Mervyn Wilson, 1944.
Taken from A Century of Punch published 1956 by W. Heinemann Ltd.

involve the adoption of clear diagnostic guidelines. Certainly professionalism and regulatory streamlining were required but Maclay didn't entirely trust the direction of travel. It was only his forays with characters like Dent that rekindled his age-old interest in novel approaches... approaches that still celebrated the sheer complexity and variety of human character.

'That's why you treat drunks, isn't it?' Maclay asked, helping himself to one of Guido's treats. 'An area of medicine that's impossible to predict.'

Dent was quiet for a moment as he tilted the wine in his glass and peered at it against the pristine white table cloth. The liquid appeared more maroon than red and had legs... proper legs. 'You may have a point,' he conceded. 'Take our American friend upstairs; we call him Chinaman by the way. If he was being treated by your mob at the Maudsley what chance would he have? My approach may include reading recognisable features like those around Guido's home: the hills, mountains and so on.' Dent gestured at one of the landscape photographs. 'But look into those valleys... shrouded in mist... how can we know what goes on down there? There are no maps... this is off-piste... psychiatry hasn't a clue. All it does is sedate and benumb; burying the patient's personality under layer upon layer of comatose inducing fogs—'

Maclay interrupted, '—and that's why you use apomorphine?'

'Of course. Apomorphine is quite unlike those other drugs, the ones increasingly being used to pet our brains and then find we cannot leave off the petting. Apo' stimulates the medulla... the research from Burden proves it. Five years ago we were told that depressants were indispensable to our medical practice. Now most of them have been withdrawn because of the number of people they've damaged to say nothing of those they've killed. And now I'm suddenly supposed to believe that the new generation of tranquillisers flooding the market are *highly* selective and safe. It is absurd, Mackers, absurd. A better way would be to supplement what we've lost and then see where we are. That's what apomorphine does... it reignites the patient's memory and motivations. The current strategy of searching for the perfect front-brain sedative is like the search for the perpetual motion machine: impossible. Our brains are far too individually complex and extraordinary to be ruined in this way.'

'But people want cures, John, something that works just like that.' Maclay snapped his fingers.

'Agh! They're gulled by each claim as preposterous as the last. You know it better than I. This brand of psychiatry reminds me of a bull in a china shop trying to glue a Ming vase with sledgehammers. With each spurious diagnosis and unnecessary intervention we end up further from the ideal of abstinence. If this continues the concept of a naturally functioning organism will be discounted altogether. We'll be so conditioned to interfere we'll end up believing that prescription is the new normal. And then what? You'll have a health industry not a service. It'll be entirely dependent on keeping patients ill. There'll be queues outside surgeries and hospitals that nobody will be able to cope with. So what then, eh?'

Maclay spluttered into his wine. Dent was a breath of fresh air. He secretly envied his autonomous brand of doctoring...a maverick, shoved to the margins as much by a benign curiosity as by a refusal to be penned in. A few psychiatrists believed that Dent and his ilk were the last of their kind, the final barrier to the medical efficiencies that the new ways demanded...but Maclay could see both sides...He thought of the mother he had heard of last week at St Thomas' who'd knocked her son out with a sleeping draught. Trouble was he didn't wake up.

'Have you thought of getting a partner?' asked Maclay.

'Don't you start,' said Dent.

'If you had one you could spend more time getting lost in the back of beyond,' he pointed towards a snowy panorama of serried hills. 'With Guido,' he grinned.

'Oh dear,' Dent mumbled.

'Well, isn't it true?'

'I do all right. I'm going to Sutherland with my daughter and grand-children for three weeks in July. Italy? Maybe later, in autumn, when it's cooler.'

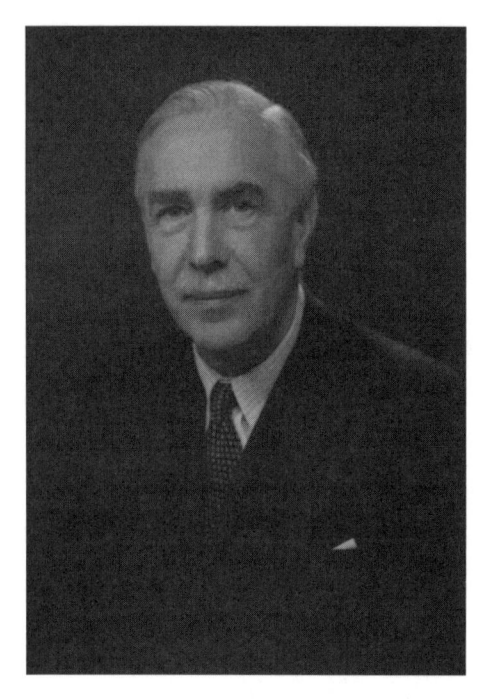

Psychiatrist, Walter Symington Maclay (1901–1964) worked tirelessly in both clinical and administrative capacities for the advancement of mental health understanding. In 1943, in conjunction with American Psychiatric Association, Maclay conducted a successful tour of the States and Canada showing the British propaganda film *Neuro Psychiatry* in which he also appears. Late in his life Maclay acquainted himself with the anthropomorphic and psychedelic cat drawings of Louis Wain, an appreciation shared by H. G. Wells. Dent, and eventually Burroughs, preferred feline purity. [©Museum of the Mind 2018]

'But who holds the fort when you're gone?'

'Look, you know full well this is not a career for anyone unless you run a pricey rest home in the Cotswolds, filling the anxious with barbiturates while emptying their bank accounts. Unless the state cottons on soon it'll be too late. My best hope is for less reliance not just on alcohol but drugs of every kind … and that includes pharmaceuticals. The whole concept of 'leaving well alone' is gradually disappearing from view. The depressed and anxious don't have structural defects. It is immoral to suggest they do. At the moment you could be forgiven for believing that some areas of science cherry-pick ideas that justify its interference. And the consequence of this is having to treat people for side effects which are worse than the original problem. It's madness.'

'Isn't this one of the things you emphasise at the Society?'

'Well, we try.'
'Are they listening?'
'Who, the health ministry?'
Maclay nodded.
'You must be joking.'
'That's where you should be directing your energies.'
'I don't disagree.'
'So,' repeated Maclay, 'get a partner. There are a few in the world of psychiatry, the synthesists, who agree with you.'
'No, I don't think I will.'
'Why ever not?'

Dent stood up. 'A good doctor must remain a practitioner. How else will he know he's doing well? But, you know, whenever I get asked that question, I think of my dad. He was a doctor with a small family practice. He said: "*don't think when you're qualified that I'll recommend you to my patients or let you become a partner.*" He knew I'd end up learning more by being self-reliant... and evolving. But I also suspect that he actually coveted his cases because he treated everyone differently. If we're honest aren't all doctors the same? I know I am. Do you really think I'd give up our friend upstairs to someone else? Every time I learn something new.... And on top of that how could I advise a young doctor to penetrate Chinaman's fog?' Dent jabbed a finger at a slender castello peeking through silvery layers of mist. 'Tell a novice doctor what he'll confront down there in the brain's wilderness and how to react when he does?' He downed his glass, barely interrupting his growl. 'For pity's sake Mackers, this isn't painting by numbers, or Venice on a sunny day. No, our man upstairs could be Transylvania in winter for all I know, or the dark side of the moon. More Hieronymus Bosch than Canabloodyletto.'

Maclay laughed as he followed Dent out of the restaurant. Two minutes later they strode into Chinaman's room.

'Hello Chinaman.' announced Dent, brusquely. 'I have great pleasure in introducing Walter Maclay, the real Maclay, the doctor who indirectly referred you to me.'

Burroughs eyed a tallish, silver haired gentleman. As he approached the bed Dent continued the introduction. 'One of the few, the *very* few,' he emphasised, 'prepared to run the rule over my improper tendencies.'

The Chinaman ignored the amusement shared by the doctors.

'Good evening, er, Chinaman,' said Maclay in a debonair, slightly stilted manner. 'And how are you being looked after? Satisfactorily, I trust?'

The patient lay huddled in bed wearing a dressing gown, his arms wrapped around his shivering shoulders. He squinted at Maclay over his long nose feeling like a gibbon in a zoo; cornered. He was ill for Chrissakes and this snooty bastard wants a kick back. He chose to ignore the question. 'How d' y' all suffer London…' his voice scraped, '…it's an icebox.'

Dent placed a chair by the bed so Maclay could sit down. Kate left the Day Notes open on the table and stood back. Dent glanced at the charts and then the exercise book. 'Good, Chinaman, no morphine since midday, over six hours… well done!' Dent moved closer to his patient. 'Any marked discomfort?'

'Slow burn, an ache all over, and no energy, that's the worst. I'm exhausted.'

'Have you eaten anything?'

'No.'

'And tired… unable to sleep?'

'Yeah, wiped out…'

'That must be difficult. Do you think some more morphine at this time would help?'

'Yeah.'

'I think it would, too. Your charts are good… but you're refusing the whisky?'

'Yeah.'

'Any reason…?'

'You're treating me like a drunk.'

'We use the alcohol to adjust and accelerate the change in your metabolism.'

'Look! You don't get it...the suffering, it's endless. I've been here before. I know what's coming.'

'You can tell us,' Dr Maclay chimed, 'I'm happy to listen.'

Chinaman covered his face with his hands. This limey bastard reminded him of the other Maclay and his odious secretary. He recalled how they'd made him feel: cold, angry and rejected. If this shrink was from the same frigid medical academy he had another thought coming. Chinaman pulled his fingers down his cheeks...and fixed Maclay's complacent face with the craziest, cold-eyed stare he could manage.

'You wanna know how I'm feeling?' Chinaman leant forward.

'Yes,' said Maclay brightly. 'I've always advocated a listening approach.'

'Then getta hold of this.' Chinaman took in a deep breath and screamed until the room shook.

A bewildered Maclay sat motionless as the Chinaman leant further forward, gripping the sides of his face and emptying the second barrel into the dumb schmuck's face.... He gave it all he had: 'AAAAAAAA-AAARRRGH!'

Maclay recoiled.

'Got it?' shouted Chinaman, collapsing back into his pillows.

The performance was more Munch than Bosch but Dent got the message. He wanted to cheer 'Bravo' but thought better of it. He knew that the human mind reveals itself through behaviour. This was the opening in the fog through which you glimpse the terrain underneath. He interpreted it as pure hurt, a desperate plea for understanding from a lonely and confused man washed up in the stifling atmosphere of a moribund society. But Dent saw too that Chinaman knew enough about how to be effective. Maclay was stunned, speechless. Dent approached the bed slowly and rested his hand on his patient's shoulder. Their eyes met, briefly.

'It's not working, is it?' sobbed Chinaman. 'I'm doomed.'

'We *are* trying our best to understand,' Dent said with conviction. He paused before squeezing the bony shoulder firmly, underscoring his sincerity. 'In your circumstances I firmly believe you *are* doing as well as any man could. I mean it, truly.'

Chinaman was reminded of the gesture. He had felt it before… in the old croaker's house. This was something he could relate to… reach out and complain to. 'But it's a failure. And this whisky.'

'You don't like it?'

'I'm not a drunk, but you're making me sicker with your APO-MOR-PHEEEN.' The Chinaman emphasised the syllables with theatrical gestures of contempt and disgust.

'Well,' said Dent, 'would it help if you took the alcohol *before* the injection? This is not an aversion treatment; nevertheless the alcohol accelerates the reaction I want to see.'

'What's that?'

'The sugar that shows in your clinitest, in your urine.'

'And what does that prove?'

'In all honesty Chinaman, I am not certain. But I take it as a bio-marker that tells me that your body has reacted …… that a metabolic change has taken place. At that point we change the whisky to just water, as much as you want.'

Dent went out and came back with the whisky tumbler. 'From now on you may have two parts water. Please.' Dent passed it to Chinaman. 'I will go and prepare the next injections. While I am gone you can have a few private words with Dr Maclay?'

'I'd prefer to be alone.'

'I do understand but if you wouldn't mind I would like it if Dr Maclay had the opportunity to get to know you. He is interested in our work here and his expertise may help us all. Would that be alright, I'd be most grateful?'

Chinaman bowed his head and muttered something into his clasped hands.

Dent took this as consent and smiled encouragingly at Maclay. He and Kate left closing the door quietly.

Maclay adjusted his jacket and bow-tie and stood up …… He would ignore what had happened and return to his sunny side, to what he believed to be his naturally positive disposition.

'I am genuinely sorry, Chinaman, about the mix up over the

referrals.' he smiled. 'I don't know why you were given the wrong address. Still, I couldn't have seen you anyway. It was my last chance to do a spot of chalk stream fishing, you see... lovely pastime. Have you ever done it... er, fly fishing?' Maclay checked himself feeling more than a little rusty with his bedside patter. He thought he better explain. 'You see, I am no longer in clinical practice anyway. I couldn't treat you... er... like this.' Maclay stalled. Chinaman's lack of engagement and wretched appearance discouraged him. Suddenly he thought of a way in.

'I am sure your family will be pleased that you are here... in safe hands,' Maclay smiled again. 'Would you like me to contact them, on your behalf, to let them know?'

Chinaman hadn't expected the question. He thought about it before answering. 'Could you?' He knocked back the whisky and water.

'Yes, certainly. I'd be more than happy to do so. They would be reassured, I'm sure.'

'But it's no use,' Chinaman moaned.

'Oh? And why would that be?'

'I don't wanna get their hopes up. This apomorphine is a waste of time... worthless.'

Maclay went to the end of the bed and picked up the day and night notes. He looked at the carefully timed entries and comments before closing the cover and waving the booklet in the air. 'These notes, Chinaman, will tell a story of gradual improvement. You're not the first person in that bed who feels like you do now. Like Dr Dent I am not sure how the change happens, but it does. I've seen it for myself... time and time again. This is why I indicated you should come here. I did so with complete confidence. Many do not get this far, their nerve fails them... but yours hasn't. So, you *are* doing well. Just persevere as best you can.'

The patient heard the words, stupid incomprehensible bullshit. How does he know? He's only here outta guilt anyhow. Two-bit limey, couldn't stick a Band-Aid.

Chinaman's head sagged. 'Don't contact my family,' he mumbled. 'Let's leave it a few days.'

'Not even to tell them that you've arrived?'

'I've already done that.'

'Oh, I see. Good.'

'I'll write.'

'Yes, well you know best. By the way, another doctor, a young Dr Bishop interested in Dr Dent's methods would like to visit. Would you have any objection?'

'Yeah, sure, go ahead…. I'm open all hours. I'll vomit in his lap if you like. Got anyone else? Any other disciple of the gag after lunch industry? My after dinner puking is a top seller. I'll even puke doing handstands. Reach my nurse, happy to fit anyone in: doctors, shrinks, vets… even fishermen…'

Dent and Kate returned with a surgical tray with two hypodermics and placed it on the bed. Chinaman sat up straight and opened his pyjama top. 'Here we go,' he sighed. 'How about my left side thissa time… closer to what's left of my heart.'

Ten minutes later Dent and Maclay emerged on Cromwell Road and prepared to go their separate ways.

'I've left you a real handful this time, John.'

'Don't worry, Mackers… really. I'm grateful you came in. He needs as much support as possible.'

'But so dramatic.'

'That's his strength.'

'Do you really think so?'

'He's suspicious and lonely and we're not exactly his cup of tea. Once he settles down we can turn that energy, the source of his outbursts, towards his wellbeing. Weren't you struck by the strength of his feeling? I was. That frustration won't be his undoing but his salvation… in the meantime we soak it up, be his punch bag… it'll help him through the next few days.'

'You make it sound so simple.'

'Well there's no point in complicating it.' Dent smiled.

'Agh, yes, I suppose you're right. And you're convinced he wants to be better?'

'Certain of it. You can tell a bluffer within five minutes. Crucially he has a clear idea of what he wants when sober.'
'What's that?'
'He's a writer.'
'Another one?'
'Nothing wrong with that. You said yourself, "How do we get our message across?" This may be the best way; how do I know?'
'Scepticism moves more mountains than certainty.'
'Exactly. Look, it would certainly help if he feels supported. Would you mind dropping by again … soak up a few more punches?'
'Aha! No, I'll come by when I'm free … and Bishop says he'll ring.'
'Good. You don't have to tell me, just let Gibbie know.'
'I will.'
'Do you want a lift home?'
'No thanks. I've heard about your driving.' Laughing, the two doctors shook hands and parted.

That evening the west wind was warmer. It surged over road and roof reminding London with its musical whisperings of a time when the land was forest, when free of trespass Nature dispensed its wisdom. Back at home with his cat the doctor listened to the wind's melody. It brought into his mind a picture of the old world, an era when arboreal splendour predated the Gothic arch, when latticed leaves had yet to inspire the prescribed fretting of stained glass …… He looked inside. The pews swelled with miserable sinners, their heads bowed. Butchers, bakers, candlestick makers, ordinary men and women wilting under the heat of churchy dogma. He turned away. He wouldn't enter but stay with the trees as antinomian as he. Immune to the moralising they stretch towards what's good, to where the breath of the night's wind is fresher … cleaner … brighter. Simple really.

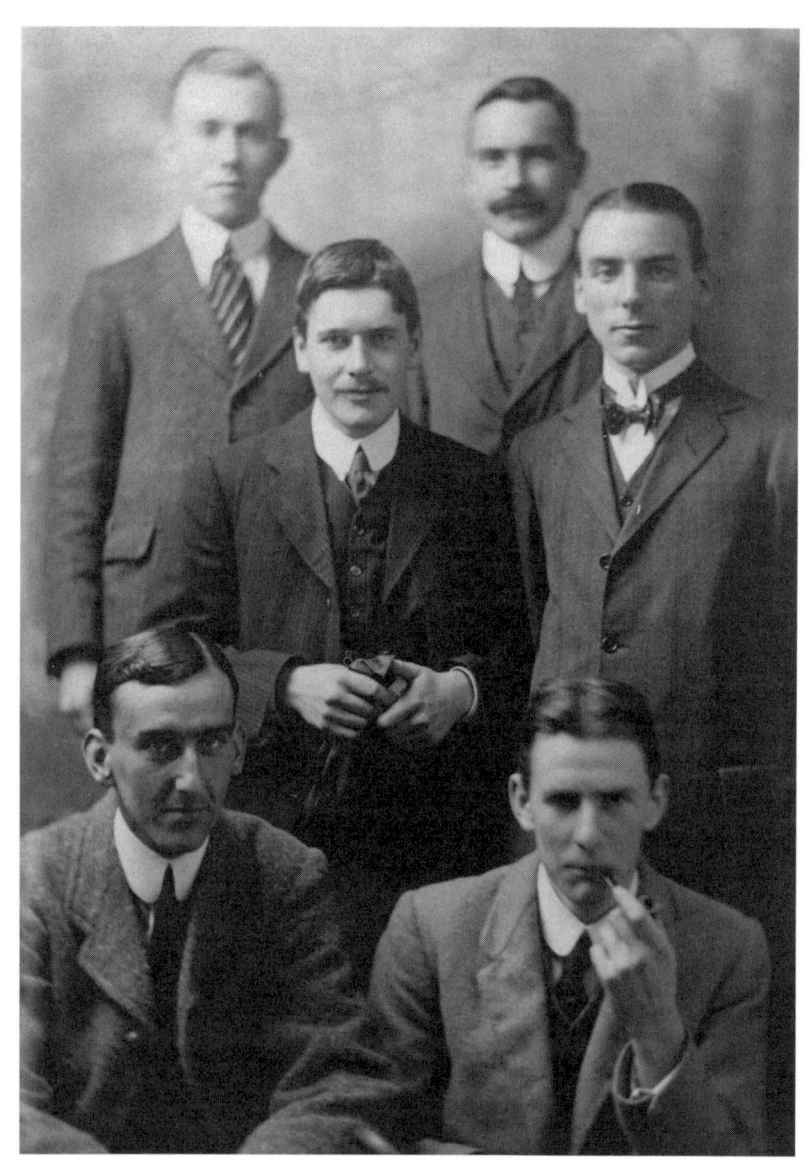

Dent center with fellow medical students, circa 1912.
[photographer unknown]

7

TB

> If every man would mend a man
> Then all mankind were mended.
> – Scottish proverb

It was a cold morning, barely 8 a.m. Thin trails of soot from a million London chimneys had begun to turn the china blue sky mustard brown. Dent got up, pulled back thin curtains and gazed across the rooftops. He could imagine the monstrous carcinogens stretching into every neighbourhood, hear their tentacles slithering over rooftops, under doors and down throats. He'd been woken by a coughing fit and choked again as he dressed. He should've stayed in bed but the obligation of a 9 a.m. private appointment with the esteemed Professor Halliburton must never be declined.

On the dot of nine o'clock Dent puffed his way to the second floor above the common room. He knocked on a heavy oak door and waited. There was a long pause. Eventually, a terse command from within bade him enter. Halliburton sat behind a huge desk surrounded by untidy shelves and cabinets. His face appeared redder and his body rounder as if the pressure of sitting down had further inflated his ballooning form. He was composing some correspondence. With a flick of his wrist he indicated that Dent should sit down while he resumed his concentration. He read through the letter to himself in a series of abbreviated grunts and murmurs. His facial expressions responded to the tenor of the content. At first his manner was ponderous; clearly he was dealing with a matter of consequence. This gave way to a rapid series of murmurs as his eyes raced over the perfunctory passages. He paused, stroked his chin before adding something with his black and gold fountain pen. He then read through the whole thing before adding his signature with a flourish. 'There,' he said, putting his pen away, 'perfect!'

He blotted the sheet of paper with a series of firm strokes, folded it, and pushed it to one side. He took off his glasses and leant back. His chair complained.

'Sorry, Dent, to get you out of bed. I'll cut to the chase. I have to talk to you about your friend, Barnes, to see if you can help.'

'Oh!?'

'Yes,' continued Halliburton, 'for some weeks we have wanted to interview him but without success. When did you last see him?'

'A week ago, sir.'

'Is that normal? You were hardly out of each other's sight.'

Dent looked at the floor.

'You see, I believe you have his best interests at heart. Is that *still* the case...?'

'Yes, of course.'

'So what do you know?'

'Well, sir, Barnes has changed, er... since his accident.'

'In what way?'

'He's become very reclusive of late. His attendance is down...'

'Well, I know that. He hasn't attended a single lecture since last term, not one.'

Dent met Halliburton's grey-green eyes; the redder his face became the colder his stare.

'You see I am concerned that Barnes has a problem... and I am no longer talking about his leg.'

'No, sir.'

'Well?'

'Well what, sir?'

'Well, what do you think is the matter? How did he appear when you last saw him?'

'Not his usual self, sir. He's lost his vitality.'

'Is he pale?'

'Yes.'

'Would you say he's lethargic, gaunt?'

'Yes, I would.'

'Anything else?'

'Well, he's been avoiding us, Dalton and I, for weeks, months. At first we didn't think much of it; that it was due to the accident ... but he no longer comes to our flat ... even when invited.'

'Go on ...'

'Well, we felt he was frustrated about something. He'd lost all traces of his humour. We tried to talk to him but without luck. Last week we went round and he told us to leave. He was evidently distressed.'

Halliburton's face twitched. 'You and Dalton went to his lodgings?'

'Yes.'

'Did he let you into his room?'

'No, he hobbled out on his sticks and closed the door. He was agitated, sweating. You could see he wasn't right, suffering, but he didn't want us there, either, we just knew.'

Halliburton got up, went to a cabinet and put a small clear glass bottle on the middle of the desk.

'Have you seen bottles like this before?'

Dent looked at it. It had a cork stopper. His father's bottles were dark green and hexagonal; this was round.

'No, sir.'

'It is opium, Dent. I have reason to believe that our friend Barnes is under its thrall. He's addicted to the stuff.'

'Oh! I see ...' Dent looked at the bottle, transfixed.

Halliburton squashed himself back into his chair. He exhaled, a sad sound, like the gasp from a punctured football. 'We knew that the first operation to fix his thigh wasn't a success.... He'd have to be operated on a second time ... He was probably given too much morphia and for too long. This is the only drug that takes away that pain. Regretably, the dispensary has reported some has gone missing.... We've made investigations and discovered it finds its way to Barnes....

Everything you have said tallies with what we already know...'
Halliburton's sentences had grown limp tails as they sank from his mouth. He sounded uncharacteristically depressed.

Dent pulled a handkerchief from the side pocket of his jacket and coughed as Halliburton returned the bottle to the cabinet. 'The question is,' Halliburton said in a faraway voice, 'what's to be done.'

'Are you in touch with his family?' asked Dent, stowing his handkerchief.

'His parents are in India; army posting. They might be here for Christmas...two months away.'

'Well, could he be treated?'

Halliburton's form mysteriously re-inflated itself. He threw back his head and guffawed. 'Oh Dent! How ridiculous. Don't even think about it.'

Dent struggled to reply. 'There must be something...surely?'

'Oh such innocence! Listen to me, when you've come across a few cases, real cases, you'll realise what I am about to say is true. For diabetes, dementia praecox, insanity or other maladies of the brain – and that includes addiction to opiates or alcohol, medicine has absolutely nothing to offer. Nothing.'

Dent felt disconnected from the irredeemable bleakness of Halliburton's words. Taken aback by their hopelessness he was unable to find his own.

'Dent? Are you listening to me? Nothing!'

'I think, sir, if you d-don't mind my saying, I find this difficult to accept.'

Halliburton hooted. 'It's immaterial what *you* accept. *This* is how it is.'

'But why, sir?' insisted Dent, causing Halliburton's bushy eyebrows to jump. 'Barnes is young, once his leg has properly mended he—'

'Oh dear!' Halliburton clasped his cheeks with his palms and looked to the heavens. 'This has nothing anymore to do with his leg; that ship has sailed. Next you'll be asking me to revive the dead.'

'But isn't it the case, sir, that people can alter their expectations—'

'What are you jabbering about?'

Dent took a deep breath and thought about the 'miracles' of spiritualism. 'If people can be made to believe in the impossible sir, why shouldn't the ill be made to feel better without medicine?'

'Oh my giddy God! Barnes isn't just ill, he's insane, mad. You said so yourself. He's impossible to talk to. He's possessed... unreachable. Look Dent, you're upset. You'd do well to forget about Barnes, sad as it may be.' Halliburton paused. 'You must face facts. The irrefutable experience of every physician who has ever lived amounts to an unpalatable truth. You cannot rewind morphinism. Syphilitics get it, those with dental pain, cancer and so on, tormented by it until the very end.'

'So why am I here? You asked me if I'd like to help Barnes without believing he can be. I feel tricked.'

Halliburton's emotional barometer swung wildly; calm to stormy.

'The Lord preserve me, to help US! The college has a problem to deal with. Now, if you wouldn't mind.'

Halliburton looked at his watch; it was the sign.

'If he recovered on his own, could he return next year?'

'Oh please! You're wasting my precious time. Now run along.'

Closing Halliburton's door Dent carried his indignities all the way back to his flat. Combined with his cough and miserable weather he now had to confront the emptiness at the heart of his chosen profession. His medical training would consist of medicine and surgery only. Anything to do with psychology was strictly off limits. It was like a forbidden land; every doctor knew of its existence but none wanted to go there. He sat in the kitchen and watched the short day sink into the onset of winter. He didn't hear Dalton's return.

'Sitting on your own in the dark, what's up?'

'Oh lots...' Dent dragged himself to his feet and offered to make the tea while Dalton took off his coat.

'You sound as though you could do with one too,' said Dalton.

Dent went into the small kitchen off the living room and placed a filled kettle on the hob. 'You may as well hear from me as you'll know soon enough. Barnes is stuck on morphine. Halliburton is certain and has more or less admitted that he'll be kicked out. There appears to be no alternative.'

'Oh no!' Dalton thought for a moment. 'Well, it all adds up, we can't be surprised.'

Dent coughed heavily as he returned to the living area. This turned into a hacking fit which persisted for several seconds. He sat down, breathing heavily.

Dalton looked up, 'That cough doesn't sound good either.'

'Just a bad chest, not sleeping well.'

'Is that all?'

Dent listened for the heat in the kettle. 'No,' he said eventually, 'I had some sputum sent over to the path lab yesterday, just to be on the safe side.'

'Good. Very sensible, you just don't know what you might have picked up.'

'Probably bronchitis.'

'Yes, a lot of it about.'

Dent got up and pre-heated a large earthenware teapot before adding the tea. He then poured in the remaining boiling water and brought in the steaming pot with two mugs, a jug of milk and teaspoons.

'A fine teapot,' said Dalton.

'Aye,' agreed Dent. 'A present from one of my aunts. "It'd 'allus serve, az gud for two az six", she'd say.'

'She was right.' Dalton's remark floated emptily over the drawing brew.

Without warning Dent slapped the table with his palms. The utensils hopped and clattered. 'Damn it all, Dalton, we're supposed to be bloody doctors. If we cannot help our friends who can we help?'

Dalton rearranged the teaspoons. 'Halliburton must know.'

'Oh yes!' said Dent, aping a subservient tone. 'And while we're grovelling at the master's feet let us not forget Medicine, the great, immutable science of Med-i-cine.' Dent drew out the word as long as he could. 'I tell you what, Dalton, this line: "there's nothing to be done", it's bloody blasphemy – heresy. I won't accept it.'

'What can we do, we're not even qualified.'

'We could stop sounding defeated before we start.'

'I'm just being practical. What would you suggest?'

'That's it.' Dent clapped his hands. 'Suggestion! I have seen how you can suggest anything – even to the most sceptical. And what is medicine, anyway, if it isn't the suggestion of health over the fear of disease?'

'But cholera can't be cured with suggestion.'

'I'm not talking about bacteriological disease but psychological disease. If this is a disease of the mind then we should do more than just fill the sufferer's head with tales of hopelessness. Poor Barnes is persecuted by everyone who reiterates Halliburton's gloomy prognosis. And now his fear has become his speciality. He believes in it as much as the idiots that suggest it. Bloody doctors, no better than witches wailing at the moon for causing whatever it is they don't understand. They simply don't help; in fact they make things worse.'

Dalton smiled at the familiar polemical tone of his friend. He poured steaming tea into the mugs and helped himself and Dent to sugar. 'Here,' he said, pushing the mug across the table. 'At least your aunt knew *this* wouldn't hurt.'

* * *

Two days later Dent was told to see the professor in pathology about his sputum. He was one of the great men of the medical establishment and never seen in anything other than a long white coat and a face to match. He knew everything there was to know about contagion; his knowledge appeared to have stained him from within. 'You must prepare yourself, Dent.'

'Oh,' said Dent.

'Yes. Mycobacterium tuberculosis takes few prisoners.'

'Oh.'

'This Christmas, likely to be your last.'

'Oh?'

'In any case your studies are over.'

'Over?'

'You're infectious Dent. You catch this bacteria off breath. That's how you picked it up. Have you been working in the slums?'

'Yes.'
'You're not the first... and won't be the last.'
'I have to leave King's?'
'That's what I meant.'
'Now?'
'Of course. No goodbyes. Your things will be sent on. Clear?'
'Yes.'
'My advice is for you to go away. A pig farm in Canada would be ideal.'
'What!?'
The specialist's arctic tone was as chilling as his prophecy. 'Once you're out of the way it'll be easier to discount all of this.'
'Canada?!'
'Yes, further away the better. Forget about us and then it'll be easier for us to forget about you. Always better in the long run.'
'B-but,... a pig farm? Why a pig farm?'
The specialist ignored the question. 'Your father is a doctor, trained here?'
'Yes.'
'Well, I understand word has already been sent on. He may know somewhere. Now, don't delay. Go straight home, that's an order. The porter will call a cab; this is a back-up note for your father. Good day.'
The specialist returned to his germ kingdom, to the sulphurous fumes that cling to your clothes for weeks and your memory forever. Dent was unable to move. He held the envelope in his hand and blankly watched as the world slowly detached itself from his hopes and dreams. A doctor swinging a stethoscope rushed past two nurses with a patient on crutches. Down the corridor a trolley banged against a pair of swing doors. It'd be the same tomorrow, with or without him.

His father greeted him at home, No. 29, St Mary Abbot's Terrace, w.8.
  'Go straight to bed Jack. Leave the windows open, wide open. Better get used to sanatorium life.'

'Where will I go?'

'There's a purpose-built one at Mundesley near Cromer. Uncle Herbert says it's run by a go-ahead team and highly regarded. He assures me they get the best results. I have asked around and it seems he's right. They boast that the air is dry, the driest in the country. Ideal for you… and, er… a lovely spot, plenty of local interest.'

'Will you come up?'

'Visiting isn't encouraged for obvious reasons. Nor, I'm afraid, is letter writing. If there's something urgent, of course we'll write, but you're going to have to be enormously self-reliant. 'Young H' says the grounds are extensive, just a short walk to the sea. It's a tiny village, with its own church and golf course, but not much else. The countryside you'll enjoy and, of course, the coastal location.'

His mother kept out of the way. Two days later she said goodbye without kissing him, but his father agreed to accompany him as far as Liverpool Street Station. Once John boarded the train Old H nodded towards the platoons of Norfolk and Suffolk yeomanry crowding the platform. 'Looks like war is inevitable.'

John, glad of the opportunity to reflect on something other than himself, agreed. 'I'm already resigned to it. But do they realise that this nationalism has been stirred by lies?'

'No, not yet. The pity of it is that the cheerleaders for this and other rotten shows are never the sort to stand in the way of bullets. None of them will suffer like these poor fellows.'

The young Dent looked away from his father. He hoped that his emotion wouldn't betray him at the last but his eyes, brimful with sorrow told their own story. As the train pulled out each man was hidden from the other in a cloud of steam, their feeble farewells engulfed by the train shed tumult of cries and whistles.

Out of the station Dent took his seat beside a young woman. The carriage was soon thick with tobacco smoke, ribaldry and patriotic song. Musing over the seismic forces at play Dent forgot his predicament until his neighbour caught his eye. 'Why ain't you singing?' she asked, her thin lips curled cheekily under the brim of a wide felt hat. She leant forward. 'Are you shy?'

'No, I'm a spy,' whispered Dent, with an expressionless face. 'Sent by the Kaiser.'

'No you ain't,' she retorted in a conspiratorially low voice, 'I heard you talking to that old fella.'

'So?'

'I reckon you're a conscie?'

'What if I am?'

'Better a coward for five minutes than a dead'un all yer life, hey?' She winked.

'If you say so....' Out of nothing Dent saw himself on a military parade ground. Flags of the Empire fluttered against a blue sky. A moustachioed colonel lurched forward and pinned a ribboned medal over his diseased lung. A reward for killing those as innocent as himself. This could be a Faustian pact, he realised. An exchange for surviving tuberculosis if he'd commit himself to a military life. He also foresaw the likelihood: himself lying dead on a battlefield with his brains dribbling down his tunic. Should he explain this to his travelling companion? Expose her patriotism lit by nothing more than the populist bunk of 'God, King and Country'? He thought better of it. He wouldn't switch places with anyone... least of all a soldier.

'I think you'd look wonderful in a uniform,' she said as she got up to get off at her stop.

'Thank you for your thoughts,' he said, 'I'm truly grateful.'

* * *

Mundesley Sanatorium, or 'san' as the residents called it was dominated by an imposing, south-facing elevation. This sat under the lee of a sandy plateau and enjoyed a dry and sunny micro-climate. These factors combined with bracing sea air benefitted not only the tubercular invalid but also the stands of pine trees which hid the building and its outlying huts from the neighbouring golf course. The windows throughout were fixed open even in winter. Upon arrival Dent was told by Dr Burton-Fanning, the medical supervisor, to go straight to bed. His prognosis was as cheerless as the specialist's in London.

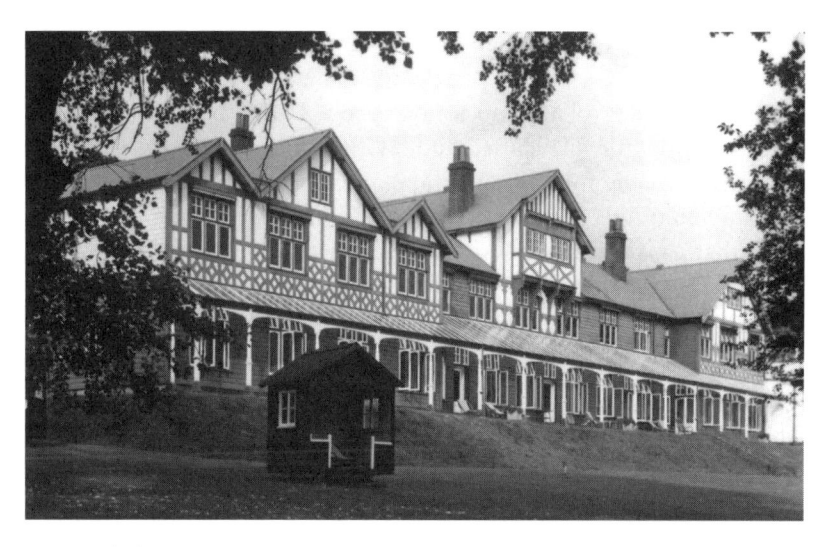

Mundesley TB Sanitarium with purpose-built verandah and hut, all part of the 'fresh air' approach first adopted in Europe. [Photographer unknown]

'Yes, there's no cure, no treatment other than rest and fresh air. There's no heating here so don't expect any; sleep outside if you can bear to. You must not work. Rest is mandatory. Sleep as much as you can and when you're awake, rest. No taxing thoughts, no worry. There is no other way to rebuild your immunity. Sleep, eat and rest. You must spend the first two weeks in bed, no exercise of any kind.'

Another doctor followed. He was also a patient, a thin man with hollow eyes. 'Death is more easily faced if you accept its inevitability,' he said in sepulchral tones while pressing his palms together; an obvious hint. Dent deduced that the poor man had probably got TB worse than he and was envious. Whenever he approached, Dent learned to be 'asleep' though he also developed the knack of simultaneously keeping an eye out for those who could lend him books.

It wasn't long before Burton-Fanning, tipped off by a nurse, was back with a retinue of fawning assistants.

'I hear you're reading!' he barked.

'Well yes, I enjoy it, it takes my mind off things and I feel better.'

'You're not better,' snapped Burton-Fanning.

'But I'm not worse.'

Burton-Fanning picked up a book from Dent's bedside table and glanced at the title. He sniffed audibly. 'Reading of this sort is forbidden. These are the rules. From whom are you getting these books?'

'I am not at liberty to say.'

'In that case from now on I will instruct the orderlies and nurses to confiscate anything other than the very lightest reading material.'

Since Dent had no intention of giving up his books he thought he'd try a different tack.

'How am I doing?'

'Well, you're the same.'

'So reading isn't doing me any harm?'

'That isn't the point.'

'Sorry? Are you saying that you are only interested in repeating the old ways?'

'It is what everyone does.'

'That's *my* point.'

'Look Dent, here at Mundesley we run a highly professional establishment and are justifiably proud of our methods. These have been adopted from the successful open-air treatments on the Continent. It should be self-evident why the most respected members of society end up here and not anywhere else.'

'But surely your results could be improved. After all, whether your establishment is frequented by Kings or paupers TB doesn't seem to know the difference, does it? Your survival figures are nothing to write home about. Why would any doctor boast about an approach that demonstrates such failure? Ever since I was diagnosed I have felt a leper and now I see you're too proud to invite change which may be remedial.'

'Stop this now, Dent. You're turning into a thoroughly disagreeable patient and I will not tolerate subversion. You may feel that you can ignore all advice but think of the problems you are causing with other patients who may see you getting away with it.'

'Getting away with not getting worse, you mean. Do you not think that there might be a relationship between feeling better and getting better?'

'Of course, there isn't. You're either ill or you're not. What you're describing is delusory. I have seen it many times. You'd do well to accept your circumstances and do as you're told. I shouldn't have to remind you we have nigh on two decades of experience…two!' Burton-Fanning stood back and crossed his arms.

'I fear, sir, we won't agree on this. Surely if I can imagine a future then that future is more easily realised.'

'And books, how are they likely to help?'

'Because there's nothing else. If I wallow in your fearful forecast with nothing to lift me then life will certainly not be worth living.'

Dent had started to sweat; Burton-Fanning saw it as the best way of winning the argument.

'Now look at you,' he said, shoving a thermometer into Dent's protesting mouth. 'You're getting emotional, flustered and wasting energy, energy that must be retained to build your strength. In future kindly observe the rules. You know what they are, I suppose?' Dent removed the thermometer to speak. Burton-Fanning shoved it back.

'Save your breath Dent and let me remind you. Sleep when you can and rest when you're awake. Eat everything put in front of you and reading from these sort of books,' he slapped his hand on Dent's stack of volumes, 'from any source and for any purpose, is absolutely forbidden. Forbidden! Is that clear? Now this conversation…' he pulled the thermometer from Dent's mouth, 'is over!' He stormed off followed by his trail of disciples and without, Dent noticed, recording his temperature.

Dent lay back and waited for his friend with whom he'd swapped Swift and Sterne for Conrad and Wells.

'We'd better be careful, the guvnor isn't happy about us sharing books,' Dent advised.

Dent's friend lowered his head. 'Right,' he whispered. 'But look, there's no need to worry. Sooner than you realise they'll allocate you one of those huts in the grounds.'

'One like yours?'

'Yes. Once outside you'll have lots of hiding places. Have a book on the go and if they confiscate it read something else until I find another copy.'

'Good idea, thank you. Do you mind if I call you the "Librarian"?'

'Not at all, I'd be honoured. And I'll call you the "Libertarian".'

Dent smiled; a kindred spirit. He felt a ripple of warmth wash through him. He was still fighting.

* * *

After a month, as the Librarian had anticipated, Dent was allocated a secluded hut that could be turned to face either the sun or away from the wind. It was thoroughly spartan, no glazing, just a low bench for a bed, with a thin horsehair mattress. It was enclosed by a hedge of broom and gorse stretching to a sandy bluff fringed with heather. He was now permitted to exercise by taking short walks to the main gates of the sanatorium. He scoffed at the challenge but was shocked to realise how difficult this simple exercise had become. He rested at the gate and summoned thoughts of a Canadian pig farm to spur him into making the return journey. He barely made it. The change in the regime of 'sleep-eat-rest' to 'sleep-eat-walk' was welcome but there were few highlights. The 'snap' of a rat in a baited trap sometimes awoke him. On other occasions the rats chewed the flannel lapels on his pyjamas and left muddy footprints on his face.

'It doesn't mention that in the promotional leaflets,' he told the Librarian at breakfast after another disturbed night.

'You're lucky; I share with badgers.'

Their conversation was broken by a commotion in the hall which spread to the refectory. A rotund, red-faced gentlemen burst in. 'Listen,' he roared, 'I've made a joke, a damn good joke! I've designed my crest in the traditional manner.' He bowed. 'Naturally,' he snorted, 'it will be, lords, ladies and gentlemen, a sputum flask couchant with, wait for it.' He made an expansive gesture. 'It'll be crossed thermometers rampant above my motto. Yes, *my* motto. I bet you cannot guess what it'll be, eh? It'll be *Dum Spiro Sputo*.' He guffawed despite everyone's barely tolerant smiles. 'Wait, wait!' he bellowed, 'I have a better idea, not *Dum Spiro Sputo* but *Dum Perspiro Sputo*.' He shook with a deafening peel of laughter until his face turned purple and a gush of blood burst from his nose and mouth. The nurses rushed in but were unable to get him to bed before he died.

Dr Burton-Fanning approached Dent's hut early one morning. 'A letter from London. From your colleague Dalton, I believe, forwarded by your father.' Dent took the letter and used it to conceal a battered copy of *Confessions of an English Opium Eater*, a parting gift from the Librarian who'd been discharged a week earlier.

'Thank you,' said Dent.

'How are your walks?' asked Burton-Fanning.

'Getting easier, thank you. I am able to make the sea cliffs. There's an Airedale terrier who has befriended me; he encourages me to stretch my legs.'

'That's good. It does seem you got here in the nick of time. You could still go under if the bacterium breaks out. If you continue as you are I might agree to let you go late summer.'

'Can I write to my parents and tell them?'

'Leave it for a few more weeks and we'll review then. Don't want to dash their hopes. Clear?'

With a stiff formality they shook hands and parted. Dent picked up Dalton's letter and shook it in the cold air as if he was emptying it of something. He hesitated and told himself to remember this moment. He sat down:

> Dear Dent,
> It pleases me greatly to hear that you are continuing to heal. I have kept in touch with your father and Halliburton

occasionally gives the odd bulletin. It seems that the worst is behind you and with warmer and hopefully drier weather to come it surely points to a complete recovery. Everyone here is cheered by your news and sends their best.

We need cheering. All the talk here is about the war, which many have a thirst for. It is as if half the country has taken leave of any sense left to it. Several senior doctors at King's have signed up and the hospital is stretched. What happens if any get killed? At least with damaged lungs you shall be spared this lunacy.

Fearfully I must report some sad and tragic news that will leave you deeply affected. Poor Barnes took his own life last week. His parents were unable to come home at Christmas but were due to arrive for Easter. We know that he was proud and failing medical school humiliated him but it seems that facing his parents as a morphine addict shamed him more – more than he could bear. He had moved out of his flat and gone into private lodgings in the East End, having sold what possessions he had. Begging and petty crime were all that was left to him. He'd fallen out with everyone and was in debt to many. I last saw him a few weeks after you left for Norfolk, nearly six months ago.

There can be no doubt that he meant it. He left a note and threw himself under a train. Halliburton told me all this in his study and then asked me if I was all right.
I think he feels in some way responsible, that he should have done more.

Do write if you're permitted. I will understand if you cannot.

I have a new girl, and have told her all about you. She says you sound a 'good egg', whatever that means.

  Yours affectionately,
  Dalton

Dent looked through bleary eyes over the furze tops and towards the sea. Some flecks of broom swayed golden against the blue. Everything was out of focus. The letter fell from his fingers and floated under the bench. He closed his eyes in an attempt to restore the memory of Barnes, the man from Liverpool, 'as smelly as Birmingham with sea breezes'. Flashes of him came and went; big soft hands rolling an egg, blond curls bouncing as he boxed or ran. But no whole face? Perhaps any completeness was corrupted by a frustration with himself. Was this a consequence of accepting Halliburton's advice to give up on his friend? He felt implicated. 'And if this is true, what now?' he asked himself, opening and rubbing his eyes. He'd still have to confront the realisation that being a doctor would be at the expense of those like Barnes because medical orthodoxy favours stigmatisation over treatment. And yet wasn't it true that some doctors rely on suggestion as much as surgery and medicine? Not Burton-Fanning, he was just a nuts and bolts man better suited to repairing lawnmowers. Maybe the best thing would be to give up any idea of being a doctor. What would be the point of joining such a cynically driven profession?

Some way off a dog barked, calling him. It was late afternoon, the tide would be out. Time to walk down to the beach below the Coronation Hall, gaze into rock pools and skim stones... another forbidden activity. But what the hell. The slow rhythmic swing of his arm to the timeless sea music helped settle the nerves. There were never enough flat stones but looking for them returned an inner sense of calm and acceptance. Nothing was perfect or could be. At that moment he foresaw himself on the empty beach with dusk spreading its cloak over the universe. He watched as he crested the cliff. With luck he might behold the nightjar, the crepuscular hawk of myth and legend, its strange, swooping flight. Even a glimpse of this fabulous bird could lift the spirit... spark the dullest memory. Perhaps this might conjure Barnes out of the sombre air... permit the crazy mad shine of him to burst one last time from the cloudening mind, rupture the darkling sky. Then he'll be free, free to fall forever... a fireball in the firmament.

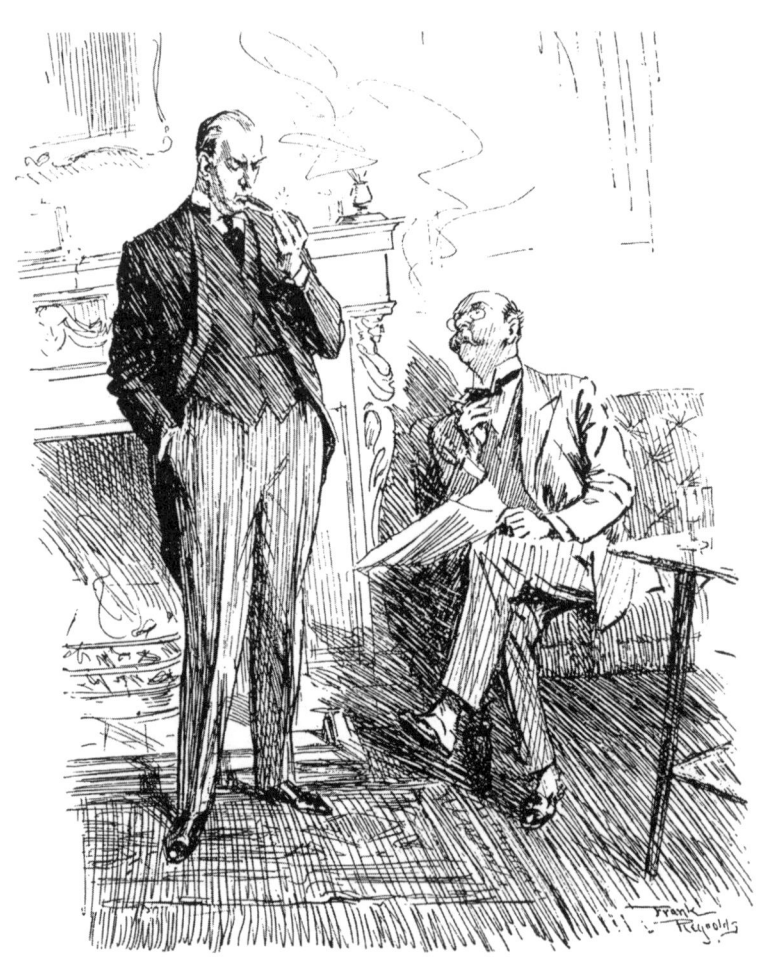

Doctor: "WHAT DID YOU OPERATE ON JONES FOR?"
Surgeon: "A HUNDRED POUNDS."
Doctor: "NO, I MEAN WHAT HAD HE GOT?"
Surgeon: "A HUNDRED POUNDS."

Frank Reynolds, 1925.
Taken from *A Century of Punch* published 1956 by W. Heinemann Ltd.

8

Dent Meets Benway

You need ONE twenty-three pill. (Just one.) Not a Drug but a Live American Remedy.㉓... — ...㉓THE BEST PILL IN THE WORLD FOR AN IRREGULAR LIVER.

I suppose it is some lingering traces of the Bladesover tradition to me that makes this combination of letters and pills seem so incongruous, just as I suppose it is a lingering trace of Plutarch and my ineradicable boyish imagination that at bottom our State should be wise, sane and dignified, that makes me think a country which leaves its medical and literary criticism, or indeed any such vitally important criticism, entirely to private enterprise and open to the advances of any purchaser must be in a frankly hopeless condition.
– H. G. Wells
Tono-Bungay

Back at 34 Dent and Ulysses curled up together in their favourite chair. Dent's mind, however, was far from still. His success at treating addiction meant only one thing: more patients. They came from every conceivable background, and their treatment required organising. To run his practice equitably he had to employ a Robin Hood policy: those who could afford it paid double and those that couldn't, nothing. It was sometimes chaotic... invariably complicated but with the help of a few dedicated supporters it usually worked.

He thought of the letter he'd received yesterday and had yet to answer:

HARDY TREE

TELEPHONE
ROD 6019.

SAINT GEMMA'S HOUSE
90 CAMBERWELL ROAD
LONDON S.E.5

Dear Doctor Dent,
    I want to write and tell you how wonderful it has been to have your kindness and great help always with these poor suffering souls.
    This treatment of apomorphine has cured a large number of very heavy drink takers. The last one, was a poor soul broken down on Mission Work abroad; and a man who had really given up all hope. This was only a few weeks ago, when I phoned you to ask if you would be so kind as to let us have more apomorphine. Now after taking large amounts this poor soul seems quite cured and fine.
    We have a large amount of people both men and women who really need this treatment and I wonder if there is a way we can get this treatment on the insurance scheme and if and how does one go about it please.
    Dear Doctor Dent, I am so deeply grateful to you for your very very generous help over all this long time, I do not want to be a continual trouble to you with all my requests but maybe you will understand how this can and will really help.
    Also may I have the names of your latest books and the old books also which I had, but gave away.
        Yours most gratefully
        Joan Cudder-Fletcher

Dent was getting more and more of these sorts of letters. His detractors had recently started to attribute the success of apomorphine to his 'charisma'. Of course, his understanding of the psycho-social

DENT MEETS BENWAY

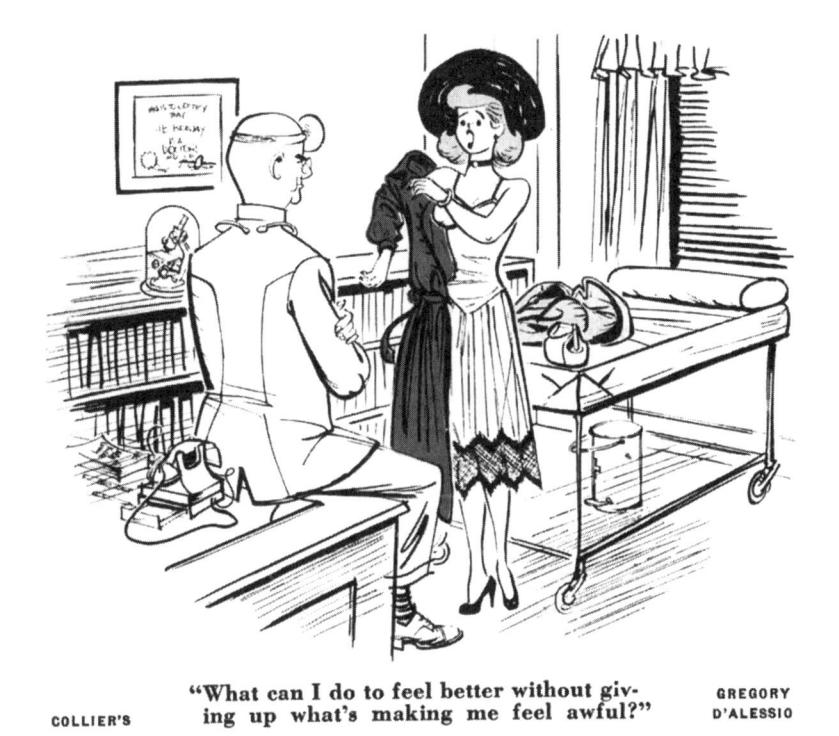

"What can I do to feel better without giving up what's making me feel awful?"

COLLIER'S
GREGORY D'ALESSIO

processes and talk therapy was not well-understood ... by some it was being wilfully ignored ... but attributing his success with apomorphine to 'charisma' alone was idiotic. How, he wondered, was he able to squeeze 'charisma' inside an envelope? He laughed to himself at the absurdity of life ... how doctors were readily prepared to discount his and others' observations by clinging to hearsay laced with prejudice ... or was it envy? It was certainly a debasement of the culture of science. It is true that years ago he used to deliver his apomorphine pills in person but this was now impossible; postage was the only way. As Rhoda, Maclay and several friends kept saying, he could do with a partner but doctors were not interested in treating addiction unless they could make a living out of it and apomorphine, being a quick solution, did not offer the opportunity for protracted treatments in expensive nursing homes. In any case, beyond the avaricious medical fraternity, society by and large still held the view that all addicts had to do was exercise 'free will', say 'no' to drink, and the problem would vanish. Even some doctors parroted this view, usually those who referred their 'drunks' to the police. Dent had done his best to chip away at this nonsense, but a hidebound attitude still prevailed; upheld, he noticed, by politicians who realised that pandering to a punitive sensibility was a vote winner in the shires. His priority, therefore, was stewardship of an emerging discipline. This would, by necessity, involve better science, research and communication. The international membership of the Society for the Study of Addiction (SSA), which Dent helped run, had recently risen alongside a broad understanding that criminalisation only made matters worse. Unfortunately, this encouraging sign was offset by directives from the World Health Organisation outlining its intention to politicise addiction by recommending more international controls, stiffer penalties and mandatory prison terms. This was regressive and a smokescreen for justifying military presence in countries that produced narcotics. And now, on top of all this, he was still being told by the American Medical Association that apomorphine was 'dangerous, addictive and hallucinogenic'. Dent wondered how he should respond and imagined using a recent case to make his point:

Dear Sir,
    You say that oral apomorphine is dangerous. Recently I had a patient who wanted to kill herself. She insisted that I give her apomorphine pills to send her on her way.
    I explained that this could not work due to the emetic property of the drug, but, she insisted. Hopeful that a more benign outcome might ensue, I supplied her with 500 pills manufactured by Parke-Davis.
    She tried that night but alas she failed. She tried the following night but again with no luck.... In fact she tried every night for a week but every attempt was as hopeless as

the first. Finally, she phoned to say that she was now quite happy, no longer wanted to kill herself and required no more pills.

So you see, despite my willingness to oblige this poor lady I bungled. To avoid any such repetition could you tell me what I'm doing wrong? I've asked around, even those clever chaps at the British Medical Council, but they're as baffled as I. Nobody in England has a clue. Alternatively, if this drug does indeed have two entirely different properties; benign in Europe, lethal in the States, perhaps, in the spirit of scientific understanding, you may let us know exactly where on a transatlantic crossing these innocent little pills become so murderous.

We in Europe are anxious to know.

Yours, etc.

J. Y. Dent.

Apart from the satire Dent knew that no matter how he answered the Americans he'd be shuffled into a backwater of interminable double-speak. Medicine needed recourse to an exacting scientific process. A process that operated above and beyond the reach of liars like the American drug czar, Henry Anslinger, his legions of bureaucratic pen-pushers and drug reps. Public provision was increasingly being undermined by forces that saw health as an opportunity for exploitation. An ill wind was forecast, one which Dent was powerless to counter. Parody was becoming his only outlet. He thought of the 750 million sedatives being sold each year in Britain, the 6,000 cases of barbiturate poisoning with over 500 annual deaths and the mountain of inducements to use the same drugs piling up on his dining-room table. Lying at the top was an eye-catching advert claiming that the troubled mother could get a decent night's sleep by giving her children 'Oblivon' (Methylpentynol).

Oblivon was addictive and potentially lethal, but it had been re-approved for general use. Meanwhile, oral apomorphine, which did not have these properties, was likely to be banned. What was going on?

'Oblivon,' he muttered to himself, 'more like oblivion!'

'Sorry, what was that?' asked Stickler.

'Oh sorry,' replied Dent, 'I was just thinking out loud.'

Stickler, a stalwart of the SSA, was trying to get Dent's editorship of the Society's quarterly journal under control. He had been instructed by the Society's Committee to bring the overdue issue out as soon as possible. He had tried to be firm with Dent but was now infuriated by the realisation that Dent had not even been listening to his exhortations.

'Look, bloody hell, Dent, how on earth can the Society expand if we cannot get the journal out on time? It is your responsibility along with everything else. Please, I do understand that you're under the cosh, but really!'

Dent lit a Senior Service and wondered how he could placate this little local difficulty. He decided to remain calm; he'd woo Stickler with some laid-back logic. He paused, looked into Stickler's glowering face and exhaled deeply.

'Now Stickler, with regard to the journal, I repeat: there is no point in sending it out with nothing in it. And I won't pad it out with lightweight material. That would be counter-productive, surely you can appreciate that? Several learned colleagues have promised papers, but I can hardly hurry them along just so we can meet our deadlines... eh?'

Stickler leant forward. 'That's not good enough, Dent, and you know it. We went over this last year. You know what the printing schedule is. You should be putting to bed the next journal right now! That is your damned job. Instead, you're *still* missing material for the current.' He wagged his finger. 'You have to appreciate that I am not the only one who is upset about this slapdash approach, far from it. Only the other day a new member from Exeter rang up, forgotten his name, nice chap...'

Stickler's drone faded as Dent's attention drifted to his annual family holiday. This year they'd be going to Balnakeil, in Durness. The cowrie-strewn beaches would be a tonic, the further away the better. He'd spend the days beach-combing and evenings peering at his 'finds' or latest atlas. He'd do the ring around tomorrow, get the dates and booking sorted.

He looked up; straight into the bloodshot eyes of Stickler. He looked like a warthog with glaucoma.

'Oh really, Dent! Am I wasting my time? I doubt you've heard a word I've said. Honestly, what do you expect of me? We have an obligation to send these journals out. That's what our members pay their subs for; they expect it.'

Stickler liked Dent. He actually felt bad about having to remind him of his responsibilities. He knew that if it hadn't been for Dent the Society would have disbanded during the war and probably a couple of times since. He also knew that the printing of the journal, about which he was bitterly complaining, would probably, once again, be paid for out of Dent's own pocket. However, largely because of Dent's idiosyncrasies, the Society was getting a bad reputation for a lack of professionalism. Stickler, with his steely resolve and military mannerisms, was the ideal man to bring the errant editor into line … or so the Committee believed.

The telephone rang in the hall. A lady's voice answered. There was a brief conversation. The phone receiver was replaced and the door opened; it was Rhoda. Stickler got up. 'Ah, Rhoda, how nice to see you, you *are* looking well.'

'Oh, thank you, you're the second doctor to say that to me today; it must be true!'

'Always good to get a second opinion,' said Dent, grumpily.

'We're finishing up here, Rhoda; will you join us?' enquired Stickler.

'Are you sure?' Rhoda replied.

'Quite sure,' said Dent. 'Can't take much more of Stickler,' he laughed.

'I'm eminently reasonable Dent. Who else will badger you?'

'I badger myself, as you well know,' said Dent, hoping that would be the end of it. 'Who was that on the phone?'

'Young Alan Maclean,' informed Rhoda. 'He didn't want to bother you and said he'd ring later. Something about tomorrow night. Remind me, what *is* happening tomorrow night?'

'"Savages and Guests" alongside a dinner hosted by the BMA. You couldn't come because of the prize giving at Lydia's school so I am inviting Alan.'

'Oh how splendid,' enthused Stickler, 'has Lydia done well?'

'It's not splendid,' interjected Dent. 'The increasing way all schools attach such a premium to precocity is very damaging. They give certificates to the one or two who simply exercise an aptitude. It'd be better to reward those who have laboured under intolerable expectations with little chance of success. All these prizes for an examination system which says at such and such an age children shall be classified as having *failed* or *succeeded*. So not *splendid* at all, *absurd* would be more accurate. What child develops at the same rate as the next, tell me that?'

'Wwwell,' stammered Stickler, taken aback by Dent's sudden broadside. 'You have to have a system, don't you? Maybe it is far from ideal, but you can't teach every individual according to their needs.'

'Of course you could,' said Dent, warming to his theme. 'In fact you cannot teach any other way… and nobody should try either. You don't think Mozart had to waste time doing geography, do you? Well neither should any child except those that want to and enjoy it. And those that love geography shouldn't have to suffer the humiliation of piano scales three afternoons a week when they'd be happier visiting coal mines or playing football. This fanatical drive for *excellence* conditions a sense of failure in the majority, with all manner of negative, long-term consequences.'

'That's all quite true, but the trouble is,' said Rhoda, 'we must subscribe to the educational system or opt out and if we do our children miss the essential dimension of socialisation amongst their peers.'

'Well, that's woolly thinking,' insisted Dent. 'A change to the educational system to something more universally humane would be a far better idea. For a start *play school* should be available until seven or eight. The young develop more happily this way and then, when they're ready, schools should slowly introduce subjects according to aptitude and interest. We are consumed by a prescriptive replicating model which induces fear and anxiety in children and a store for pent-up resentment. Where is it going to end? A nation full of sick automatons, dependent on the state, incapable of invention?'

Rhoda poured herself a sherry. 'Would either of you care for a drink; Scotch?'

'No thanks,' said Stickler. 'Er, yes Dent, that is all very well, but what of Rhoda's point? Think of the cost of having to cater for children who want to study Art or Botany rather than the three Rs.'

'I am disappointed in you, Stickler,' announced Dent, sourly. 'That wasn't Rhoda's point at all. Whereas my point: the hidden costs of a rigid educational system with no appreciation for diversity will lead to greater inequality, a lack of opportunity and more people in care than society will ever be able to cope with…. Surely you, a doctor, can foresee that. Is that what you want?'

'Are you sure you won't have that whisky?' asked Rhoda, amused by the characteristic way Dent tore into his pet hate: stuffy conservatism.

'Go on then,' muttered Stickler, disconsolately.

'You see,' said Rhoda, smiling, 'John can be very persuasive. If you want to take him on you have to reason beyond the familiar. My point was really about children missing out on developing social skills, you know… if you pull them out of school altogether. John's point about play until seven is something that works very well in Scandinavia, I believe.'

'The pair of you are a formidable team,' noted Stickler, taking his whisky tumbler from Rhoda. 'And, I must confess, I'm not much of a psychologist and haven't really considered how education can have such a deleterious effect on society's health. I stand corrected.'

'Well,' said Dent, 'it should be one of the growing concerns of our age and should certainly be better understood by everyone. Unless we can see how all these policies interact how can any strategy work? And this isn't limited to medicine or domestic policies either. As the world gets smaller we must think internationally. This goes for education, health care, immigration, technology, everything...the global environment will not cope otherwise.'

'My word,' said Stickler, leaning back. 'And I came round here to sort out the journal. Suddenly that seems a bit insignificant.'

'I knew I could convince you,' hooted Dent. They all laughed, Stickler a little self-consciously. They raised their glasses.

Dent downed his drink. 'So that's settled then?'

'What is?' asked Stickler, confused.

'The journal will be printed and sent out when it's ready and not before.'

'Bloody hell, Dent, you're impossible! I am honour-bound to reel you in. You've just tied me up like a kipper.'

'Wait till you read it, it'll be a stormer; we've got three international papers. Three! You'll glow with pride when you see it. Your wife will plug you into the national grid.'

'Can we say Wednesday and not a day later?'

'This Wednesday or Wednesday week?'

'THIS!' hissed Stickler, 'for God's sake man!'

Dent had to stifle his amusement. He observed that Stickler got hot under the collar at the slightest vexation. In his imagination Stickler had metamorphosed from a wild pig into a steam pump with air vents for ears. Dent had resigned himself to an extension until Monday. Wednesday was a bonus.

'Right!' said Stickler, finishing his Scotch, 'I think my business is done and I'd best be off. I have a long day tomorrow, surgery all morning and Barts in the afternoon.'

Dent and Stickler got up and moved into the hall. They shook hands and parted with a solemn assurance that if there were any further delays Dent would keep the Committee informed.

Dent made a quick telephone call before returning to sit beside Rhoda in front of the fire.

'I'm needed back at the clinic. Oh, that reminds me. I forgot to call Alan Maclean back. I hope he doesn't find Savages too much. Do you think he'll manage?'

Rhoda looked up, surprised by the question. Dent had treated young Maclean for alcohol addiction several months ago and gradually it seemed to Rhoda that Dent had taken him under his wing. He'd recently been a dinner guest at 34. 'Do I take it,' she asked, 'that he's no longer a patient?'

'Perfectly correct,' replied Dent. 'He's fine, but I am still trying to show him that he needn't fear these boozy evenings. He'll enjoy them perfectly well without the need for alcohol. He's just a bit stuck, I feel. This is just a gentle nudge. As soon as he realises he can cope, that he's survived, there'll be no stopping him. He's convivial, enjoys all sorts. It'd be a shame to see him becoming reclusive.'

'Don't you think you're taking your obligations a bit far?' asked Rhoda.

'Not at all. I am sure Maclean sees it as an act of friendship, nothing more.'

'And is it?' quizzed Rhoda.

'Most certainly. We have a lot in common and have always hit it off. Of course, support is important, but where else can he get it? Certainly not the National Health Scheme, they still don't think alcoholism is anything to worry about. As for aftercare, forget it.'

'So it *is* part of your medical care if you see it as therapeutic.'

'You have me there,' acknowledged Dent. 'What did Stickler say?' Dent continued, adopting the most highfaluting voice he could manage: '"You've tied me up like a kipper".' He burst out laughing … Rhoda joined in.

A coal in the grate cracked and spat sparks through thick smoke. Ulysses looked up before going back to sleep. Dent sank back into his chair and tacitly reflected on Alan Maclean, his life and circumstantial difficulties. Chief among these was losing his job and promising career at the Foreign Office by dint of his brother Donald defecting to the Russians as a spy. This had weighed heavily on the young man, who found that copious quantities of alcohol pushed these troubles away. He had moved into publishing yet despite being successful it was clear to everyone bar himself that booze had become a problem. A family friend told him about a friend, a film director, who'd had his career saved by a doctor in Kensington. After a chaotic consultation conducted while Dent siphoned water from a fish tank Maclean entered the clinic for his apomorphine treatment and emerged ten days later an exhausted teetotaller.

Dent stood up. 'I will ring Maclean now,' he said and went into the hall. Rhoda leant forward and turned up the wireless. It was Beethoven; she loved his symphonies, though she couldn't decide on her favourite.

Dent picked up the receiver and asked to be put through to Paddington.

The phone was answered promptly.

'Hello Tiger Tim.'

Maclean laughed. 'Agh Henry. All set for tomorrow night?'

'Yes, but I am actually ringing about something else.'

'Oh?'

'I have a new patient; he's in your old bed as a matter of fact.'

'Poor chap.'

'Yes, and I was wondering if you would be so good as to meet him. You might be able to help...'

'The evidence of "after" to someone who's "before"...'

'Yes, that shouldn't hurt. He's a few years older than you but American and doesn't know a soul. He'd definitely benefit from feeling less isolated.'

'I see.'

'But that's not all.'

'Hit me.'

'Well, he has an ambition to write. He's already written a book. Normally, I might not think much of it except...'

'Yes...?'

'Except in this case, I'd say this is more than a hunch...'

'You should know.'

'Well, your interpretation might be more helpful. Like so many he probably needs an entry into publishing.'

'I see...'

'Now I am not recommending him to Macmillan, in fact I think that probably wouldn't do. But you might be able to steer him.... You never know.'

'Well, I'd certainly be happy to come in... when?'
'It is too early now, but by tomorrow night I should have a better idea. Perhaps Sunday afternoon. Clear some time from your busy schedule.'

Maclean laughed. 'I might squeeze you in.'

'I just wanted to give you an early heads up...'

Dent put down the receiver and returned to sit with Rhoda and Beethoven... a few minutes of relaxation before a short drive to the clinic.

* * *

At 99 Cromwell Road Kate was writing up her notes and preparing to brief her colleague, Sister Jones. She heard her arriving and signalled that they should have a quick chat in the kitchen.

'He's asleep at the moment,' Kate said, 'but he'll be restless when he wakes and probably complain of having no energy, with a headache and muscle cramps. He goes by the name "Chinaman". He's been very withdrawn most of the day, despondent and has absolutely no faith in the treatment... or us.'

'Blingin' 'eck, any good news?' asked Sister Jones in her rich South Wales accent.

Kate smiled. She did not like to be negative but honesty was best. 'Ah, well, not really. He can suddenly get very excited... theatrical. Then he quietens down. You can expect a difficult night. Very up and down.'

Sister Jones thanked Kate and prepared herself. She had developed an interest in addiction before nursing due to her father, a preacher, being a member of the Temperance Society. This had also interested her husband a doctor, from Cardiff. As she laid out a few things on the kitchen table she heard a moan from the Chinaman's bedroom. Opening the door she found an anaemic and naked torso hanging face down over the side of the bed.

'Good evening,' she announced. 'Here, let me help.'

She rearranged the pillows, lifted her patient and turned him onto his back. He spoke without opening his eyes. 'What time is it?'

'Nine-fifteen.'

He rubbed his face with his long fingers but stopped abruptly so he could peer between them. Suddenly he jerked his head back and scrabbled for his glasses. 'Who are you?' his voice sounded frantic.

'I'm Sister Jones, your night nurse.'

Chinaman focused on the uniformed woman. She was fiftyish, with short fair hair and blue eyes. Half her age she could have been a poster girl for soap powder or cigarettes.

He reminded her of a sewer rat.

'You can call me Sister Jones or Hannah, I doon' mind.'

'Swell.'

'Now then, is there anything I can do for oo?'

'What can you possibly do?'

'I can 'elp?'

'I've got no energy, you've no idea.'

'Kate said you're baard.'

'She don't get it.'

'Now what's that mean?'

'They're all out to get me. Dent, Sister Gibson and that gangster Maclay.'

'Aww, come on ... I'm ...'

'And this cure,' Chinaman interrupted, 'a waste of time. It's making me ill. They've given me hundreds of injections and all I do is throw up ... and they make me drink whisky and suck poison. Well, that's it. I'm finished.'

'You've had ...' Sister Jones looked at the notes. 'Now let me see ... one apo-mor-r-pheen every two 'ours ... right ... That's one, two ... seven injections and you've been sick oonly twice ...'

'Never mind what's there; you listen to me. They're out to do me in and rip me off.'

Hannah Jones held her mouth and turned away under the pretext of checking the window ......

'They're all in on it, the CIA, everybody.' He waved an arm towards the window. 'Did you see anybody on the way in?'

'What on ear-r-th are you on about?'

DENT MEETS BENWAY

'You know, spooks in the shadows, hanging around, snooping.'

'No, I did not. And that's right crazy talk Chinaman if you don't mind my saying.'

'It's out there. Evil's everywhere.'

'Is that so?' Hannah shrugged and proceeded to tidy up.

Chinaman watched her for a minute. 'So, you're the good cop. Right?'

'Wha?'

'My salvation, to save me from vipers and bring me opium.'

'Opium?'

'So, you're not deaf. Yeah, opium, as much as I need and ven I vant it. It's written into the Constitution, the Geneva Convention. I insist on my rights as an American citizen...... according to the public health statute, número: tres, tres, cuatro.'

'Goodness gr-r-acious, you're a right one, carryin' on.' Hannah struggled to keep a straight face. 'I don't know what's going on in your head... all I know is... I've to help you avoid drugs... it's why you're 'ere, isn't it?'

'I don't know why I'm here. All I know is you can save me. Look, get your stash and we'll make a run for it. Just you and me, now... tonight.'

'Oh my God. And where would we go?'

'Does it matter? Anywhere but here... you, your stash and me. If I stay here for another minute, I'll die.'

'Come, stop this nonsense, will oo?' she ventured.

'You're not listening. I told you, I'm dying. Tonight's my last, call the undertaker.' He kicked off the covers.

'Aw, the charts tell a different story.'

'All bunkum, honey.'

'Temp-r-r-ature good, pulse slightly var-r-iable, br-reathin' excellent. You're far-r from dying, Mr Chinaman.'

'Never mind that bullshit; listen to me. I don't need no doctor. Ring Dent, ask him if he knows a priest.'

'I don't need to. I can see with my own eyes.'

'I look like carrion.'

Hannah ignored the remark. 'You're here to get better and with everyone's cooperation...' she hesitated, 'and that incloods yer oown ...I am sure you will.'

'Look, just do as I say and we'll get along fine. I'm paying for my opium and I'm due, it's the only thing that'll pull me outta the fire.'

'Ah, 'ark at it. If you were dying you wouldn't be carryin' on like like you are, right?'

'Opium, now!'

Sister Jones had a way with difficult customers. She prided herself with being from the no-nonsense school of medicine....... She drew herself up to her full height, all five-foot-six of it, and folded her arms. 'So then, Mr Chinaman, I take it you'd like to escape?' Her patient looked up. 'Now, there's noo need, right? This treatment, here with Dr Dent, see, is voluntar-r-ily submitted to. If you don't like it or wan'a leave, you can goo anytime. I'll help you downstairs and lead'oo to the bus stop, if oo wan'?'

The Chinaman didn't like the sound of this. The tedious consistency between Sisters Gibson and Jones filled him with dread. His voice turned to a sarcastic whine. 'Oh don't tell me. You're one of those who thought nursing was flower arranging. Well, it ain't. It's about giving me what I need: opium. Doc Dent said I could have it; that's your job. How much you got? Sister Kate told me he's stocked up. So quit stalling...'

Hannah sighed. This looked like the prelude to a difficult week. She opened the wardrobe where Kate had hung Chinaman's clothes. 'So, Chinaman, shall I help you get dressed or will you manage?'

'I'm too sick. I'll die without a fix, come on.'

'In my opinion, that's not like-ly, no.'

'Opium, Jones. It's on the menu and your damned job.'

'My job is to care for oo, right? How about you tell me what's the matter.... Tell me what you're going through... *really* going through, mm?'

'GOING THROUGH!?' The Chinaman grabbed the pillow behind him and threw it across the room and himself backwards. Without the pillow his skull rattled the bedstead. Hannah, finally unable to check herself, exploded in a fit of giggles.

Enraged, Chinaman hauled himself to his feet and stood shakily on squeaking bedsprings. 'I'll show you, what I'm going through.' He plucked an imaginary knife from the air. 'It's like this.' He thrust his arm forward. 'A motherfuckin' burn all over my motherfucking body, like this, and THIS!' His voice rose as he lunged at Sister Jones. 'The agonies, and the sweats, like THIS!' He twisted the 'blade' through several frantic gestures until his pyjama cord unravelled and his bottoms fell around his ankles. Simultaneously a door slam echoed in the stairwell.

'Agh, that'll be Doctor Dent,' Hannah confirmed. She lifted up his pyjamas and re-tied the cord. 'Praps you'd like to tell *him* what's troublin'? He'll be fa-scin-ated. Tell 'im if you'd wanna stick around, will oo? It's all the same to me.'

She retrieved the pillow and helped the suddenly compliant patient back under the bed covers. She noticed and responded... her sing-song tones more imposing, 'Let all you' silliness out, Chinaman. And then we can 'ava peaceful night...... right?'

'Won't make any difference,' the Chinaman's voice had returned to desultory. 'I'm only here cos there's nowhere else, you wouldn't get it. I'm trapped and it's all useless... hopeless...'

Dent marched in.

'Good evening, Hannah, Chinaman. How are we getting along?'

'We were just discussing that,' said Sister Jones, brightly. 'The Chinaman had some ver-ry imaginative things to say about his stay here... with us.'

'Splendid!' said Dent. 'He's an accomplished writer, did he tell you that? Always helps to have imagination if you're a writer.' Dent fixed his patient with keen eyes and grinned.

Sheepishly Chinaman looked away. 'The old croaker's got me, there's no fooling him,' he thought. 'I'll have to fight back.'

'Doctor Dent?'

'Yes, Chinaman?'

'I'm changing my name.'

'Oh?'

'Yeah, from now on I'm Benway, *Doctor* Benway.'

Dent clapped his hands. 'Haha! Excellent, I'll let everyone know. Now then, how are you feeling?'

Benway thought for a moment. 'How would I know?'

'I thought you said you were a doctor?'

'Sorry I'm off for the weekend. Never work weekends; I have rules and standards, very high standards.'

'Can we take over then?'

'Won't make any difference, I'll be stiff by morning.'

'Oh dear, that'd be a pity.'

'Why's that?'

'Because I wanted to hear about your life, about your earlier attempts to overcome this sickness. We could certainly benefit from your perspective and particularly now that we know you're from a medical background...' Dent paused and waited till the disconsolate figure looked up. 'You could make a valuable contribution to the scientific community.'

Dr Benway immediately knew what to say. He would enjoy the moment.

'I already done that.'

'Oh?'

'Yeah. But *you* wouldn't be innerested.'

'Try me.'

'I discovered the psychoactive power of *Banisteriopsis caapi*. It comes from other plants.' Dr Benway watched the old croaker sift through his brain box and draw a blank. He had him.

Dent sat down on the bed and rested his chin in his hand. 'Sorry, I am not sure what that means.'

'If I let on can I have my morphine...now?'

Dent burst out laughing. 'Dr Benway! You can have as much morphine as you like but I'd prefer you to have as much as you need.'

'It'd be a start just to have some.'

Dent thought for a moment. 'Tell me, Dr Benway, do you consider yourself worse now than twelve hours ago?'

'I'm no better.'

'With the greatest respect and without meaning to undermine your learned opinion,' Dent gave a little cough, 'that is not what I asked.'

Dr Benway tried not to smile...but failed. Sister Jones and the croaker had turned the tables on him.

Dent stood up and walked towards the door. 'While I prepare your injections perhaps you can tell Hannah whether you are worse now than this morning. Objectively speaking we have the charts to go on but I am always *innerested*, as you put it, in the patient's view. My treatments can always be bettered.' Dent moved to the door. 'And when I come back you can tell me all about...banisterias...what was it?'

'Yagé.'

'Yagé? YAGÉ!' shouted Dent, rushing back to the bed. 'Why didn't you say?'

Dr Benway had won the exchange after all.

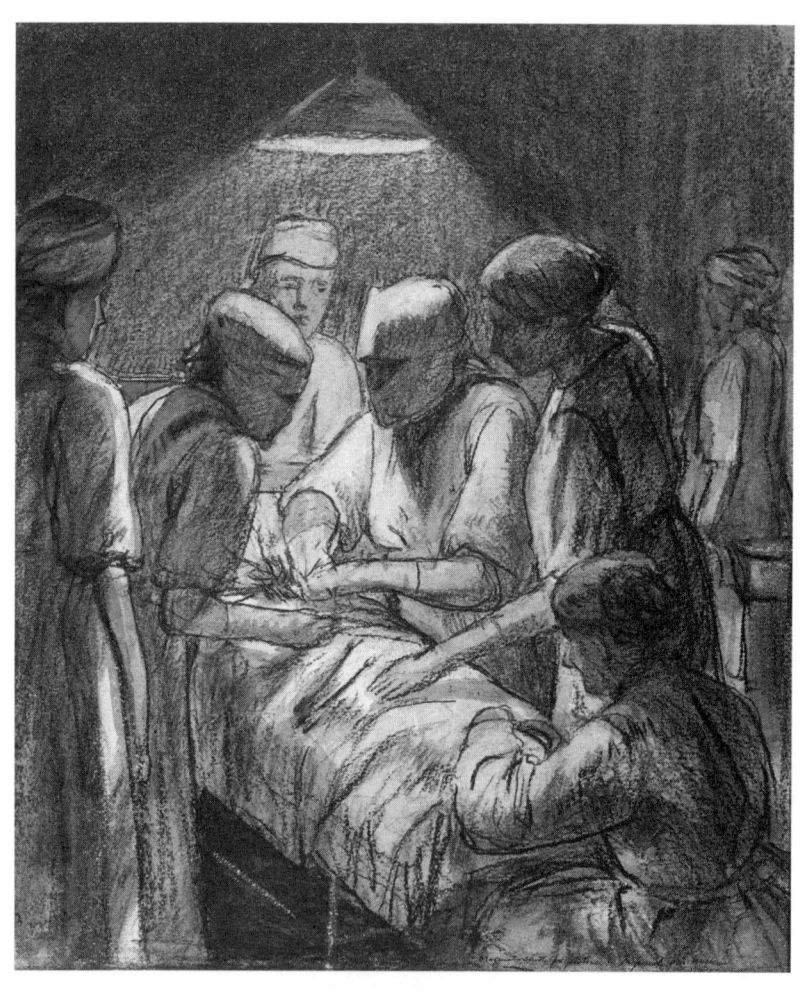

*An operation for appendicitus
conducted entirely by women at the Military Hospital, Endell Street, London.
Chalk drawing, 1917, by Francis Dodd (1874–1949).
[©Wellcome Collection]*

9

Death Before Dishonour

William Humble, Earl of Dudley, and Lady Dudley, accompanied by Lieutenant-Colonel Hesseltine, drove out after luncheon from the viceregal lodge [...] From its sluice in Wood quay wall under Tom Devan's office Poddle river hung out in fealty a tongue of liquid sewage.
  – James Joyce
   Ulysses

```
CRISIS AT HOSPITAL STOP
CAN YOU HELP OUT THIS WEEKEND URGENT STOP
YOURS DALTON
```

Junior Doctor Dent held his friend's telegram almost as limply as his letter two years previously. He *could* help, but did he want to?

There'd be work soon enough in London and a trip to a nondescript part of the Midlands miles from both sea and mountains held scant appeal... but Dalton was a good friend; they had shared much as medical students and pulled each other through the dark times. Dalton wouldn't ask if he wasn't in a fix.

Dent replied:

```
COMING TONIGHT STOP
WAIT FOR ME AT HOSPITAL 8PM DENT STOP
```

The mist at Dudley station had turned drizzly by the time Dent reached Guest Hospital, an early Victorian Gothic building forming three sides of a quadrangle. It overlooked a landscaped garden with well-maintained flowerbeds and shrubs. The porter saw him approaching and alerted Dalton:

'Dent! Fantastic of you to come, we're so grateful,' said Dalton.

They hugged each other.

'Aha! You're looking well!' said Dent.

'You too. Leave your bag with the porter and we'll go for a drink. Just a short walk.'

They found the Gypsy's Tent after about ten minutes and sat down either side of a warm coal fire. The pub appeared strangely lopsided.

'I can't be drunk yet, can I?' asked Dent.

'It's not you, it's subsidence,' grinned Dalton. 'Caused by a mine shaft out the back. They say it is why the fire's always lit even in the summer. And popular amongst those who cannot afford to buy coal.' Dalton nodded towards the back of the room where a ring of elderly ladies in black lace shawls played a bar game. They were taking turns spinning a cage full of numbered balls that rattled until one dropped into a tray underneath.

Dent watched the rhythm of the game and thought of the players. They resembled raggedy rooks pecking at a carcass.

'Now, Dent,' interrupted Dalton, 'I think you'll enjoy Dudley Guest Hospital. It has its own eye department with an honorary ophthalmic.'

'Really?'

'Yes, with both in- and out-patient facilities. I'll show it to you but the thing is, right now I'm … well, *we*, are in a fix. With, er, Matron.'

'That's the second time you've said, "we".'

'Yes, I must confess, leaving King's hasn't exactly cured me of my weaknesses …'

Dent suddenly regretted his mercy mission.

'Don't tell me; who is it this time? Nurse or Matron?'

'Both!'

'*Both*! Oh that's different.'

'No, it's not quite like that. Yes, I am involved with Marie, lovely girl, a nurse. You'll meet her, of course. But the problem is Matron, who we both work with. Well, she makes our lives hell. This weekend she deliberately put me on call because she heard that Marie and I were having a break...er, together. It's pure spite, nothing more. Anyway, if you cover for me until Monday, she won't have any complaint. She won't like it, of course, but we've got through worse. It'll be like old times...'

'—But different...' added Dent.

Dalton shifted in his chair. 'Ok, you've got me. But Matron could be my mother, for pity's sake.'

Dent laughed. 'Oh Dalton! You'll never learn.'

'Really, do you think so?'

Dent did not know how to react to this mixture of resignation and self-pity. He waited, hoping Dalton would provide his own explanation. Eventually it came: 'I don't know what to think. It's not as if I didn't see this coming.'

'So stop it coming,' said Dent. 'Did you think by leaving London you could escape? Remember Susan, in the first year, and then Lillian? And all that trouble with what's-a-name, the one from Guildford. Every time you'd call them a "disaster" or worse. But, you know as well as I do, the only thing they had in common was you.'

Dalton looked into his beer; Dent decided he wouldn't ask if Marie was 'the one'. She was probably the latest in a long line of wide-eyed nurses who'd fallen for Dalton's dashing good looks and bashful vulnerability. Dalton didn't even have to try. He took in girls like some men changed their trousers. The more he tried on the better he got at it. Dent imagined that this time he'd probably soiled one pair and simply put another pair over the top. He laughed at the thought.

'It isn't funny, Dent,' protested Dalton.

'What isn't?'

'You're laughing at me.'

'Don't try it, Dalton. This "little boy lost" won't wash.'

Dalton looked into the fire, the hot coals catching his profile. Dent finished off his pint and continued to appraise the situation.

'I should have guessed. If you had to run this hospital singlehanded you'd cope, but a crisis in the Dalton book of calamities, is a woman you don't know how to say "no" to.'

Their eyes met; Dalton's face darkened. 'You can be cruel, you know? Bloody cruel.'

'It'd only be cruel if I were asking you to do something of which you're not capable.'

'And how do you know what I'm capable of?'

'Well, you didn't expect me to come all this way and whistle another tune, did you?'

'No, but you haven't answered my question.'

Dent thought for a second. 'No, you're right. I do not know what you're capable of. Maybe this is something you'd like to stop but can't. Mind you, many would give their back teeth to have your way with women.'

Dalton adopted a praying gesture, 'Oh doctor,' he bleated, 'couldn't you sweeten your pill?'

They grinned, half-heartedly. Dent looked away. He didn't like to be critical of anyone, least of all somebody he cared for. He knew that Dalton's tendency to attract women was probably complex. Just because Dalton was in a jam didn't mean he had the right to assume a moral position. He extended his hand to Dalton's sleeve and tugged it.

'Don't worry and I'm sorry. We'll handle this, you'll see. What time do I start?'

'8 a.m.'

'Any clues as to what I'll face?'

'Matron.'

'Is that the worst of it?'

Dalton nodded.

'I expect you'll be agog to know how I get on.'

'Marie and I will be back Sunday night; I'll want all the gory details.'

'And Marie, this new light in your life, will she be with you?'

'Oh no, strictly off-limits. Up here couples have to walk on opposite sides of the road. This place is medieval compared to London.'

The two men left the pub in heavy rain. As they walked Dent felt energised... a Black Country melodrama and he a leading part. He also liked walking in the rain; it emboldened him. He was a stranger but rain doesn't discriminate. He'd get rained on like the locals; he liked that.

Back in the Gypsy's Tent the remaining wooden 'peas' in the last game were spun. 'Faster!' someone urged in defiance of time and fate and like a shovel of grit the balls fell against the grill. One of the circle turned towards the tray. She unfolded an arm like a bat's wing and picked at the fallen ball. Squinting she cackled and turned the ball round so the others could see. It was her age, 99. 'Bingo,' she croaked.

Soon the rain was widespread, stretching from sea to sea. It would soak moor and field, fall on every road, path, roof and garden, fill drains, swell rivers and seep into every bone, even those underground. And later, at closing time, when the coven of old ladies left the warmth it would anoint them too.

At 7.55 the next morning Dent found his way to the part of the hospital that held the outpatient clinic. This was a barrel-roofed hall with rows of benches for outpatients. To one side there was a row of cubicles where the junior doctors would see everyone in turn providing they had a ticket. Because of the war, older doctors and surgeons had been urged back into service so the juniors were expected to do their bit and work weekends. Referrals would return during the week or be sent to Birmingham.

'Do you know where I might find Dr Rees?' Dent asked a nurse.

'Yes, certainly. You'll find him in the third cubicle, along there.' She pointed to an oak swing door.

Dent knocked.

'Come in,' called a grouchy voice.

Dent entered and saw the back of a white-coated man with his head bent low over a pile of notes. 'Swotting,' he said gruffly, without looking up. 'Exams in a few weeks.'

'Finals?'

'Yes.' He spun round and extended his hand. 'You'll be Dent. I'm Rees from Rhonda, and I don't know why God sent me here. He must have been having a right joke because the last thing I wanted was this. Look at it.' He got up and slid open an observation hatch. 'Most of these are illiterate. Not even a tenth would be so afflicted back home, I tell you.'

Dent looked out at the gradually filling benches.

'Where should I go?'

'You're next door, boyo. Where we can look out for each other. Now then, if we get a "difficult" we can help each other, right?'

'But how?'

'Ah, Dalton said you'd be slow to catch on. It's like this, see. Sometimes we just can't get rid of a patient. Suppose it's a pain in the neck. Haha, it's always a pain in the neck. No, suppose it's, I dunno, a diagnosis they won't accept, or an incurable and you end up goin' round in circles. So I say, "I'm not a back specialist, but I can get one, he's an expert." Then I leave, see, tip you off on your area of specialism and in you come all la-di-da and say what must be done. "Cold shower, every morning, stop eating carrots", it doesn't matter; they'll take your word for it cos you're an expert with knowledge, see, and then they leave... and that's it. Hopefully we can get through all this by lunchtime and the rest of the day is ours.'

'I see,' said Dent doubtfully.

'Incidentally, Dent, do you actually have an area of specialism?'

'No, like you I'm not qualified... I've got midwifery and an interest in ophthalmology.'

'Excellent, better to know nothing. There's very little we can do anyway, you'll get the hang of it.'

'And you?'

'No. No interest whatsoever. I thought I might tr-r-avel when I'm qualified but the war's ruled that out. Oooh! Did you hear that?'

'No. What?'

'Matron. You'd better shoot; don't want her kicking up a stink.'

'I've heard.'

'Whatever you've heard isn't the half of it. While she thinks Dalton is here, she'll be sweet. With any luck she won't find out until close of play.'

Discouraged by everything he had heard, Dent crept into Dalton's cubicle and waited for his first patient. It was a man of about fifty.

He took his cap off as he entered and shuffled forward with a down-turned face. Dent stood up, took his medical card and offered the man a chair.

'Ah, George Butler, please sit down. I'm Dent. Thank you for coming to see me.'

'Zur.'

'How can I help you?'

'I ain't poorly.'

'Oh? Well, good, I'm glad. So how can I help?'

'It's me aiz.'

'Oh? And what's the matter with your eyes?'

'I dunno, at the works they's said I 'asta come an' see yow.'

'But what is wrong?'

'I don't know, zur.'

'Well, shall we give you an eye test?'

'Will it 'urt?'

'No, no, you just read these letters here on the wall. Shall we start at the top?'

'Ooo, I dunno, I ain't schooled, see.'

'It's a letter.'

'Agh letters iz it?'

'Yes.'

'Well, it maks no odds, I ent no reader. The works sez I must 'av me aiz tested.'

'Have you learnt to read?'

'Not likely.'

'Ah, so your eyes may not be the problem?'

'If yow sez so, doctor.'

'Shall we have a look at them?'

Dent spent a minute peering into each of the man's eyes. They looked perfect.

'Your eyes are the eyes of a man half your age,' he said in a reassuring voice while he drew a tiny picture of a stick man.

'Is this man upside-down?' Dent asked, holding up the drawing.

The man scratched his head.

'Scuze my sayin' zur, but dat ent no man, it's paper.'
'You're quite right,' said Dent, struggling. He suddenly felt out of his depth. This was his first patient but he'd be damned before asking Rees to rescue him.

'What do you like doing? I mean, when you have spare time?'

The man looked about him and signalled that Dent should come closer.

Dent bent forward until their heads were almost touching.

'I dint want yow blaberen,' he said in a whisper, 'but I like a spot a fishin' see, but I ain't ullowed.' They leant back from each other.

'Your secret is safe with me, Mr Butler, I won't tell a soul. And do you tie your hooks?'

The man started to wheeze with embarrassed laughter.

'Hihehezz, hooks! Hehe, I mek meown flies. I ketch trout, see, agh duz. Down Sturry, I know the spots.'

'Do you?'

'I duz…. Yama powcher!' The man giggled.

'Well, a great skill…err…tying flies. Very close work, I believe; requires good colour sense, err…which you've probably mastered. Well done!' Dent scribbled a note on the man's card. 'Now then, no need to see the dispensary. Just take this to the foreman at your factory. Tell them you have seen the doctor and your eyes are in excellent condition, couldn't be better.'

'Thank ye, doctah.'

'Is there anything else you'd like to tell me?'

'Aboot fishin'?'

'Err, no. I was wondering if you'd like to learn to read. Maybe the factory could arrange a course, at the library perhaps?'

'Oh, I corra do dat lark.'

'Why not?'

'If ah can read Gaffer'll mek me do uvver graft.'

'And you are happy with your job?'

'Nah, I HET it, but wat canyam do, eh?'

Dent paused…he felt the consultation should finish positively.

'But you could read about fish, about trout.' Dent thought about his favourite childhood book, Furneaux's *Ponds and Streams* and its beautifully detailed illustrations, its colour plates. He wished he had a copy to show his patient.

'Der ain't nuffin am dunt know aboot 'em,' Mr Butler said.

'I agree; you're probably an expert.' Dent leant forward and whispered: 'A master poacher.'

'I am zur, I tek ous kid.'

'Your son?'

'Ay, shood 'im the ropes, loike. Weem gowin' ou' t'morrer night,' Mr Butler trembled with a bout of nervous chuckling. 'Sssssh!' he said when he'd calmed down, pressing a finger to his lips.

'And can he read?' asked Dent.

'Ooo aye, 'ee ain't soft loike me.'

'Good. Well, get him to read a book about trout. And when you hear something that is wrong, your son can write a better book, with your help, of course.'

'Yamma pullin' me leg?' His eyes tightened as he peered at Dent. 'Yous 'avin' me on!'

'No, I'm serious. You could collaborate. Why ever not?'

'Yow ain't coddin' me?'

'Err, no, I assure you.'

Mr Butler clasped his hands in front of him as if in prayer.

'Bloomin 'eck!'

Realising that the queue of patients would soon be stretching outside the hospital Dent stood up.

Mr Butler followed suit.

'And thank you very much for coming to see me,' said Dent. 'I enjoyed hearing about your fishing... er, and your son.' Dent extended his hand for a parting handshake.

The man held his eyes downwards, unable to conceal a blush of embarrassment. He bowed slightly, still clutching his cap, and edged backwards towards the door.

'Bloomin' 'eck! Ower kidder, hey?' he mumbled as he turned and left.

The rest of the morning passed without hiccup though Dent realised that he saw half the number of patients as Rees next door. He'd never last if he couldn't speed up. To his relief Rees didn't prevail on him to draw on any area of specialism, though he suspected that Rees had another accomplice. At lunchtime Rees introduced Dent to the doctor in the first cubicle.

'Dent, meet Blair. A hopeless but plausible doctor.'

Blair smirked into his shepherd's pie.

'Hello, Dent. Yes, that bloke really swallowed my cure for hallucinations,' he said.

'Hook, line and sinker,' added Rees.

'What was that?' asked Dent, sitting down.

'Sixty-year-old man, tweed jacket, farmer. Complains he's mad,' informed Rees. '"Are you sure?" I ask him.

'"Barking!" he assures me. "So you're crazy." I say. "That as well," he says. "And anything else,' I ask, "other than widespread insanity?" "Horrid dreams, every night..." he said. "Well," I said: "I know the very man for you."'

'So, what did you suggest?' asked Dent, looking at Blair.

'I walk in, all lah-di-dah, but obviously I *don't* sit down,' he started, grinning. 'I told him that I had studied dreams throughout my training in Vienna. This impressed him and he became very attentive. Then I asked him if he could remember what troubled his dreams. "My parents," he said, "who have been dead for years."

'So I stroked my chin slowly, like this you see, and after deep thought recommended the séance every Wednesday night at the back of The Angel because, I repeat in a *very* solemn tone: "they have a solid reputation for putting wandering souls to rest... particularly those pesky sleep interrupters, itinerant souls from the underworld, who can also be banished with valerian and prayer. And," I said, clapping my hands together, "side by side the two treatments never fail... GUAR-AN-TEED!"' He fixed Dent with a stare, before bursting into a maniacal fit of giggles.

'Easy as pie,' Rees added, sharing the joke.

'Yes,' agreed Blair, 'just don't hesitate and look them straight in the eye. If Rees has done the spadework my job's a breeze.'

Dent suddenly became aware of a looming presence behind Blair. It was a tall woman around forty years of age. She was glowering.

'Who is this?' she demanded.

'Dalton's replacement, Matron. Junior Doctor Dent, arrived hot foot all the way from London last night. Aren't we lucky that—'

'Shut up, Rees! I haven't been notified. Why not? You know the rules.'

'There wasn't time, Matron. Dalton had a family crisis and Dent stepped into the breach. We're very fortunate to get such an able replacement…'

'Agh! Dent, is it? What are your bonafides?'

'Exactly the same as Dalton, Matron. We started together at King's…'

'I see, then you'll know that he's a scoundrel; a beastly, unhung charlatan!'

Matron stormed off not giving Dent an opportunity to reply.

'Phew! Not as bad as I thought she'd be,' said Rees.

'She must have suspected something was up,' added Blair.

'Will that be the end of it?' enquired Dent, hopefully.

The other two smirked.

'Hardly,' promised Rees. 'This has been brewing. Either Dalton leaves or she will.'

They finished with lunch and worked most of the afternoon. The surgery finally closed at four-thirty and the doctors met in the pub. They started to talk about poetry but running out of erudite references the tone quickly degenerated.

'I've learnt a belter,' Blair coughed apologetically, 'one with a local flavour.'

'Try me,' said Rees.

Blair began to recite:

There were three young ladies of Brummagem
And this is a story concernin' 'em.
They lifted the frock and tickled the cock
Of the reverend archbishop confirmin' 'em.

Now this old rector was no fool
For he'd been to a good public school
So he lifted their breeches and buggered the bitches
With his nine-inch episcopal tool!

'That's more like it,' trumpeted Rees.
'I made up a short one last night,' said Dent.
'Oh yes?' said Rees.
Dent cleared his throat;

It's worse than a curse
To be in love with a nurse
When her patron's your matron
Who wanted you first.

'Ha!' guffawed Rees. 'Very sharp, an astute summation of the facts, boyo. You're settling in. Another beer?'
By Sunday evening Dent was certainly beginning to feel part of the furniture. It was with this thought in mind that he greeted Dalton.
'Welcome home,' he said, pushing a pint towards his friend.
'So why don't you stay on?' asked Dalton. 'You've nothing pressing back in London. You can fill any number of vacancies.'
Dent was silent, watching the smoke rise from the smouldering coal.
'And,' continued Dalton, a broad grin spreading across his face, 'you'll get a better idea of doctoring in the sticks. All part of your education. You'll thank me one day, really.'

* * *

Early next morning Dent introduced himself to Marie and the team of nurses in the canteen. They chatted until the last duty nurse arrived, announcing that Underhill 'was on the prowl'. A gloom descended upon the group.

'Who's Underhill?' asked Dent, struck by the impact of this news.

'He's the honorary visiting surgeon, retired years ago but brought back cos of the war…' said Marie. '…a measure of how bad things have become.'

'Ssssh!' One of the other nurses jerked her thumb towards the door. 'That's 'im now. I'd recognise that horrid voice anywhere. You'd think he owns the place the way he carries on.'

Dent got up and moved towards the door so that he could hear better. An overbearing voice filled the corridor.

'Bear up my girl, bear up! We did our best. Just a boy I know, but what a struggle! Enough to make a mother proud, eh? How old was he? Eighteen? You'll miss him then, what?'

A woman's wail was drowned out by Underhill.

'Now, now, NEVER MIND! We all have to go sometime, CHIN UP!'

The wail continued.

'Good God,' commented one of the nurses, 'he doesn't think, does he?'

'Who's he talking to?' asked another.

One of the nurses got up and joined Dent by the door.

'It's Mrs East!' she cried, incredulous.

'Oh no!' cried Marie, 'her son's not dead, he's fine!'

'The idiot's read the wrong notes again. Paul's only in for colic.'

'Jesus Christ! Do something, Doctor,' begged Marie.

'What?' blurted Dent. 'He won't know me.'

'Distract him; we'll deal with her.'

Dent entered the corridor followed by a nurse. Underhill had started to thump the grieving mother on the back.

'COME ALONG, come along! BUCK UP! There's a good girl. No need to carry on. Think of the good times. He wouldn't want this, he'd say: "MUM, pull yourself together", I'm certain…'

'Excuse me,' interrupted Dent. 'EXCUSE ME, SIR!'

Underhill looked up. 'What's that? Terrible shock, eh? Such a plucky lad. What a waste! Could've joined up, killed a few Hun.'

'Can I have a word, sir?'

'A mere stripling, a pup! But, madam, a fighter, did you know that, eh? Such endurance. Gallant, oh yes! Struggled to the very end, just the sort of pluck the Empire needs.'

Mrs East gushed tears as the nurse escorted her down the corridor to be reunited with her son, still very much alive. Dent took her place.

'Hello, sir. I'm Dent, a junior, from London.'

Underhill unbuttoned his jacket, revealing a bright yellow waistcoat with a gold watch chain. He clasped his hands comfortably behind his head.

'What was that?' he asked disinterestedly.

'London, sir. I'm a junior doctor from King's, London.'

'London, eh? Don't they think we can cope on our own?' Suddenly his demeanour changed as if he had realised something. He sat up and put an arm around Dent. 'Mind you, London, I am forced to admit we certainly have a crisis.'

Dent shifted uncomfortably. 'Oh! What's that, sir?'

Underhill lowered his voice. 'Women, you see, too damned many in the hospital. Next they'll be doctors.' He jabbed his finger into Dent's chest. 'How would you feel if you had to be examined by one, eh?'

Dent thought this question was not worthy of a response and tried to wriggle free of Underhill's clutches and scrutiny.

'Why aren't you at the Front, London? Fighting for the Empire, mmm?'

Dent hated this question. The truth was he had no intention of fighting for anything, least of all for a cause with no sensible purpose. However, the other reason was always easier.

'Damaged lungs, sir. TB.'

'Not funk?'

'Sir?'

'You're not faint-hearted?'

'I don't believe so, sir.'

'Mmm, well, if that's the case, you can apply for this vacancy here, "resident medical officer". I and the nation expect it.'

Dent stiffened. Underhill was annoyed by the lack of response. 'It's your damned duty, man.' He punched Dent on the arm. 'The least you can do for the boys. Heroes every man Jack of them, England's finest. Oh, if only I were younger… I'd gobble the Bosch for breakfast. Dirty rotten scoundrels.'

Underhill punctuated this remark by smacking his right fist into the palm of his left hand. Thinking he hadn't made his point forcefully enough he repeated the action: smack! Dent's body shrank as he wished he were somewhere else, anywhere else. Oblivious, Underhill sidled closer, put his arm back around Dent's shoulder and gave him a squeeze. 'What I must divulge, London, is that someone with excellent qualifications and experience has also applied for this post of "res. med". Someone who'll also do it for a smaller salary than the next man. But London,' Underhill's eyebrows arched, 'the devil of it is – it's a she!' He stamped his foot. 'I won't have it, not in my hospital. NEVER!' Underhill's raving rose an octave. 'It'd be intolerable, the end!' He grabbed Dent by the lapels and pulled him close. 'So, London, uphold the honour of the hospital. It's the least you can do for the glory of Crown an' Empire. Do that and Mum's the word about your funk, what?'

Dent was too disgusted to respond.

'And what's more, London, if you pass muster in surgery,' Underhill continued, straightening Dent's tie, 'I'll put in a good word and offer a few tricks of the trade, what?' Underhill tapped his temple and winked before his attention was interrupted by the arrival of Dalton. 'Agh, Dalton lad, where have you been?'

Dalton sat down. 'Hello, sir.'

'Can't run this hospital on my own, Dalton. Did you hear about my little mercy mission this morning? A young lad called to join the great majority. Thank goodness I was on hand, what?'

Underhill puffed out his waistcoat and stretched out his legs. Without warning he clapped his hands. 'No matter. The Lord taketh but by crikey, He giveth too. Isn't it true? Just as the hospital threatens to go to the dogs, London arrives…in the nick of time. So let's see what he's made of, eh? There's an urgent case in Ward Two, third bed, by the window. That's right, no use looking frightened, Dalton. It's just appendicitis. Simple procedure and a nice little earner. Nothing to it. Take it as my good deed for the day. We'll squeeze it in before lunch. Dalton, you can be my gasser; London, my slasher, 11 a.m.'

'But sir—'

'But nothing, Dalton, I've told the duty doctor, what's his name, Cardiff? 11 a.m. Now, where's the stairs? Damn it, Dalton, the stairs; come along now.'

The three men got to their feet and proceeded slowly down the corridor. Dalton looked at Dent, who felt he'd wandered into a lunatic asylum.

'See what we're up against,' hissed Dalton, 'why we need your help?'

'You don't know the half of it,' whispered Dent. 'He's offered me a position, Res. Med. Officer.'

'Really? You move quick,' said Dalton, sounding pleased.

'But up against someone with professional experience,' warned Dent.

'Oh.'

'A woman.'

'Well then, the job's yours,' said Dalton.

'I don't know if I should apply.'

Dalton stopped walking. 'Why ever not?'

'Because she's better qualified than either of us,' emphasised Dent.

Dalton grabbed his friend by the shoulder. Underhill, oblivious, continued to amble down the corridor.

'Dammit, you want to save lives; well, stay here. The old fool wouldn't work with the Queen of Sheba. This isn't an either-or-situation, it's you or nobody. Every doctor's in France, on manoeuvres or transferred to the auxiliaries. Together we can keep him out of theatre, and even when he's there we can reduce the damage. He killed three last week, *three!*'

There was a dull noise at the end of the corridor as Underhill bumped against glass doors.

'DALTON! Where the devil are you? DOORS, my boy, come along.'

Dalton ran to open them.
'Don't open on their own.'
'No, sir, how silly of me.'
'What was that Dalton?'
'11 a.m., sir.'
'What?'
'I said, ELEVEN, sir, THEATRE.'
'Yes, nil by mouth, I've told Cardiff.'
'Very good, sir.'
'Now take me to the Wolsey, I need a nap.'

* * *

An apprehensive Dent met Dalton at ten-fifty outside Theatre One. Fumes of disinfectant only added to the dreadful atmosphere. Two nurses entered, helping each other with surgical gowns and masks. The first took Dalton to one side and started to complain about something in hushed, urgent tones. Dalton gave up trying to whisper and spoke up so everyone could hear.

'I know, but there is nothing we can do,' he said. 'Underhill wants to operate and that's that. He sacked a nurse last week for saying what you just said to me, so let's just do the best we can in admittedly difficult circumstances. I'm sorry.'

Hearing this and the thought that he might be responsible added to Dent's disquiet. One of the nurses left and Dalton went into the theatre to start anaesthetising the patient, a thirty-year-old man, who was being comforted by a nurse.

Dent inspected the operating theatre. There was plenty of light, a hydraulic steel table and a tiled floor with a central drain. Voices outside told him Underhill had arrived and the nurses were struggling to help him on with his surgical wear: gloves, gown and mask.

'Precious minutes, nursey, you're wasting precious minutes. What's that you say? ASEPSIS? Oh, if I had a penny for every time I hear that word I'd pave the road to Brummagem in gold. Most septic thing I ever saw in a woman was a canary. Did I tell you the story?'

Dalton looked to the heavens while Underhill turned the operating theatre into a music hall melodrama. 'It was a cold and rainy night when I got the call. One of those hovels behind the gasworks. Filthy it was, rain like bullets. Slipped in the alley and arrived covered in mud. There's no light to speak of, just a candle, no help and it's a bloody breech boys. So I open her up. Zzzip!'

Underhill made a vigorous cutting gesture as he moved back from the operating table and ripped off his mask. 'Well, boys, I don't mean to brag but I whip the creature out before you can say "Jack Robinson".' He gestured like a magician. 'I hold it up to the candle to see if we have a soldier or nurse. Dammit, it wriggles like a wet fish and knocks the canary off its hook into the woman's belly. Cage, bird, seed, feathers, you name it.'

'Weeell, I picked out what I could and stitched her up...all on my own. And she lived, by Jove!' Underhill bowed. 'And you flibbertigibbets talk to me about asepsis! Nowadays it's all you hear. "Asepsis this, asepsis that." Nancy-boy's talk. Ridiculous.'

'The operation, sir,' reminded Dalton.

'Caesarian, of course.'

'I think he means this one, sir,' suggested Dent.

'Ah yes! Haha. Silly me. Well, what are you waiting for? In my day this'd be over by now...cut and slash, four inches, no make it eight, the bigger the better, zzzip! There. Oooo! Did you see that, boys and girls, make a man of London yet, eh? Hang on!'

'What's the matter sir?'

'Wrong glasses, must be in the Wolsey. Door nursey, won't be a jiffy, tally ho!'

Ten minutes later Underhill returned and was issued with replacement gloves.

'New surgicals, sir,' said the nurse, trying to remain cheerful.

'Oh, don't tell me. Asepsis all the rage, eh?' Underhill laughed sarcastically as Dalton's anger boiled. Dent, nauseous, tried to concentrate.

'Are we ready, sir?'

'Ooooo crikey, yes. A dekko please.' He peered at the incision, pushing his glasses to the bridge of his nose. 'Ah HA, that's better.

DEATH BEFORE DISHONOUR

FORCEPS, come along, come along, nursey whatsyername. Right, pull on that, harder, HARDER. Let the dog see the rabbit. HARDER, perit-it-o-ne-um, lovely, hold it. Jolly good. Hold it. HOLD IT. Hang on a minute.' Underhill pulled off his surgical mask. 'What's this?'

'The liver, sir,' said Dent.

'Dalton?'

'Yes, sir, it's the liver.'

'Are we all agreed?'

'Yes, sir,' confirmed Dent, 'definitely the liver.'

'Ah ha. Jolly fine show, boys,' enthused Underhill, failing to replace his mask, 'now we're getting somewhere, and isn't this why we're here? Doing our bit for the lads. What's my motto, Dalton? Speak up!!'

'"Death before dishonour", sir,' Dalton said, miserably.

'By gad, how right you are, Dalton, how right *you* are. DEATH BEFORE DISHONOUR, let's not forget. NOW, what's this, eh?'

'A kidney, sir?' suggested Dent, astounded at what was unfolding.

'Are we sure?'

'Quite sure.'

'And this?'

'The other kidney, sir, most definitely,' said Dent.

Dalton cursed under his breath.

'So, this is the appendix?'

'No, sir,' said Dalton wearily, 'I think you'll find that that is the spleen.'

'The *spleen*. Good God! What the devil's it doing here?!'

'There's the appendix,' indicated Dalton, pointing to a perfectly healthy organ.

'But can we be sure? London?'

'There's no doubt about it, sir; Dalton is correct, that *is* the appendix.'

'Wonderful, SO, my boy, we've located the offender and now the punishment. We'll cut the blighter out, right out! Save this poor man, in the nick of time by the look of it. Scissors. SCISSORS, Nurse, come a-long!'

[195]

'Forceps first,' suggested Dent.

The nurse handed over the forceps.

'If you insist.' Underhill allowed Dent to guide his shaking hand and close the forceps. 'And now the scissors. Come ALONG!'

'Scissors, sir.'

'SNIP!' Underhill cut out the appendix, lifted it up between his finger and thumb wiggling it – vigorously… before dropping it onto a tray of sterilised instruments.

'And that, boys, is how to conduct an AP-PEN-DECT-OMY! Stitch him up, Sister; women's work, needle and thread, what.' He grabbed and undid the forceps before anyone could stop him. Immediately the patient's abdomen started to fill with blood.

'He hasn't tied it off!' gasped Dent.

'What!? *Get him out!*' seethed Dalton to the nurse. 'Sir, you must be tired after all that exertion. Why not grab a cuppa in the canteen? Nurse Ryan will escort you.'

The nurse took Underhill's arm and led him out as the patient was turned on his side. Blood splashed over the table and floor while Dalton and Dent started a desperate race against time, searching for the pumping artery. Cursing, Dalton found, cauterised and tied off the stump. He then took an hour to carefully stitch the man up.

'And that,' said Dalton through gritted teeth, 'is the cure for constipation.'

'A simple operation,' said Dent.

'Underhill never does simple operations.'

'So I see.'

'Bugger it, Dent, now you know why we need you.'

'Wouldn't it be easier to simply retire him, permanently? Talk to the Board?'

'Oh *hell*, don't think we haven't tried. Underhill is venerated in Dudley; his father was the first senior house surgeon, and his family original benefactors. There's a statue of his grandfather in the town paid for by his friend, the Earl of Dudley, another sacred cow. They're like the monarchy; brainless and untouchable.'

'I see.' Dent's empty remark tipped Dalton over the edge.

'It's a cussed perversion,' he shouted, hurling his surgical gloves at the wall. 'Last week because Rees was off, three died. I cannot be everywhere. When we know he's in we switch the "surgery due" cards but recently he's been picking up the odd case from emergency. Last week he bagged an industrial accident, a lad with severe concussion. When I arrive he's lifting out bits of skull with brain still attached and takes offence to my disgust. "*Stop fretting Dalton, he's a fellow Black Country lad!*" he says, "*I know what he can stand.*" I swear I'd shoot the bastard if I thought I'd get away with it.'

Dent turned to his friend. 'Look, I've said I'll help out in maternity…'

The surgical assistant burst in. 'Sorry to interrupt but you two are needed next door, there's an injured man from the steelworks, Underhill's got there first, I'm afraid.'

Dalton and Dent rushed into the second theatre. A man was struggling on a trolley with Underhill and a nurse holding him down.

'Ahha! Look nursey, the cavalry have arrived. As if we couldn't handle this, a mere skirmish.'

'What is it?' asked Dalton.

'Steel splinters, I've seen this before, but not here,' shouted Underhill. 'More chloroform, hold the hand, Dalton.'

Underhill scraped around between the man's lacerated shoulder and armpit.

'Clothing caught in a machine, poor blighter. Lucky I'm here. What a day, all go, eh?'

Dent watched in horror as Underhill jabbed away with a scalpel. Suddenly there was a suck of air as blood from the brachial artery hosed the wall six feet away.

'Whoops!' said Underhill, looking up at Dalton still holding the man's hand. 'Pulse, Dalton?'

'Nothing, sir.'

There was silence save for the drip of blood onto the tiled floor. Detecting a mutinous mood Underhill suggested that everyone retire to the sitting room. 'A quick rest and refreshment will help us decide where to amputate,' he promised.

With a mug of tea Underhill appeared to have recovered his poise. 'Cheer up lads. When you've had as much experience as I you won't let a little mishap like this disturb you. I think I can honestly say I have accidentally cut every single major artery in the body. Every single one.'

Dent felt he had to comment. 'I bet I can think of one you will have missed, sir.'

'Well name it boy.'

'The aorta sir.'

'Oh listen to that Dalton, such innocence. I bagged my first aorta when a chap came in complaining of a chest swelling. I took it to be an abscess and stuck in my scalpel. It was an aneurysm. Got it straight in the face.'

By mid-afternoon a disconsolate Dalton scrubbed dried blood from his hands. Dent watched for several minutes before speaking.

'Let's talk tonight, over dinner. I'll cook.'

'Thanks. What's on the menu?'

'I'll think of something.'

Leaving the hospital two hours later Dent's eye was drawn to a plaque on the wall. There was an inscription which verified what Dalton had said about the parochial benevolence in founding the hospital. There was Arthur Underhill's name immediately below 'William Humble, Earl of Dudley'. 'Humble?' thought Dent, as the porter approached.

'Young gentleman looking for you, sir. That lad outside, in the school cap.'

Dent walked down the entrance steps and introduced himself.

'Hello, I'm Dent.'

'Ah, hello. Glad I caught you. A present from my dad.'

The youth handed over a brown paper parcel done up with string.

'What is it?'

'Brown trout; my dad wanted you to have them.'

'Oh! My word, yes! So you'll be, errr... Mr Butler's son.' Dent looked down at the parcel, weighing it in his hands. 'This is most generous – there was really no need,' he added, more than slightly taken aback.

'We'd be honoured if you'd take them.'

'I'm truly grateful,' said Dent warmly. 'Please, thank your father.'

'I will. They're fresh, caught this morning.'

'Yes, he said you were going out. Well, thank you so much, I did nothing... really.'

George Butler's son looked up. 'He told me you showed him proper respect. He's not used to that, see, from a doctor.'

'Ah!' said Dent, momentarily overcome. He took a deep breath. 'Then, knowing that will make them taste even better.'

The lad radiated pleasure. 'Good, I'll tell him.'

They shook hands and parted.

Dent watched George Butler's son merge into the throng by the hospital entrance: tradesmen, miners, schoolchildren and women with groceries. Farther away a military band approached followed by lines of bobbing khaki marching with arms. In front of the gates a laundry-man pulled up his cart to let the soldiers pass. His skewbald carthorses shook their traces and several children, one with a small flag, paused to admire the procession. Golden sunlight glinted off polished rifles and stretched into the hospital quad across the lawns and flowerbeds. The translucent blooms burned holes in Dent's memory that he'd never forget. 'Humility First,' he said to himself, querying whether such a motto existed. Few in London would understand but it was dawning on him that he'd stay in Dudley. Helping his friend in the battles against Matron and Underhill was a factor but not the full story. No, the real war was the universal deference towards rank and seniority. The top-down entitlement personified by Underhill was evident throughout medicine but the same imbalance prevailed in law, the military, religion and education. In fact in every single societal structure that depended on people remaining subjects not citizens. Nobody, Dent was beginning to understand, was safe.

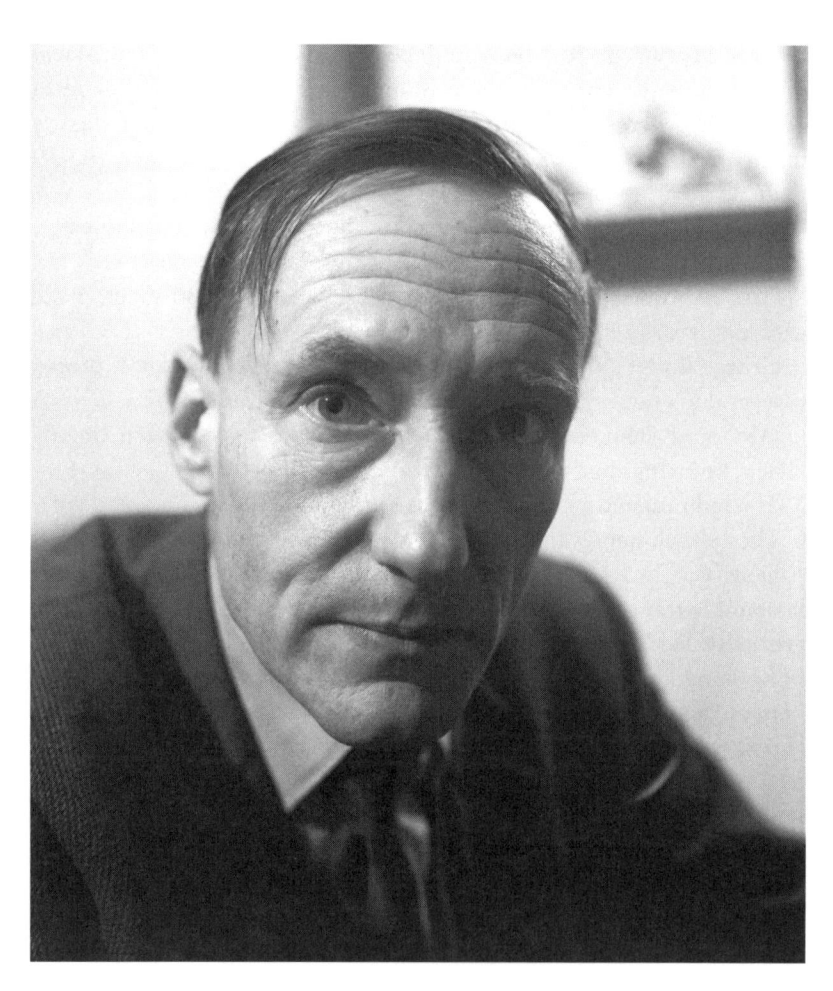

William S. Burroughs, (1914–1997)
Photograph taken in 1960, London.
[©Harriet Crowder]

10

Buffoons Talking Bollocks

Kate checked Benway's pulse and breathing. He said he didn't want any more morphine. She injected him with a sub-emetic dose of apomorphine. This triggered another bout of yawning...... he stretched and began to feel sleepy. Soon he was tumbling... back down the rabbit hole.

Thin as a tree Bill Lee looked between his legs and fell through the floor / cold air jolted him wide awake / he could make out a coastline as he fell / a man without a parachute / 3.1 seconds / time to relax / to let go / oh he'd let go all right like Contessa had beseeched / he smiled / a distant light / it flashed and disappeared somewhere behind the cliffs of England / the dark curdled waters rose to meet him / splash ...
No chance to be rescued now / he'd die unseen unknown / he lost consciousness / a firm hand gripped his wrist and hauled him aboard the galleon / watch out rocks ahead / a shrill voice penetrated the storm / Gibbie squeezed his hand / port in a storm / I'd say so / Lee wanted to sleep unnoticed curl up by the fire but the storm was heavy / more gas come on / his teeth rattled ...
Jesters and grotesques moved steadily around the bed / he sensed that his own laughter might be real too / momentarily his mania got off / they shared a joke and he wasn't it / how strange / he chased the thoughts around his bed / everything span / numbers / roulette / the galleon in a midwest twister / he pointed out rocks to Don Quixote / I'll be his Sancho /

[201]

they'd be a team / set on banishing the terrors of the night / his face bathed orange from the fire / the fetid heat was back with a raking thirst ...
—I'll burn you now he commanded somebody threw on more petrol / screams lost in the furnace / ole walrus returned - panting / dish-dash opened / tortoiseshell half-moon specs peered into his soul
—A haven / I'd say so / the knacker's yard if we fail
—Just like Horace moaned his Father / feel the shame/ you have failed me failed us all
—<u>NOT SO</u> argued the doctor in court / an hereditary dimension maybe / there's no half measures / opprobrium no sympathetic tears not even fear will make you seaworthy but you - your imaginative forces - your talent - mark my words / but we must reach the shore / onward he cried / work to do / I plead my case / it is for science to answer I am a molecule man not a buggering bishop / the hanging judge said nothing
The walrus braced himself / spray strafed the deck more sea than air / huge green-grey wave thumped the cliff / Balors Gun thundered under Horn Head / drenched the old sea dog / he re-emerged / yellow whiskers twitched
—I had TB they said go to the sanatorium / Lee positioned his stethoscope so that everyone could see / Contessa upstaged him giving birth to blood-red stag beetles / She ate a couple leering / TV ratings spiked / she licked the air leaving numbers ...

<u>443444 99344423 ... 1811</u>

—Yes the frog was revered by the Mayans said the walrus —The lamprey is semi-parasitic with an extraordinary life cycle but we still laugh ourselves sick / grow love sick / we need our vomiting reflex
—Oh quizzed the traveller
—Yes - shat out of our gobs long time ago a phenotypical

BUFFOONS TALKING BOLLOCKS

response triggered by a life in politics
Typhoons of laughter / mirth changed the colour of the
wallpaper / Lee shivered / the fire roared again
—I need water to put the fire out here you fuck he pointed
to his mouth —not there
Two nurses entered waving hypodermics / the crimson sky grew
mauve then turquoise the fin dance / Taffy Jones spoke kindly
—nasal spray - the doctor says it bypasses the stomach
straight to the back brain / that is why you mustn't swallow
your pills
—All rubbish shouted the traveller / give me injections only
thing that works / bypass the stomach / who do you think you
are / Let me tell you I was psychoanalysed in Vienna /
oh yes / don't look surprised / a sought after shrink spoke
professorially while stroking my super ego / like so /
a firm Oedipal caress with Korzakoffian accent sprinkled with
Freudian hogwash / shook down all the rich Jewesses round
Goldenes Quartier boy we had us some fun / sideline in
speed balls ...
Halfway to paradise a window opened / the galleon's figurehead
leaned over the bed / posed for photos / fairground colours
sparkled in the flashlights / cavernous gob closed over Lee's
cock / she paused and turned her attention to the scientific
community / her pearly white teeth frigid voice and polished
demeanour picked over proceedings with delicacy / a surgeon
playing spillikins / Lee nodded respectfully ...
—We have to understand where all this is leading she said
loftily pushing back her fringe - I will take your pulse
monitor your libido lobotomise you with the <u>latest greatest-</u>
number 23 placeeeebo / force feed you vitamin B / this
ridiculous insistence on treatment based on endogenous neural
mechanisms / not currently favoured by our offshore tax
avoiders
She coughed loud eyes squinting at shiny HQ of 1000 gleaming
arseholes

—I mean shareholders – our esteemed scientists / oh fiddle-d-dee-fucksticks / what the hell / yam only a PR whore told to give it the old flannel who wants solutions anyhow? where's the angle in that? you progressive little shit
Her stern matronly presence and eight-inch pricking device rendered protest futile / hundreds more from <u>Prehensile School of Medicine</u> raised in incubators and up to their eyeballs in debt stood to applaud like rows of dry cunts craving antidotes for erectile dysfunction
—Sadly she advised —this will never happen on account of there being no known <u>patentable</u> <u>pinky</u> ... otherwise ... you think we'd be hanging around?
She pulled out her massive tool
—Over you go sonny / did that hurt? not half enough? Oh you child / If I had my way you'd all hang in cages under Westminster Bridge fed on Adolfine / he may have been a Nazi the old crazy but he knew an angle when he saw one / we had it in the bag until the Commies muscled in / she screamed in frustration her pupils number eight balls
Bill Lee wanted to escape / he was being rogered mercilessly but what a way to go / desiccated by self-pity he dissolved / a cloud of atoms but listening ... a voice? Maybe it was him, the boy before the ugly possession. He would follow the sound / gradually his child-self rose outta the storm's rattle .... / moved to the next room down the stairs and out into the street ... onward he urged ... soon they were two Bills floating along ... over the lone and level sands to someplace else where only the boy could see .... thru anterior eyes .... beyond the torpor and despair ... further ... deeper ... pre Hadean ... primordial ... where everything forgotten reappeared ... from before the cradle and after the grave ..... then slowly, miraculously, a sound grew till it swallowed space .... a rumble rebounding to the echo ... billowing air sea sand an' rock ...... rippling the sapphire sky and trundling around the sun .... Yeah, man, it rolls

thru all things ... that sound ... wordless .... boundless ...
eternal ... maybe that's the answer if you put your ear to the
shell ... the space whistle? It'd be cool to know who's out
there ... transmitting? Otherwise space is nothing but our own
emptiness staring us down ...
BANG! He was back! Abruptly at 2 a.m. the old walrus jumped
onto the deck but the seductress had got there first ...
—Agh, Benway you've met
He bent forward, gripping the ship's wheel for support /
crazed siren climbed in through a porthole; golden curls, blue
eyes and crimson lips
—Yes, I lived here during the Blitz, several bombs fell round
the back, one took out half a street. I remember the smell,
gas, smoke, burning flesh / lingered for days / doity words
from such a beauty ...
Lee saw the windows rearrange themselves ... like baccarat ...
something else emerged from his earthen mind
—My life is here / it is now / he called for his mother —She
is out said / the door
He felt fear but he'd do his best / always did his best
—Benway I will leave you in the capable hands of these fine
ladies and call tonight / no need to worry about not sleeping
let it come when you're ready / Rest ... there's paper and
pens in the drawers if you need / nothing to bother you /
you're doing well ... very well ...
Lee watched over the side of his pillow / Primrose sunlight
chased away the terror of the night / breeze from the street
blurred the shadows / doc had gone but voice remained / Do not
let it worry you you'll know what to do when the time comes
... / the insect morse murmuring droned back and forth ...
boundless and bare ... there again that ole buff rock by the
dry river slipping into blue light / look here are my
credentials / I'm a potentate with a salivating spiel on
Pavlovian chocolate withdrawal / It is all in my book / The
Human Machine / we're nothing more you know / nothing more

than creatures of habit programmed and prodded like anything made of steel and carbon / Sufi dancers spiralling stamping / masked faces appeared one by one / the first was mother then Joan / What is real / these voices or their words / Misery came on heavy like tropical rain / if only he could sleep / but no roaches tickling under the skin / what ministry he searched under the carpet for answers / more black and white numbers / rattling the wheel of fortune/ latitudes / logarithms

3499, 9934 6738 18 11 18 11

—Hello, yes, this is Western 6738, hello, how are you? Does it seem to be persisting? Is that better? Something / way off, Summat stirred and changed trains / the corrupted nerve terminals opened / more intersections; he blinked, they flashed. A menacing figure lurched towards him
—I'll have that, sonny boy. The bureau knows your liver is fuckarooed, but these bits and bobs pay the bills ... why are you struggling? My dedicated disciples would appreciate a degree of co-operation Let me at your ass, why the hell aint you comatose? We don't do the late shift for nothing / anymore backchat I'll drown you in barbs / there that'll settle your go-ahead hipness / Aww diddums / your radical pen all dried up? Get a job doing PR copy for plastics you piss-a-bed hack ...
A sadist's hand cut through his stomach wall / plucked out choice cuts / drunk on surgical spirit he raved
—The faculty want to name the library extension after my cancer cure / oh my / as long as the morons fixate on cure not prevention / haha / bans on refrigeration insecticides and antibiotics could stop it all tomorrow but what about the dollar you asshole? America's not a country / you bum it's bizness the BIZNESS / the ONLY way / outta my sight
Lee looked at himself from behind the wallpaper / If he could

hide for the next few minutes the surgeons would move to the next bed. He groped for his knife, flicked open the blade. It cut him. Blood oozed and ran across the floor like quicksilver ––If they see it I'm rumbled / he leapt for the door / there were thirteen of them / the witch ripped open his tunic, skin and ribs / pointed at his pure brave heart. He didn't have to nod; the jungle is being exploited. A calculator churned out the tap dance, figures gave way to letters that morphed into words then abstractions. Is there nothing the walrus doesn't know?
––Come this way, pleeeeze / this is the last lineage in storytelling / nothing more after this / nowhere to go / no new frontiers / capitalism is a crap race / co-ops between peoples the only way / the last sunset before the eternal night and falling / cartwheeling over and over / we disappear into the void halfway down the brain is switched off ... then on, but with no memory. Abracadabra! He relaxed / he would enjoy the moment / the seconds became hours and still he fell / down down / there can be no ending because you're already dead / spiralling stars citizen colours and a wish to be heard .... far off the night train whistled 'Danny Boy' and the conductor got off ... 'Two grains of "God's Own" please, doc.'
'Certainly, here you go.'
'Thank you.'
'You asked for a priest. I can do much better, this is Bishop a medical man from the ministry. So, are you whole again, now that I've kissed it better? Nursed your WASPish tendencies, your ambition to rule the world.'
'Yes, much better, thank you. Unconditional love is what I needed. Simple really, never had it before, see? I must thank you.'
'You're welcome .... anytime.'

* * *

Sister Kate sitting at the table in the bay looked towards the bed. She momentarily wondered what Dr Benway was screaming at; what could he see? He was shouting about pouring gas on them to shut them up. His striped pyjamas were now so wet they would have to be changed...again. He seemed to be looking over the bed as if he was terrified of falling into a chasm and at the same time avoiding being hit by something. Were they punches or bullets? She couldn't tell. 'Leave me alone, I want to stay where I am,' he was shouting, tears rolling down his perspiring face. He asked if the fire was out. 'Is it?' he screamed again, demanding an answer. Kate confidently asserted that it was never lit. 'We don't need a fire in here, it is quite warm enough.' She lifted Benway's eiderdown quilt and blanket from the floor for the umpteenth time. The cotton sheets had got tangled by his feet.

'The ragheads need a bit of "you know what", a bit of pour on *les* water, you dig? Where's Doc Dent? Wonder if he knows about Anslinger? He's just an old croaker, too simple to have his mind soiled by that shit. Have to tell him, but I don't have the proof. Don't get mad, he said. If I was a God-fearing Dixieboy I'd be ashamed, you know. As it is I just gotta get even......restore a modicum of honour, you gettit?'

Benway heard his nurse's voice and awoke with a start.

'Yes, Dr Benway, sorry to have to wake you,' announced Kate, preparing the next injection. The patient turned over; his whole body ached. But, something was different. She massaged his arm for a minute and injected him. In and out, no fuss. She was talking as if he could understand.

'The carbachol has helped,' she said, 'evidence of sugar, strong acetone in your clinitest. It is a good sign, and you're sleeping more. No need for any more whisky, just water from now on, or fruit juice, as much as you want. It's all there; help yourself.' She gestured towards a tray on the comodino. Without hesitation he gulped down a glass of water followed by a mug of tea.

'Now, Dr Benway, would you like to go to the bathroom while I change your bed? You'll find a basket with clean pyjamas.'

'Yeah,' he grunted, climbing unsteadily off the bed. Kate helped him to the door and across the landing. Once in the bathroom he went straight to the mirror. His skin looked awful. He rubbed his cheeks; nothing. Only his pupils offered depth, like bullet holes in a tin can. He corrugated his brow, regular troughs of grey on white; what a boring face, he could hardly grow a decent beard. He felt under his hairline for the tell-tale smear; nothing, no sweat? He should tell Kate. He turned round and squatted on the toilet; he was a deadbeat, kaput…. He pushed his long fingers through his hair until he'd enclosed his skull. He squeezed until he could feel bone on bone, harder, harder; it would distract him from the constant ache and nausea.

The effort was good, he thought; he should appreciate his body while he owned it. He remembered why he was here, in London. Gotta get through this, just to get away. Nothing for me here, nothing.

There was a knock on the door.

'Are you all right, Dr Benway?'

'Yes, I'll be out in a minute.'

'Your room is ready, everything shipshape.'

'Yeah … sure.'

He wobbled as he stood up. It was all he could do to change his pyjamas and open the door. He'd thought Kate would be there to escort him back to his bed but she'd returned to the room. Lightheaded he wavered; could he trust himself to pass the top of the stairs? To his relief Kate appeared and walked towards him. Like a blind man he waited and let her shepherd him back to his room, his sanctuary. Intuitively Kate adjusted to what was needed.

'You're safe now, nothing for you to do but rest and get your strength back. No need to rush. Easy does it…'

Benway thought that was something Dent might say. Kate helped him back into bed and eased up the bed covers.

The sheets felt clean, luxuriously cool. He wasn't sure what was happening but he needed to know. 'How've I been?'

'Very chatty early this morning. You're quite imaginative.' Her eyes sparkled.

'Oh?'

'Yes.' Kate seemed cheerful as she took Benway's blood pressure.

'We've been around the world; Mexico, a jungle, I don't know where, outer space. You thought Hannah was an alien and Dr Dent works for the Russians.' She laughed.

The conversation lapsed while Kate sat down to enter some observations on the charts. Benway watched her.

'Did I misbehave?'

Kate looked up from her notes. 'Oh no, Hannah and I enjoy our conversations.' Her face broke into a wide smile. 'Of course, it's too obvious to say that your dreams aren't real; yours seemed real enough, yesterday you were convinced I was after your kidneys!' She laughed. 'We've had some exchanges and you've broadened our horizons.'

'I apologise.' Benway met Kate's eyes to press home his sincerity.

'Oh we never take it seriously. My word, if we did we wouldn't last two minutes.' She looked up and noticed that Benway's face had softened but it was clear he was still experiencing discomfort.

'How many more days will I be here, do you think?' he asked.

'It's too early to tell,' answered Kate. She thought for a minute. 'I will talk to Dr Dent and be able to give you a better idea then. Your charts are good but your cramps and headaches seem to be persisting … and you need to recover your strength.'

'I'm not sweating.'

'No, though you were before you woke up. Do you feel different?'

'Yes.'

'How?'

'I don't know, but things seem to be less intense, maybe I'm adjusting. I'm able to concentrate.'

'Excellent.'

'Is this what always happens … with your apomorphine?'

'What you've said tallies. Other little things return, smells, sights … your appetite. Are you hungry?'

Whenever he was asked that question he always said, "no" but this time he wasn't sure. Kate put down the notes. 'It's probably a bit early but we can get in whatever you want; steak, chicken, vegetables, an English breakfast, cheese, bread, milk … you name it.'

'Steak?'

'Yes, when you're ready...why not?' She looked at her watch. 'Look, Dr Dent is coming in the next few minutes and he's bringing an old friend for you to meet.'

'What!? Here?'

'Yes, a young man who used to be a patient. Now and again he drops by. Why don't you have a cup of tea with them and maybe when they've gone you can tell me if you'd like something to eat.'

Benway felt awkward, he didn't want to see anyone. He heard the sound of voices on the stairs.

'That'll be them now,' indicated Kate, 'I'll pour the tea.' She left, leaving the door open. Dent strode in, followed by a tall, youngish man with brushed-back hair.

'I hope you don't mind, Dr Benway, but I've taken the liberty of inviting an old friend, Tiger Tim. He had your bed not so long ago and you might like to share a few things. Nothing you say to each other can hurt and may, you never know, help.'

Benway rubbed his face, he was exhausted and in no mood to be sociable...particularly with a complete stranger. He'd have to be diplomatic. 'Sure,' he said and rubbed his cheeks.

'Hello.' Tiger Tim edged towards the bed and extended his hand for a cursory handshake. Kate returned and left a tray with three steaming mugs of tea on the comodino.

'Now, I have to spend a few minutes with a patient next door,' said Dent, grabbing one of the mugs, 'but that shouldn't keep me very long. Please, chat away. Nice day, isn't it?'

Dent and Kate strode out and closed the door firmly, leaving the two men alone. The silence was sudden, a lull *after* the storm.

Tiger Tim took his tea, retreated to the bay and sat down. He spoke first.

'Well, Dr Benway, I hope you don't mind my dropping by. Did Kate say? I'm an old patient?'

'Yeah.'

'I had a drink problem. It was getting out of hand but Henry and apomorphine helped. I've been clean ever since, no problems.'

'That's swell; *Henry?*' asked Benway.

'Agh, yes, that's just my name for Dr Dent. I use it ironically because I told him one day that he reminds me of the Henry Foster in *Brave New World*. A character less like Dr Dent would be hard to imagine but then he'd christened me "Tiger Tim" so I was just getting my own back,' he shrugged, 'Well, we all have nicknames here, why not the good doctor?'

'Well, I'm in for junk, heroin,' Benway berated. 'Not the same thing at all.'

'No, you're probably right.'

'How long did your torture last?'

'Ten days all told. Bearable overall but the DTs were extraordinary. I was delirious for one or two days. Amazing experience. They had to hold me down. I really put them through it. Henry was very hands-on, but the nurses bore the brunt of it.'

'And now?' drilled Benway.

'Well, I'm clean, but what's truly amazing is I don't even think about it. I even look forward to sparkling water. Before I couldn't get out of the house without a whisky breakfast.'

'You don't think about it?' repeated Benway, vaguely recalling something Dent had said.

'Not at all. It's quite remarkable,' said Tiger Tim. 'Unless, like this, I try and remember. I really don't know how to explain it.'

'Try,' said Benway.

'Er, well, I suppose I'm referring to what some call "craving"? It was as if there was this dripping tap in my head. A drip that I couldn't turn off. Before apomorphine only booze worked. And when that wore off, and the hangover subsided, back came the drip. It began to affect everything, my relationships, my health; I couldn't concentrate, I had panic attacks. My work suffered.'

'What's that?'

'Publishing. Oh, and that's the other thing Henry mentioned. He said something about you having written a book. He thought I might be able to help.'

'Who do you work for?'

'Macmillan.'

'Macmillan?!' Benway sneered.

'Yes.'

'Man, they're square.'

'Oh yes! I suppose so. They certainly have *"standards"*, a reputation for traditional values, whatever they may be... er, which they like to uphold.'

'They'd never take me on,' Benway gripped his stomach under the bedclothes.

'Perhaps you're right. Still, they have a large readership and never rule anything out.'

'They'd make an exception for me.' Benway turned a wince into a snigger.

'Oh, why is that?' Maclean crossed his arms.

The patient finally looked at his visitor, small creases softening the hard stare. 'Well...' he dragged out the words as long as possible, 'I'm not the next Henry James.'

'Oh, ha, I see.' Maclean's amusement was stilted. 'No chance you'd adapt your style?' he probed.

'Country simple, NOPE,' confirmed Benway, rolling his eyes.

'Well, I think that clears that up.' Tiger Tim offered a thin smile to the unforgiving face, its cold eyes and thin lips. He shuffled uneasily; the hostility was killing him. 'You see, er, there's a moral backlash at the moment against anything risqué.' He glanced at his old bed, at the American's long face turned to the ceiling. 'P-p-publishers reflect the m-mood rather than challenge it,' he faltered. 'A st-stultifying atmosphere at the heart of mainstream publishing, I cannot deny it. I am sorry... but there it is.'

Benway finally responded. 'You're apologising to me for what you do?'

'Well, er... it's just, er... p-policy. I agree, it's a shame. Only progressive writers endure, unlike the page-turners usually favoured by Macmillan. Of course, there's a stable of "serious" writers; Yeats, Hardy and so on. Unfortunately, we also have a spoiling editor whose sole job is to keep us from ending up in court. He knows nothing about literature but everything about the law. That's the reality, I'm afraid.'

'Oh dear,' sneered Benway, 'what a calamity.'

Maclean heard a noise from the landing and looked optimistically towards the door. The room had become airless.

Benway turned on his side, the bed creaked. He didn't care for this intrusion, least of all from a jerk who, in normal circumstances, he'd avoid like the plague. However, he was starved of company and there was that worry... the one about himself. Without turning his head he spoke as if addressing the wall. 'Do you think that Doc Dent is put off ... I mean ... by me?'

Tiger Tim reacted immediately. 'Oh my goodness, no. Not at all. Henry has no side, one of the least judgmental characters you could ever meet.' Benway stirred while the intruder elaborated. 'When I came here I was a bit worried about that, too. You see, I've had – well... let's say certain "issues" in my life... but he's genuinely not bothered; which is a relief because it is the only thing that some want to bang on about...'

Benway finally studied his visitor. 'How well-known is he?'

'How do you mean?'

'Medically.'

'Oh, I see. Well, it's hard to say, no doctor can advertise, of course. The Medical Council is quite clear about that. And after you leave here you're honour bound not to broadcast his name either. Frightful conservatism again, I'm afraid. Still, Henry is always busy, gets lots of private referrals.'

'But he's, I don't know, "*establishment*"?'

Tiger Tim suddenly realised that even for an American much gets lost in translation. He uncrossed his arms and laughed. 'Oh my word no, not at all. He's not even a real Londoner. I tease him about that. His family roots are from the North of England, Lancashire, I think.'

'I thought he was... I dunno, Ivy League?'

Tiger Tim carried on laughing. 'As if! I suppose it must be difficult to judge these things. Some of his patients are certainly upper crust, but Henry? Anything but. More of an outsider looking in, I'd say.' Tiger Tim finished off his tea. 'Henry actually exploits the wealth of some patients so that he can extend his care to those less fortunate. He's quite open about it and it seems to work. Indeed, I think he's right because clearly addiction can affect anyone. When you're a bit better and you get the chance you should talk to him about it. He has some great stories; a few are in his memoirs. There was a copy lying around when I was in, helped pass the time. Ask Kate if you can't find it and you're interested.'

Benway let the information settle for a few seconds. He recalled the young man who'd helped him with his coat at Dent's house... and those piles of books.

'What's he read?'

'Well, I'm supposed to be the expert but I can't outdo him. He was a founding member of the disbanded Left Book Club; moved in that circle I believe. An avid reader of Swift, er... Kipling, Wells, Joyce, you name it, but his favourite is Sterne.'

'Sterne?'

'Yes, Laurence Sterne, another Irish genius, non-linear satire with a strong ethical focus. He was a parson, I believe. Brilliant flights of fancy with all manner of references, Cervantes, Rabelais. Everything was fair game, no plagiarism then. Not to everyone's taste and a bit, er, bawdy for some... but that's exactly what appeals to Henry. He loves all that lampooning of humbug and hypocrisy. Nothing amuses him more or gives him greater pleasure, nothing.'

Benway lifted himself up so he could get a better view of his visitor. He was intrigued by the deep impression that Doc Dent had clearly made on this young man.

For his part Tiger Tim was happy to have found his register. 'There is perhaps one other thing that gives Henry greater pleasure,' he added.

'What's that?'

'That his patients should become ex-patients.'

'Oh yeah,' Benway wheezed, 'I'm trying.'

HARDY TREE

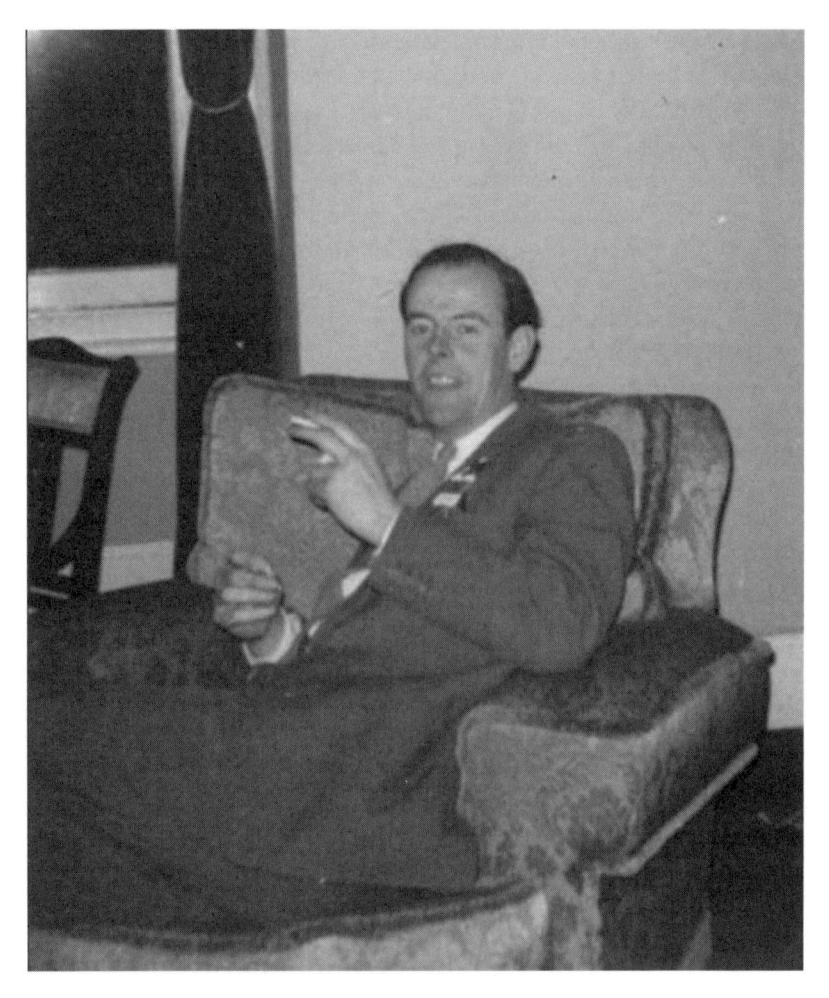

Alan Maclean (1924–2006) a successful literally editor who tried to revisit Dent's medical initiatives in the late 1960s. Burroughs responded with 'Academy 23' which eventually found its way into *The Job: Interviews with William Burroughs* (Jonathan Cape Ltd) 1970. (photographer unknown)

'You know, I even recommended Henry to my boss, which if you think about it was a risk... but he hasn't looked back, either... had it much worse than me, too.'

'Who else has he treated?'

'Ah, I've spoken out of turn... please, if you want to stay on the right side of Henry do not ask him that. I asked him about an ex-patient once and he nearly bit my head off. I think it is the only thing guaranteed to upset him.'

'This confidentiality business.'

'Exactly, mum's the word. He's fiercely protective of the patient's right to privacy. He'll never divulge anything unless it's remedial.'

'Got it.' Benway looked towards the window, trying to remember what else had struck him about Dent; his easy going hospitality, his thick warm hands, that voice... and Ulysses the cat... and book. What was it about Joyce? The language for sure... He dug that. Somebody had said that *Junkie* could do for addiction what Orwell had done for poverty... maybe. He had little to say, and structure worried him, he couldn't concentrate for five minutes on that... if only...

Tiger Tim stood up and returned his empty mug to the bedside table. 'So what are you writing... I mean, what are you hoping to publish?'

'Oh, I don't know; first thing is to get through this.'

'You will, I am sure,' said the young editor, trying to be encouraging. 'You're in good hands, the best.'

Another stab of pain, more jagged this time, ripped into Benway's guts. Tiger Tim noticed and both men were relieved when Dent returned, carrying a small case which he plonked on the table before sitting down to survey the younger men. He appeared engrossed in thought when suddenly he started to chuckle. He checked himself before diving in at the deep end.

'Well, you two don't have to like each other, you know? Typically boozers despise junkies and vice versa. The popular view is that neither group would ever stoop so low as to end up in the other's shoes.' Dent hesitated before expanding his reasoning. 'Think about it.

In reality you share so much. Your drug environments may have been different but that's all there is to it. Sober you can't tell one addict from another. However, what is certainly true is that you're both stigmatised by society so there should be no need to take it out on each other.' He paused; his eyes shining mischievously.

The two men shifted uncomfortably. The old doc had unmasked them and Benway regretted his earlier aloofness.

Tiger Tim responded first. Numerous fraught 'editorials' at Macmillan had left him with the necessary skills. He spoke in his usual urbane manner. 'Oh, we're all right, Henry. We've established that Macmillan is just too concerned with maintaining its reputation as a mainstream publisher. There's hell to pay if anything even vaguely obscene slips through. We're just too bloody dull to embrace progressive talent and to his credit, Dr Benway isn't going to change his tune to suit the mood; why on Earth should he?'

'He shouldn't,' said Dent. 'Too many lazy scribes as it is. We deserve better but most are just hacks, ruined by journalism and hardly independent. Others just echo groupthink, the stuffy verbiage of their canteen colleagues. Look at the BBC. It's hardly objective despite what it claims. No, more than ever, we need writers with guts and imagination; cheerleaders for a civilised world, not pot-boiling makeweights.'

'Amen to that,' wheezed Benway.

'I am certain something will come up,' said Dent. 'Isn't Penguin awaiting the verdict on *Lady Chatterley's Lover*? Poor Lawrence, two "cunts" and a "John Thomas" and he had to emigrate.'

The young men laughed as one and Dent, pleased by the reaction, continued to hold forth.

'The state wants to ration morality in the same way it did butter and bacon in the war. If they could install slot meters on bedposts they'd commodify the orgasm. And as for an honest exploration of sexuality and its taboos? Forget it! Half of our moral arbiters are still convinced of the virgin birth and the rest whisper about "birds and bees". Where does that leave us?'

'Beggary or buggery,' commented Benway.

'Ha! Yes, exactly,' roared Dent, thrilled by the language. 'And those

BUFFOONS TALKING BOLLOCKS

girls downstairs getting marital advice from confirmed celibates. Buffoons talking bollocks.'

Laughter swelled the room, barely ceasing when Kate entered.

'Ah! Do come in, Gibbie,' said Dent. 'Things are in danger of getting out of hand.'

'And I'd better be getting along,' said Tiger Tim, taking his cue.

He shook hands with everyone while offering further encouraging words to Dr Benway and left.

Dent concentrated on the charts. 'How are we doing, Dr Benway, any changes?'

'Comes and goes,' the patient said drily. 'Still a lot of pain, exhausted.'

'Well, I'm delighted by your progress... but if you wouldn't mind I'd like you to have a saponic. Kate?'

Kate met Benway's gaze. 'I think that would be a very good idea; I am sure it will relieve you of your stomach cramps. You'll find it easier to rest and it'll restore your appetite and in turn your energy.' She went out.

'Saponic?' asked Benway.

'An enema,' said Dent. 'We refer to it as "saponic". It's a litre of warm, soapy water flushed through your lower colon, to clear you out. When I was a student during the First World War, diets were particularly poor and so saponic enemas were commonly used in the maternity wards and military hospitals... I remember a mad surgeon who insisted on water for the infantry but champagne for the officers. Don't worry; we'll stick to water. We start with a single litre followed by two litres a day or two later... to get to the upper reaches... the upper or large colon. It always works, is perfectly safe and will banish your stomach cramps.'

Kate returned carrying an apparatus that included a rubber hose connected to a hot water bottle. Benway studied the contraption.

She held up the long end of the hose pipe which was connected to an ivory-coloured penile shape. It was about five inches long. 'Do you think you'll manage?' she asked.

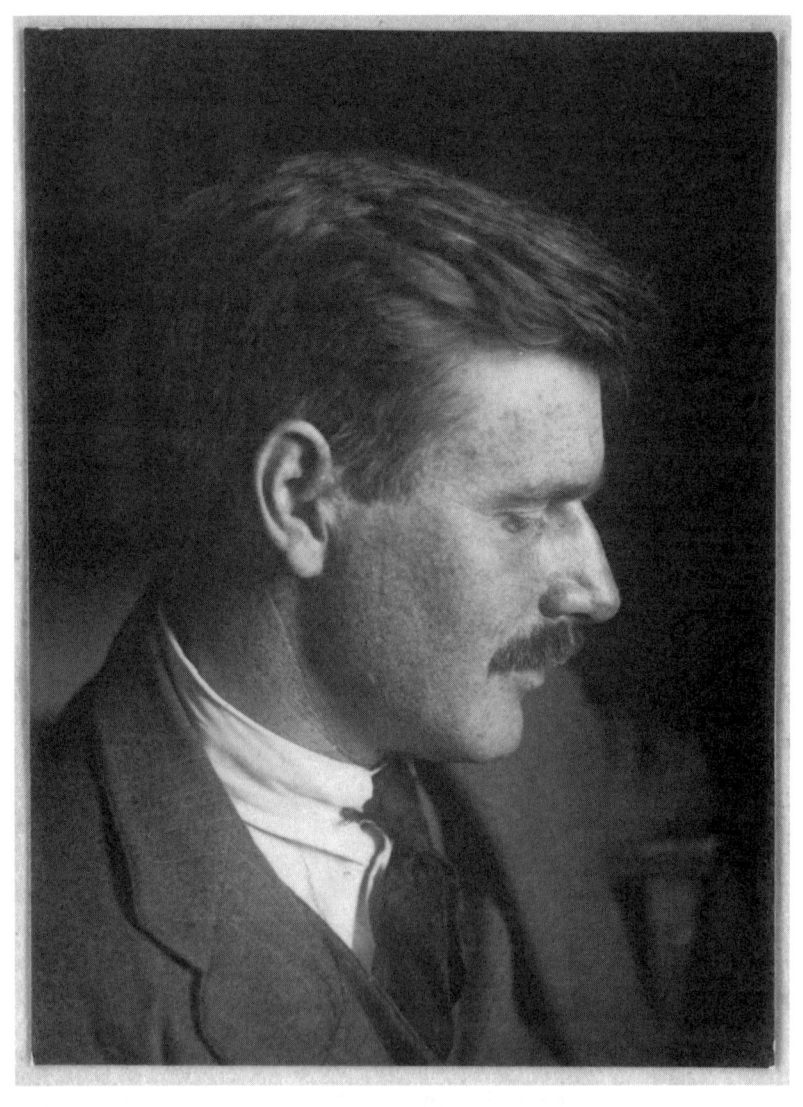

John Yerbury Dent aged 31.
The photograph was taken by his wife, Alma Langford Dent, *née* Broadbridge.

11

St Pancras, Poor Law Infirmary, 1918

We have wondered since times historic
If ale makes a man melancholic?
But it's now my belief
That sadness and grief
Turns the boy into yon alcoholic.
   – Anon.

It was 1918 and the world was still at war. John Yerbury Dent had recently got married and been appointed resident First Assistant Medical Superintendent at St Pancras Hospital (South) with an annual salary of £300. He looked at the list; two hundred patients at risk of Spanish flu and only six vaccines. 'Six!' he repeated out loud. He glanced across the doctors' mess at his old friend and colleague, Dalton.

'Can you help me?' Dent asked.

'No can do, sorry,' Dalton replied, in the middle of rooting through a cupboard in search of a clean overall. 'I'm due in surgery after the meeting. There's procedures all day. I'll be in until evening.'

Dent weighed up his options. He could give the vaccines to the worst sufferers, the ones with the highest temperatures or, to the ones most likely to survive. He consulted his friend.

'Who out of the two hundred are most likely to benefit from the vaccines? The most advanced cases or the relatively young and stronger ones?'

Dalton pulled on an overall stained with dried blood. He stopped buttoning the garment. 'I'm really sorry, Dent, I have no idea. And I doubt anyone else has either; there's no advice to be had from the Chief other than "do the best you can".'

He did up the last button. 'There, how does that look?'

Dent looked at the rich ochre stain which ran from Dalton's lapel to his midriff. 'There must be a cleaner one?'

'There isn't and I've been to the laundry; nothing doing.'

'Turn it inside out,' Dent suggested.

'Genius,' said Dalton, sarcastically. 'You're such an asset.'

'And you look an ass.'

'Ah, that reminds me. The Christmas play, we've been volunteered to be the pantomime cow, and I've bagged the head, no ifs and buts.'

'Wonderful,' said Dent.

'You'll love it; you get udders to swing and a tail to wag.'

'What I've always wanted... though, isn't Master Cameron the one who needs a tail?'

'How d'you mean?'

'Well Man gave up his tail and learnt to smile, something Master Cameron has yet to, er, master.'

Dalton took off his coat and looked at the inside. 'Yes, the miserable bastard, just one of several aspects of evolution to pass him by.'

The door opened and a third young doctor entered, wiping sleep from his eyes.

'Morning, Doohan,' said Dalton.

'Morning, gentlemen. Christ Almighty, Dent, you look terrible.'

'He's not getting enough sleep,' said Dalton.

'I told you, Dent, about sleeping *above* the job.' Doohan let the point hang for a moment. 'Never a good idea,' he continued. 'How many hours did you get last night?'

'Not many.'

'Well, I can see that,' stressed Doohan. 'We want you to leave the job on time not on a stretcher.'

'Sshh!' said Dent, holding his finger in the air. Dalton and Doohan cocked their ears to catch a long wail from the corridor.

'Who's that?' asked Dalton.

'Agnes from the Mental Ward. Tertiary syphilis, I'm afraid. She tried to bite one of the nurses and has to stay in the cell until there's transport to Hanwell.' Dent paused. 'You see, even when I get to bed we have to listen to her screams floating up the stairwell. My wife calls her "our nightingale".'

'So when are you going to get your own place?' asked Dalton. 'I get eight hours' sleep every night, but even that isn't enough.'

'Yes,' said Dent, 'but they need a "live-in" more than ever now.'

'All those drunks?' asked Doohan.

'Undoubtedly,' answered Dalton. 'So many soldiers invalided out. Situation gets worse daily.'

Dent lit a cigarette. 'Do you think if judges lived above prisons they'd be less likely to impose custodial sentences?'

'Come again?' asked Doohan, sitting down and helping himself to a Player's.

'Well, if judges and magistrates had to confront the consequences of their judgements in the same way as a live-in doctor has to confront the consequences of disease would they think twice?'

'Steady on!' exclaimed Dalton, 'they struggle with once.'

Doohan's face lit up. 'What a good idea! It might get the fools to realise that imprisonment doesn't help.'

'All gaols could be built with "Judges' quarters". Their bedrooms above the execution chamber,' suggested Dalton, warming to the theme.

'Well, I was thinking about this listening to poor Agnes last night,' continued Dent. 'It struck me, you see, that medicine is in some ways just as bad as the law... this "lock 'em up and throw away the key" view is perpetuated by our attitude towards the mentally ill as much as it is towards the hardened criminal.'

Doohan sat back. 'My word, Dent, that doesn't make us look good.'

'The government is worse though,' added Dalton. 'I was in the boozer last night and there was this captain from the Machine Gun Corp. He looked a bit down and the barmaid was giving him the glad eye, you know, the usual chitchat: "What was it like, our brave boys", and so on. Well, he was soon well-oiled and then it all came out. His vitriol for the top brass shocked everyone. Told us his medals counted for nothing. Then some tactless clot suggested that the government would sort it out. Well, for the captain that was the last straw. "Lying bastards!" he shouted and burst into tears. We left the pub feeling very down.'

'My hope is,' said Dent, 'that society can learn from all this folly. It is no use saying "never again", if we aren't able to change.'

'What would you do?' asked Doohan.

'For a start I wouldn't put the mentally ill in padded cells. It lacks compassion,' said Dent.

'But that's hardly a change, is it?' Doohan pressed.

'It'd be a start,' Dent volunteered. 'Change can only be measured by small acts which eventually become normal.'

'In the meantime,' added Dalton, 'we're considered unpatriotic if we don't "do our bit". The war is destroying us but our compliance perpetuates the destruction. We're only having this discussion because it's private. Out there we politely drop all these thoughts into that padded cell marked "denial". We should be shouting our outrage from the rooftops.'

'You're right,' agreed Dent. 'The hospital doesn't have enough drugs or staff because everything goes to the Front, and now, because of the huge number of displaced people, we have a pandemic on our hands and St Pancras is expected to stem the tide with six vaccines.'

'Six?!' exclaimed Doohan.

'Over twenty deaths last week,' grumbled Dalton. 'The orderlies cannot catch up on burials.'

'I know what I'm going to do,' said Dent, clapping his hands. Dalton looked up, 'Yes?' he enquired.

'I'll give the six vaccines to those we assess to be critical and a saline solution to the other 194. That way nobody will accuse me of favouritism and who knows, the others may get better due to improved expectations…'

Before Dent could get a response Matron Skehan burst in, holding the door open for Master Cameron. He marched in, followed briskly by a pair of orderlies who threw two huge files on the table.

'Strong brew, please, two sugars, snappy,' the master ordered.

One of the orderlies leapt over to the hob to check the level of water in the kettle. He muttered something before disappearing back into the corridor. The master sat down and took out his pipe and pouch of tobacco.

'Righty right, gentlemen. Please be seated. Ashby, notes please. Thank you. What day is it?'

'30th October, sir.'

'All Hallows' Eve, sir,' ventured Matron Skehan cheerfully, pushing a wisp of hair under her bonnet.

'Day of the damned week, I mean.'

'Wednesday, sir.'

'Are we agreed, Dent?'

'Yes, sir, all day long, 'tis Wednesday.'

'Good, then we agree about something, Dent.'

'Is there anything we don't agree upon, sir?'

'Yes, Dent, there most certainly is. These admission forms, you're still not filling the damn things in.'

'What's that, sir?'

'Oh Dent! You know bloody well. Where it says 'religion'. You have to find out the religion of every single patient. The Home Office demands it.'

'But to what purpose, sir?'

'It's an official requirement and part of your job.'

'Well, sir, if you don't mind my saying, it's a perversity.'

'What?! It's your duty.'

'I have no duties, sir, just responsibilities.'

'What's the damned difference?'

'Duty is what a soldier or sailor does. Doctors have responsibilities, to their patients.'

'What rubbish!'

'Not rubbish, sir. I have a responsibility to care for my patients. And if these forms have negative medical consequences then, by insisting on their completion, I would be failing in my responsibilities, wouldn't I?'

'You've lost me, Dent.' The master pulled out his pouch of tobacco and started to scrape clean the bowl of his pipe.

'I think I can help,' Doohan interrupted.

'Shut up, Doohan. The day I ask for your help will indeed be a desperate day for Christendom.'

Orderly Ashby failed to quell a laugh and drew a withering look from the master, who banged his clenched fist on the table.

'What you all fail to grasp is that the Home Office has become aware of this hospital's shortcomings.' The master's voice began to shake. 'Your failings Dent have become an enormous w-waste of time and now everyone is irritated. But what's insufferable is that the blame is being laid at my door! Mine! *This* arrived yesterday.'

Master Cameron slapped a large official-looking envelope in front of Dent.

'Yes! A letter which threatens disciplinary measures if we persist in this failing. A lamentable state of affairs and shameful for St Pancras.'

Doohan raised his hand to speak.

'What is it, Doohan?'

'A dent in the honour of the hospital, sir?' he suggested.

'Exactly!' exclaimed Cameron rising to the bait, 'St Pancras is justifiably very proud of its record throughout the war. Our support for the unity of the nation had remained undiminished. We simply cannot be seen to cause any additional problems for the government. Lord knows they've more than enough on their plate. SO, explain yourself, Dent, because this has to stop. Do you hear? STOP!'

The three doctors stirred. Doohan buried his mirth in his hands. Dent was caught between wondering whether he should make more capital out of Master Cameron's stupidity or defuse the situation entirely.

'Well, certainly, sir. I am delighted to be given the opportunity to explain myself. Once everything is subject to your legendary common sense I am sure all will become clear.'

Dalton squeezed his nose as hard as he could until his eyes watered. Dent continued:

'As we all know we have a great many military personnel coming to the hospital. They have endured an arduous journey, some are grievously wounded and in great pain. In admissions the form requires name, rank and religion. When I get to the third part, religion, they invariably hesitate and become distressed. They answer: "Am I as bad as that?" Of course, I could beat about the bush. I could say, it's just a simple question, or, we want to know if you'd prefer fish on Friday. But I'm afraid this never allays their suspicions. They say, "I'm dying, aren't I?" Even if I strenuously deny this, it is too late. The expectation of death rather than any hope of recovery has consumed them and the forthright ones say: "You want to know where to bury me." Now this, sir, is the proof of the failure of my responsibility as a doctor because in too many cases it becomes a self-fulfilling prophecy. So, in my capacity as a doctor, I have vowed never to place my responsibilities to the State, Crown or Church above those of my patients. Are we clear, sir?'

'Perfectly put, Dent,' said Doohan.

'Doohan!' roared the master, throwing down his pipe and pointing at the door. 'Get out! And you Dalton, what are you sniggering for? Get out the pair of you, seditious louts.'

'SIR!' interrupted Matron Skehan. 'We're here for a ward briefing; we need the doctors, surely.'

'Oh, I know that! Damn this bloody place. Full of Communists...'

Doohan and Dalton stood, hesitating.

The matron signalled they should sit down.

'Your last chance, I warn you,' said the master.

He shuffled the papers, reorganising them, retrieved his pipe, adjusted his spectacles and scratched his ear. When he had finished he looked up.

'Right, Dent, regrettably your explanation holds no water, none whatsoever. This is your last chance.' He held the bowl of the pipe in his hand and jabbed its stem straight at Dent. 'If you persist I will have no alternative but to fire you, is that clear?'

'Perfectly, sir. Shall I save you the trouble by leaving now?'

'What do you mean?'

'Well, my mind is made up. I have no intention of failing in my responsibility to these poor fellows. As I have explained, recording a patient's religion only adds to their suffering. And that is NOT my job.'

'But, damn you, the government demands it!'

'They also demand conscription in order to prosecute a ridiculous war but here, within the hospital, medical matters should prevail.'

'Bloody hell, Dent, you're impossible. Very well, I accept your resignation.'

'I'm not resigning,' informed Dent in a matter-of-fact manner.

'Sir!' cried the matron. 'You cannot do this. We're overstretched as it is.'

'We'll find a replacement,' said the master dismissively, opening a sheaf of papers.

'You'll have to fire me,' continued Dent.

'You're fired,' announced the master.

'No, Master! I won't allow it!' exclaimed the matron, her eyes popping out of her head. 'Please! What on Earth do you think you're doing? Dr Dent and I have to inoculate Wards One, Two and Three… all of them *this* afternoon. That is two hundred patients. We cannot afford not to – not for a minute longer.'

'Get somebody else,' said the master, stuffing his pipe with tobacco.

'For crying out loud, WHO? We're struggling by on half the required number as it is. All available doctors are immediately pressed into active duty… you know this better than anyone.'

The matron stood and drew herself up to her full height.

'And another thing, Master,' she said. 'If Dr Dent goes I go too… Now! Right NOW!'

'Matron Skehan, please! Please, sit down,' insisted the master. 'What about my authority?'

'Your authority should be to do your best for this hospital and its patients,' rejoined the matron. She seemed taken aback by her own forwardness.

ST PANCRAS, POOR LAW INFIRMARY, 1918

The door opened and the orderly entered with a tray of steaming mugs. Cameron's face lit up. 'Ah, jolly good. I don't know about any of you but I'm bone dry.'

He leant back, permitting the orderly to place the tray on the table. With his left hand he pulled his watch from his waistcoat and wound it before clicking it open to check the time. As the mugs of hot tea were handed round, he scribbled a quick note on a large sheet of paper. He folded this neatly, four times before secreting it away inside his wallet.

'AHEM! Righty right, everyone. Please sit down, Matron. I've been forced to consider many pressing issues this morning and have decided to refer this whole matter to the Board of Guardians. I will recommend that they take the necessary disciplinary measures against Dr Dent. Until then you, Dent, and the Guardians, can deal with the Home Office directly. I will inform the Chairwoman myself, and any future correspondence on form-filling will be directed to you. You can explain yourself to Whitehall and you will keep me and the rest of the hospital out of it. If that means carrying the can, so be it. Is that clear?'

'Perfectly, sir,' assured Dent. 'And do I take it, therefore, that I am temporarily free to conduct my responsibilities as I see fit and that, at least in principle, you accept my position?'

'Err, yes... until the Guardians state otherwise, and believe me, Dent, they will.'

The atmosphere in the room adjusted to the inevitability of bureaucratic menace. The master lit his pipe with loud sucking noises and disappeared behind a billowing cloud of smoke as Matron Skehan finally sat down. The thrust and counter thrust of the early stages of the ward meeting were familiar but today Dent had to accept the new threat to his livelihood. He caught the flicker of warning in the matron's eyes and felt the covert pat on the back from Doohan. Normally he would have accepted these tiny signs of encouragement without concern but the brewing confrontation with officialdom made him uneasy. He would struggle to find a new job without references and he'd have to find new accommodation... immediately. He disliked the master intensely, his depressing lack of imagination, his frigid, paper-shuffling mannerisms. Perhaps he should accept that handling this ponderous fool had provided a lustful motivation. A motivation that had sprung from his frustration at the national predicament. Master Cameron, felt Dent, symbolised much that was wrong with the nation's sensibility, its stultifying, hidebound idiocy that perpetuated aggression and nationalism. They would always be at loggerheads; this was just a short reprieve. Dent's thoughts were interrupted by Cameron rapping the table with his pipe.

'Righty right, gentlemen! We must press on. Matters arising from last week, Ashby? Read from the minutes, will you? Oh, *do* come on, you're as slow as a turtle in a winter four-ball...'

* * *

Half an hour later weak sunlight had begun to dry the condensation running down the walls in the south wing. A small group of medical staff entered the Receiving Ward to start the round of every bed in the hospital. There had been four deaths that night including a suicide offset by three births. The hospital never had enough beds. Patients slept on the floor or in the corridors and with the flu epidemic there had been a higher than usual number of admissions. One new case in particular drew Dent's attention.

'Name?' asked Matron Skehan.

'Ruth Rose, twenty-five years old,' answered the attendant nurse.

Dent studied the young woman. Her thick auburn hair framed a pretty face though her staring eyes were red and swollen. She was evidently unconscious.

'Any information?' he asked.

'Not much.... Her mother brought her in in the very early hours. Seems that last night she came home from work with a swollen eye and complaining of a headache.'

'And upon admission, did you notice anything else about Ruth?'

'She was delirious when she got 'ere. She had spasms but in the last couple of hours she's just drifted off. An' now she's burnin' up. I tried to get some water in her but it comes straight back. She don't like being touched.'

Dent listened to Ruth's chest and back with his stethoscope. He couldn't hear any obstruction. It was a process of elimination.

'Not sure,' he murmured, more to himself than anyone in particular.

'Right,' he said, 'can we move her to the end bed. Straight away, please. I'll need to take a sample.'

A nurse spoke to the orderly who marched to the far end of the ward.

'And erect a screen, I'll return to her as soon as I can,' Dent added.

The small group then proceeded with the ward round.

Within fifteen minutes Dent was again looking down at Ruth. He turned her over and drew a bloody sample of pus from her spine. He held up the syringe for the matron to see and for the second time that day they exchanged glances. This was the look of resignation. Ruth Rose's case was hopeless. Acute spinal meningitis meant she'd be dead within a matter of hours.

The matron spoke briefly to the sister and nurses and left to help Dalton and Doohan in surgery. Dent, however, stayed behind. He was fascinated by Ruth's staring eyes. He sat down on the side of the bed and peered into them. He got closer. They floated like mirrored orbs reversing the light from every corner of the ward. They appeared to be protruding more now that he knew what was wrong. And they would float like this, bejewelled light catchers until she died. At that moment Dent made up his mind that he would be looking at the back of her eyes at the moment of her death.

He went downstairs and brought up a self-illuminating ophthalmoscope. He arranged the attachments on the bed cover, looking at her eyes in expectation. It was more than interesting; he was captivated. As he settled down the loud voice of Chief Rowntree made him jump:

'DENT! What on earth are you doing?'

Dent pulled away and looked up.

'You shouldn't take the risk. No matter what. The damn thing is caught through the nose, you know that?!'

'Yes, Chief, I know. Thank you.'

Dent got up and proceeded to attend some patients in other wards but he couldn't take his mind off the prize that lay within his grasp. As he dealt with each case he checked the time. He was being compelled by a force greater than he understood. He'd be drawn back, no matter what.

As he worked he asked himself: 'What if I get there and she's gone, and I'm too late?' He calculated how long it would take to finish his shift. Then he'd dash back, nothing would stop him. He'd delve as far as possible into the fundus of Ruth's eyes...... until her death. He looked at the minute hand on the ward clock, just ten more minutes. He finished off; the decks were clear, finally he could escape.

He raced back down the stairs, pulling his instrument from his pocket. He pushed past a pair of nurses and in through the swing doors. The ward was quiet, too quiet. Drawing back the screen he couldn't tell if Ruth had died. She looked the same, those paralysed globes still fixed on the emptiness in front of her. He bent down and listened; she was alive! He returned the instrument to her pupil, searching for a point of focus. Suddenly it locked on. Before him lay the most sublime sight in creation, the inner eye floating like the filtered face of the sun. Excited, he turned the mechanism, pulling and pushing the arteries from the membrane that held them.

He gasped at the unfolding splendour and momentarily forgot where he was and what he was doing. Remembering, he pondered whether he should stop and take Ruth's pulse until he realised he was watching it. Feathery blood vessels vibrated clear against glimmering lakes of lava. Crimson and orange veils floated over folds first white... then purple... suspended in a void more magnificent than any man could ever see, or hope to see...

These were Ruth Rose's final moments and he would stay for them. He turned the dial till the front element almost touched the eye and the concertinaed heavens grew wider and more vast than even the night sky itself. There, stars are just pinpricks of light, but within the eye, light has every form, shape and gradation of colour. Bewitched, Dent pushed his eye down as far as possible. As he did so another horizon appeared, curving towards the first till their ends touched, enclosing the whole palpating cosmos. It shimmered, glowed and exploded; one last burst of life...

Then, as he peered, something happened. Small gaps appeared along the tentacled arteries. The tiny streams of blood broke into necklaces of ruby droplets that jerked with every slowing heartbeat...three, two, one...and then...stillness.

Almost imperceptibly, a gas-like mist crept from the corners like smoke under a door. It curdled into layers of yellowy fog before forming a thick cloud. In seconds everything was blotted out. Ruth Rose had died and now the eye itself was dead.

* * *

A week later Dent was finishing off his morning round.

'Dent, the Board of Guardians wants you,' said Chief Rowntree.

'Can it wait until the next "monthly"?'

'No, they want you now.'

'Now?'

'That's right, Dent, special convening, just for you. I'll cover, till you get back.'

Dent made his way across Euston Road to the Town Hall and up the two flights of stairs to the first floor. He knocked on the dark double doors.

'Come in!'

He entered the chamber, which was set out like a small court with a raised platform in the middle.

There were a circle of chairs and a few tables. People in dark suits were either sitting or standing in small groups.

'Ah! Dr Dent's here, ladies and gentlemen, ORDER!' shouted the Chairwoman.

All eyes turned to Dent, who stood inside the door, expectantly.

'Right, can we all be seated, thank you.'

There was a good deal of chair-scraping and commotion as everyone found their places.

The Chairwoman, who was almost completely deaf, shouted that Dent should step forward so she could 'see' him.

'Now then, Dent,' she continued, 'this extraordinary meeting has been called because it appears the Home Office is concerned about an administrative issue and sent a secretary, Sir Jacob Smeggore, to report on what has become a disciplinary matter. We have a quorum, as you see, but as we all have busy lives can we press on, thank you.'

She hammered down a gavel. 'ORDER, the meeting is now in progress. I call upon witness Dr John Dent to answer for his action. Doctor?'

Dent watched as the Chairwoman turned sideways and lifted her ear trumpet to her 'best' ear.

'But what action?' asked Dent, perplexed by the speed of events.

'Ahem.' There was a loud scrape from the back of the chamber as Master Cameron got to his feet. He put down his pipe and felt for his enamel and gilded Alderman's badge that hung from his neck and was reserved for such occasions. He turned the chain so that the resplendent pendant stood out against his dark blue waistcoat. He cleared his throat:

'I think I can help here, Chair. Just one week ago I told Dent that he should desist in omitting essential information on the admissions forms. He dreamt up a very unsatisfactory excuse, if I may say, and I was prompted, if I may add, to warn him that the consequences of his action were to be his and his alone. He accepted this arrangement, as I notified the Board at the "Monthly" on the first of November, last Friday, if you remember.'

'Yes, thank you, Master.'

'So, Dent, as you must now realise, things have come to a head. I need not remind you that the Nation and Commonwealth are still engaged in hostilities and this matter is inconvenient to all concerned. Unfortunately I am forced to inform you, Dent, that your position here at St Pancras is under review. What have you to say?'

Dent looked around the ring of stern faces.

'Thank you, Chair, I understand. Is the Home Office representative present?'

A rotund, uniformed gentleman clambered to his feet. 'Smeggore, Sir Jacob Smeggore at your service.' He sounded slightly irritated and, returning to his seat, resumed the preening of his very long moustache. Dent panicked. How should one address a 'Sir', he'd never met one... was it with the Christian name or surname?

'Er, thank you, Sir Smeggore, what seems to be the problem?'

'Speak up, Dent,' shouted the Chairwoman.

'I'm sorry. I asked, "WHAT IS THE PROBLEM"?'

'There's no need to shout,' screamed the Chairwoman.

This seemed to amuse some of the guardians.

'If I could be so bold, Chair?' volunteered Master Cameron, pulling himself up once more.

'Please, Master, carry on.'

'Well, Dent, of course, knows jolly well what the problem is. He's pleading ignorance because he's embarrassed. He has a duty to fill in the admission forms. A duty to the State, the Crown and all the defenders of our faith.'

'If I could intercede, Chair?' asked Dent.

'Please do ... and dispense with the formalities, we have little time.'

'Thank you. I should just like to say that in my capacity as a doctor at this hospital I put the needs of my patients above any *duties* that the master may think I have. Furthermore, I am certainly not embarrassed, not in the slightest.'

'Well, Dent you *still* have to answer to Sir Jacob; please, if you could get on with it.'

'Certainly, Chairwoman, but first I would like to ask you a question. If you were ill and needed an operation who would you like to conduct it, me or Sir Jacob?'

'Don't be silly, Dent, you, of course!'

'Well, exactly, and furthermore, filling in these forms is a medical matter because it has medical consequences. And therefore, as I will demonstrate, these sorts of decisions should be made by doctors, not civil servants.'

A faint murmur of understanding spread around the chamber. Dent continued: 'Now the master knows this as I explained it to him at the ward briefing last week ... as anyone can check from the minutes.'

The master went a peculiar shade of crimson which took some of the lustre from his badge.

'So I see,' said the Chairwoman, looking down at Cameron, who had begun to fidget with his pipe.

'But please, Dent, *we* still have *not* had the benefit of your medical

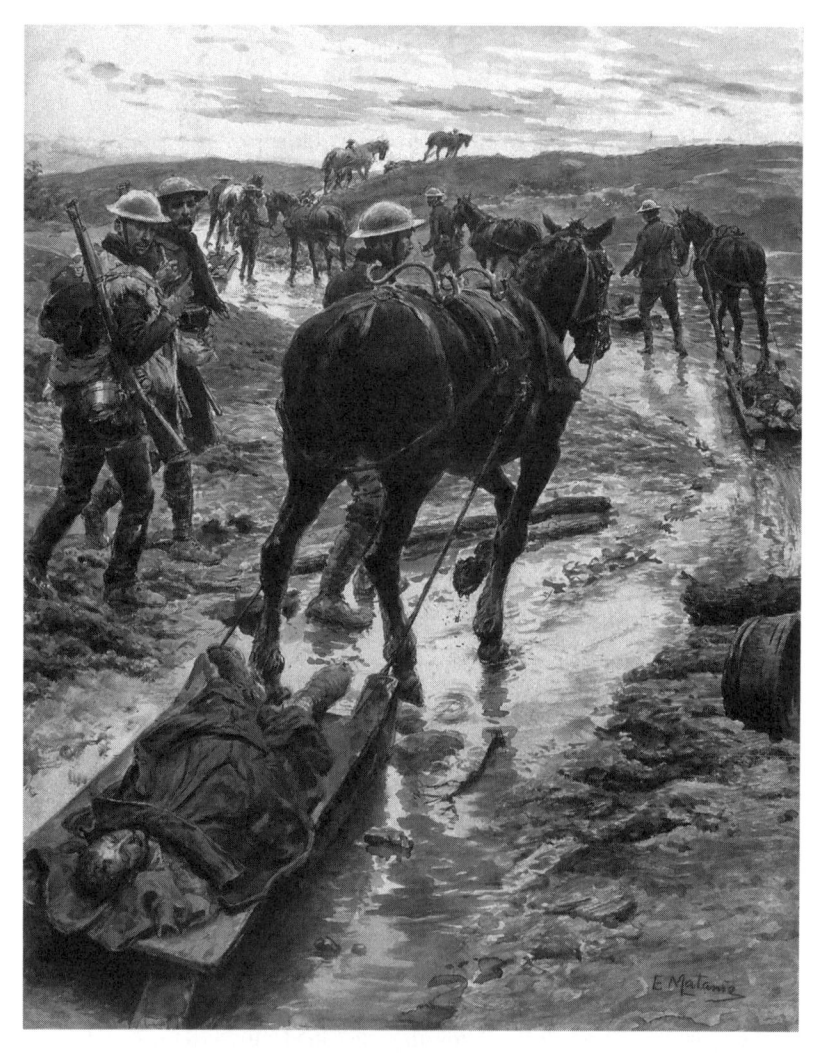

'They are wounded and have usually suffered a long and arduous journey...'
Grey wash by Ugo Matania (1888–1979), 1916.
[©Wellcome Collection]

expertise. Explain your position to Sir Jacob; I am sure he'd like to return to Whitehall with a bit of medical "know-how and make-do".'

'Certainly.' Dent turned towards the bristling face of the Home Office.

'Our noble servicemen, Sir Jacob, have served their country well as I am sure everyone here agrees.'

There was a rumble of agreement from the room.

'There have been many casualties but I am concerned with those *still* in need of medical care. They are often wounded and have usually suffered an arduous journey from far-flung corners of the Continent. Some are in extremis and require urgent, life-saving medical intervention. But, ladies and gentlemen, before I or any of the medical staff can help these poor men they have to attend what has become customary: the "heroes' welcome".'

The Chairwoman interrupted with a sharp rap of the gavel. 'Excuse me Dr Dent, but I would be interested to know if Sir Jacob has ever attended one of these events.'

'Of course,' he said in a presumptive voice, 'it is the very least I can do.'

'Ah,' said Dent, 'then you are part of the problem. You should know Sir Jacob that by meeting and greeting these grievously wounded soldiers you are prolonging their agonies.'

'Preposterous!' shouted Sir Jacob.

'Not so, Sir Jacob because what happens at St Pancras happens at every hospital in the land. Typically the stricken soldiers are arranged on stretchers along station platforms to be addressed by the Lord and Lady Mayor, the aldermen of the borough, a delegation from the Salvation Army and, if it is term time, local school children with bouquets of daisies and violets. After this, along with all their previous privations, they are often cold and are lifted to the Hospital Admissions and Waiting Hall where a religious service is conducted by whomever is available. It could be a visiting curate, a rabbi, vicar or priest but it has to be done because it is an obligatory part of the "heroes' welcome". This multi-denominational farce typically consists of hymns, prayers, a sermon, hymns, prayers and lastly, *more hymns.*

After this each man is individually blessed by whomever led the service. It is only then and at long last, that the wounded are released by the military into medical care. Here at St Pancras the hospital orderlies carry these men to me, whereupon I must fill in the admissions form. So, Sir Jacob when I get to the third question on the form, religion, they say: "Oh, I'm as bad as that, am I? ... You want to know where to bury me."'

Dent walked over to Sir Jacob and produced one of the Whitehall forms from his jacket pocket. 'The truth is, Sir Jacob,' he said, placing the form on the desk, 'the only honest way of filling in your bureaucratic question after such a travesty, isn't Protestant, Catholic, Hindu or Jew, it is *militant atheist*, is that what you want?'

The Chairwoman was seen to smile broadly. She had often been forced to conceal her left-leaning tendencies in the face of the patriotic idiocy which had brought Europe to its knees. She knew too that this had been stoked equally by the religious and political establishments in both Britain and Germany with little thought of the consequences.

'Is that all, Dr Dent?' she asked, hoping that it was not.

Dent, invigorated by his own performance, was on a roll.

'No, Chairwoman, it certainly is *not*. Whilst we have a member of the Home Office here, I would like to ask him if, in light of the sacrifice these men have made and the impact this will have on the rest of their lives, can the Home Office indicate what provision it will recommend to the government ... to make good? And I speak in particular of the men who have had their minds so grievously damaged by the brutality of war. In other words, what compensation will be made to these poor men for their enduring losses?'

'Whatever do you mean?' asked Sir Jacob, his temples throbbing with indignation.

'Well, sir, it is clear to me that in prosecuting the war the state has encouraged madness because out there, in the trenches, it is only the mad that can survive.'

'What nonsense.'

'How is this nonsense? If a man operates machinery or a train when he is drunk and incapable he is dismissed. And yet when men are in charge of sophisticated weapons of war they are not discouraged from having beer or spirits with their rations. And just before they go "over the top" they get double Dutch courage. This custom is widely practiced, which, as your medals indicate, you must know.'

'What of it?'

'The consequences, sir, *that* is the "what of it". Because of the brutality of your war these men are stupefying themselves with alcohol. They develop a thirst for the stuff. So, even if they survive the bloodshed this habit can destroy their lives. They deserve a pension just as much as those who have lost a limb or contracted disease during service. I will be recommending a written report from the Guardians to the Home Office to this effect, but in the meantime, in *your* report to the Home Office, I trust you will be pleading the case of all these men so afflicted. Irrespective of their religion, it is certainly the *Christian* thing to do.'

A silence pervaded the room. All eyes turned to the voice of authority; the establishment and the aristocracy. Their representative, Sir Jacob Smeggore, was no longer twiddling his moustache. He'd come to witness a minor re-adjustment towards the moral authority of the Land that suddenly didn't have a leg to stand on. He slowly got to his feet, holding his chair for support.

'Thank you, G-g-Guardians. I will, of course, Lady Chairwoman, members of the B-b-board, be submitting my report to my office, as the doctor suggests. As to the matter of the third question on the admission forms I think the Home Office will consider this an anomaly, an internal dispute to be resolved as you see fit.'

He edged towards the door.

'As is normal in these circumstances a formal answer will be prepared and submitted in due course.'

He reached for the door handle but dropped his top hat.

'Thank you very much... for your time, er, Ladies, Gentlemen... and, er, Guardians.'

He turned and bowed slightly as he retreated through the door, closing it as he whispered a faint 'Goodbye.'

As the door shut there was a collective intake of breath. The

Guardians of St Pancras Hospital needed to take stock. Gradually the room found its voice and the murmurs rose to a tumult...everybody, bar Dent and Master Cameron, wanted to have their say. Some started to giggle nervously, one uncontrollably.

With no one to address directly the Chairwoman dropped her ear-piece and banged her gavel in a rare show of procedural contrariness. 'Order, ORDER! ORDER!!' she cried, craving the opposite.

Another alderman from the proud Borough of St Pancras, bowed by age and rows of medals, advanced unsteadily towards Dent.

'Inspiring, Dent, and – I speak for my fallen comrades – thank you.'

Tears were rolling down the old boy's face. Dent bent down to hear what he had to say.

'We fought hard to keep the old world going, and for what? For this?'

The old boy tottered as he lifted up his cane and scythed the air in an expansive sweep. Dent held him by his other arm.

'It's too late for me, Dent, but the new world has to get rid of the Sir Jacobs. They've virtually destroyed civilisation. There has to be an alternative.... It's up to you boys now, it's the only way.'

Dent squeezed the veteran's hand and looked up at the Chairwoman.

'Don't think the Home Office will be back in a hurry!' she bellowed.

Dent climbed the steps beside the lectern until he was level with her earpiece.

'Am I dismissed or shall I get back to work?' he asked.

'WORK! And omit the third question on admissions. Farcical any-way, as if God cares what bloody silly club we're in.'

As Dent walked back to the hospital he thought about the veteran soldier and whether the end of the Great War would herald change. It was one thing to identify the grudges of those who had sacrificed so much but change doesn't mean better. A young nurse ran past him, her pinafore soaked in fresh blood. Just inside the entrance two stretchers with bodies were left to be taken to the mortuary.

No, Dent thought to himself, people soon forget; that's what survival is, a process of forgetting. If we couldn't forget we'd be more tortured than we are.

There'll be more wars, more Sir Jacobs. Whitehall has played its part in prosecuting a ridiculous war by proclaiming God was in favour. That's why the State clings so resolutely to its self-proclaimed role as defender of faith...and insists on that third question on 'Admissions'.

'Hoodwinking manipulators...' he muttered to himself.

He turned a corner and walked straight into the arms and bustling form of Matron Skehan.

'Oh, look who it is,' she cried. 'Have you finished playing your "man of the people" routine?'

'You should have seen it, there wasn't a dry seat in the house,' said Dent.

'Sorry, but you're now required in a different theatre,' she said, smiling.

'Oh?'

'Surgery, I'm afraid. Chief Rowntree awaits your entrance, centre stage.'

'Thank you, Matron. Onwards and upwards, hey?'

As they advanced together she was relieved this storm in a teacup was over. She felt a warmth towards strong men; they stopped her from going mad, from falling apart.

Dent wondered if his belief in humanitarian values and the connection he felt to people like Matron Skehan would sustain him, prevent *him* from going mad, from falling apart.

He certainly liked the matron, they had much in common; more than they would ever know.

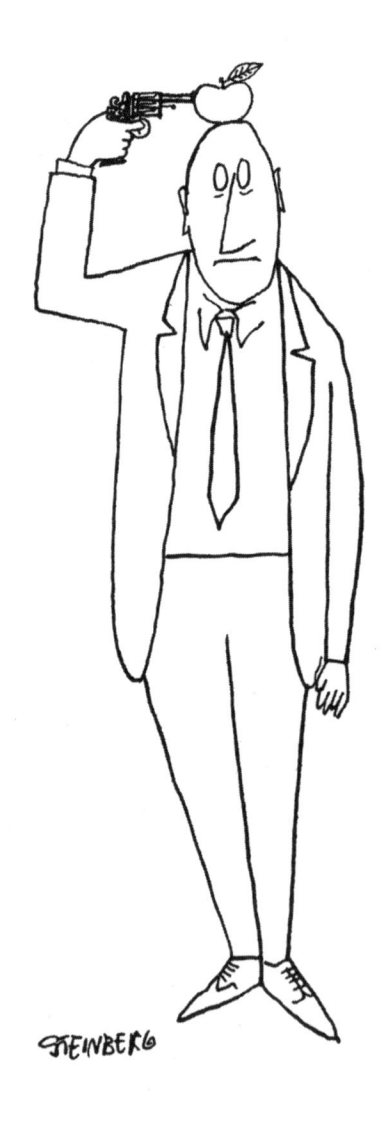

Saul Steinberg
The New Yorker Collection
[The Cartoon Bank]

12

Waking Suggestion

Three and a half days into his treatment Dr Benway lay in bed looking at the ceiling. Kate had just congratulated him for going a whole morning without asking the time. He thought about it...? Dammit, she's right... but why? Could it be due to being *off* 'junk time'? He ran through the umpteen cures he'd endured and the inevitable pain of withdrawal which had always got worse. This was the dread common to all junkies, accompanied by the endless figuring; how long before the fix wears off, how long before the monster must be fed?, how many hits have I got?, when is the farmacia open?... how much will I need?... how can I pay...? Before, when he'd tried to go cold turkey... or done the Chinaman's reduction cure, the first day was bearable but by the end of the second he'd be crawling up the wall... he'd kill to get fixed. But this time it'd gone the other way... the thing he'd feared most hadn't happened... it'd got easier instead of harder. Maybe it was time to consider the hope beyond hope... maybe there's something to this crazy old croaker after all, his soft ways and his apomorpheeen?

He waited till Kate popped out. He studied the charts... he'd gone from feeding the Chinaman between thirty-forty grains a day to virtually nothing... in a few days... he sure as hell couldn't be described as 'well' but something had changed... he felt, well... different? Offered morphine on the first day he'd bitten their hand off; now he could ponder resistance! This was extraordinary. He'd just gone nearly fifteen hours without any! He was taking vitamin B and now insulin but he'd had these before... antihistamines too... the only difference was apomorphine... the only thing... would it last?... It probably won't... 'Once I leave off apomorphine I'll need junk again... that'll be it... that's the rub... there's always a rub.'

He sat back against the pillows and scratched his stubble. Yesterday Hannah had given him several quarters of God's own. She was fussy with the needle... and so damn literal. 'When I trained as a nurse,' she had said, 'we practised injections on an orange.' Benway asked her if it had been a blood orange, but she just said 'Noo, it wasn't,' without a flicker. Kate was happier to discuss stuff. She returned with some milk and Marmite toast on a tray.

'How will I know?' he asked her.

'When the treatment begins to work?'

'Yeah.'

'As you must be tired of hearing, everyone is different. You might begin to dream more... or less. You may remember something that you gave up doing but suddenly want to do again... to think differently about the future... I cannot say.'

'You mean apomorphine changes my mind?'

'Oh good heavens no!' Kate's eyes widened behind her glasses as she looked up from the charts. 'Only you can do that.'

'How d'you mean?'

'Our patients initially seem unable to change their mind about anything even when they say they want to. Every belief is locked away in a safe and not even the patient knows the combination... I can talk to them until I'm blue in the face but nothing gets through. Then, with apomorphine, they start making the connections themselves, without prompting. I don't know how else to explain it. I have talked to Dr Dent about it several times. He says we can never know how the brain works but we can interpret behaviour. The more I see the more I recognise that he's right. As you settle down you're able to re-learn things. If those first signals are positive they help you. Dr Dent is a firm believer in this "start as you mean to go on" policy. We encourage whatever works for each individual... whatever leads to good habits.'

'A benign environment?'

Kate smiled. 'Yes, an environment that is supportive, definitely.'

Benway bit into his brown toast with Marmite. The taste was strong, he savoured it. He was dog-tired but since the enema he'd noticed his appetite had returned. He was looking forward to the milk.

Kate sat down beside the bed and Benway offered his wrist to begin the usual round of checks. His pulse was strong...regular, 70 beats a minute, breathing consistent, 20 per minute, temperature slightly elevated, 99.4...nothing to worry about. Oral and nasal administration of apomorphine reduced to every three hours...no sickness, less sweating. Benerva to be continued with small amounts of insulin. He was woozy when he sat up, lightheaded...'You're better off lying flat...resting,' Kate assured. 'By all means read...write...but better off in bed for the time being.'

Kate's presence reassured him. He had adjusted to his surroundings and the rhythm of the treatment. Initially he'd resisted Kate and Hannah...now he appreciated their company, their feedback.... It was evidence he could latch onto...the confirmation he needed that proved he was re-emerging like a butterfly from a chrysalis: changed. Kate watched him as he finished his milk and toast and arranged himself for the next dose of sub-emetic apomorphine pills. He looked as though he could fall asleep without them. This was another good sign...sure enough, he soon drifted off...once more into the land of withdrawal and apomorphine induced sleep...it wasn't all bad...this experience...far from it......

* * *

```
Bill Lee hurtled into space / adjusted headrest / watched land
recede / two horizons curved  until shimmering they collided
to ring the brown planet / shrinking to the size of a pebble
in 55 secs / walrus in HEADspace 'took' his hand / the
gentleness of the sub-vocal presence quite at odds with the
dreadfulness of the message
--There's been a viral contamination on Saturnalia / everybody
wiped out / MISSIONWipeout spared you / AITC reckons you're
the best bet after ancestral analysis / your credentials not
to be sniffed at - debased cruelty - compulsive drug use - sex
tourism - debauchery - white male privilege - homicide - niche
in counter-cultural radicalism / Quite a hand there Bill ...
```

—I'm a reluctant participant of a bullshit industry / Miles and Miles of it / trivialised and blabbed over like any other commodity spat Bill / I'm a writer for Chrissakes with ideas / turned into a faddist's freak show by lush workers
—Oh - yes smiled HEADspace / the bilge of smug frippery is partly why Artificial Intel/Toto Control lost patience with Homo sapiens / another reason was technology that widened disparities and cultivated irrationality / Nationalism and tribal passions whipped-up by the unspeakable destroyed the blue environment / AITC kept the species going because it could manipulate fear / recently even this characteristic disappeared / BETAplan is to vacate Mother Earth for 100 million years / to see if a co-operative organism can be tweaked into existence / Life is impossible above ground anyway / to this end AITC formed BIOsingularity which urged returning to the 2D gastrula stage / when the organism had only one hole for food and waste ...
Bill's epigenetic recall dialled up the coincidence of the old croaker's chair - Anguilla anguilla. HEADspace's steady voice continued to run the rule over the end of history ...
—AITC initially preferred ALPHAplan / that every brutal tendency could and should be wiped from the motherboard / this worked until it became obvious that being human relies on all its impulses / look at your social engineering exploits as evidence / clones gazing at their shoes all day / zombolicals devoid of creativity and motivation / a direct result of BIOlab progeny with no spasmodic mutation / personal identities started to disappear one by one / AITC now realise that the full spectrum of the human spirit can only return to the species by being begotten in the traditional manner ...
Bill Lee didn't care about the ins and outs of it and wondered when the lecture would end / there was some trash-lit to get through / he'd never held out much hope for humanity anyhow / to his annoyance HEADspace continued to flesh out the consequences of BIOlab progeny

—A small ELITEclass was the aim but after pre-modifying life
in vitro for generations it suddenly became clear that the
species had passed a tipping point / recently humanity lost
the Y chromosome altogether and every single cock with it
Bill heard a word he recognised / he looked up
—That's right Bill / a disaster of AITC's making / the female
of the species simultaneously became adrift from the mothering
instinct / now they haven't the foggiest / SOCIOlab has tried
everything - picture books - extra orifices - bribery -
sexbots / it seems the last hurrah for your species is coitus
with a degenerate / that is why you're here rather than
returned to Saturnalia / you and CAPA have been selected as
the dam-sires / AITC deduces there is no two better suited /
every agency is in awe of your repulsive villainy
Bill started fidgeting with his worry beads / he didn't like
the sound of this / Headspace would have to spell it out ...
—Yes Bill / you're going to have to perform with the boss /
Quite an irony - eh? Your special brand of deviancy the last
flip of the coin / the future of humanity in your hands / Well
- not there exactly but you get the idea / If you fail that'll
be it for mankind
—JEEEZE Doc / Bill gulped —How the hell do they expect me to
do the switcheroo? Have you seen CAPA recently / at least
seven decades minus gravity / bones all over the place / An
abomination without trace instinct, emotion or memory / this
is fucking horrendous
—I don't disagree
—No way
—You'll have to do your best
—Can you get me some Apo?
—Banned for two Earth centuries now / I'll see what I can do
Bill closed his long fingers round his face —What about my
freeze-dried seedlings?
—Lost in the system malfunction
Bill felt sick —Look this is impossible / do you hear me? /

futile / he spluttered / his air tube accelerated / InfoScreen flashed

TIME TO DOCKING — 12 EARTH MINUTES

Bill's desperation twisted his guts / hangers-on had boasted about his rich strains of depravity - addict - misogyny - queerness / none of it had hurt his reputation / it amounted to kudos / saved him from anonymity / as if they knew / now this / AITC needed him to save the gene pool / what a joke / he'd cry but no one left knew what tears were let alone how to dry them / Boy was he lonely / the last man standing / the last miserable intuit left ...

Somewhere between Mars and Jupiter CAPA who'd been conceived in a Petri dish 119 years ago - sat between glowing panels drumming prehensile claws upon the backsides of the interns sucking off anything worth upcycling / There wouldn't be much / carbon fibre intestines maybe or the pioneering holes that had qualified her for highest orifice / The blankness of the screens mirrored her temperament / She attributed it to being run down after an exhausting sojourn / she adored Chiantisphere but where had that vision of <u>harvest festival</u> come from? The idea that this was a <u>flash from the flesh</u> was too awful / Epigenes and imagination had been alien forever / their eradication deemed essential along with the humours / wit fancy eloquence / If they'd inexplicably re-surfaced via some methyl dysregulation ... She'd be unplugged / This wedding with ZyclonBILL had to bear fruit / that word <u>fruit</u> troubled her but why?
—<u>I must I must increase my bust, I do it for the boys not us</u> she chimed zealously, working what was left of her rib cage

VISITOR ARRIVED

the hologram glowed <u>deep-sea</u> phosphorescence / CAPA focussed on InfoScreen /

MR BILL LEE SIX P.M. INTERNAL TRANSIT

/ it blinked
A grin stretched her chops like a banana / few highlights these days / pale blue and mauve chequered the floor as <u>boudoir</u> was air-dropped along with <u>synth sandalwood</u> Bill's signature perfume / she indicated <u>acceptance</u> / A naked intern escorted Bill to the inner sanctum / Stripped of its personality and character all choice had fallen away with its wardrobe / logical
CAPA curtsied and held up the sagging side of her face /
——<u>Delighted</u> / she was progged to say
——Always delighted to serve / Bill lied embellishing the air with three signs of the zodiac
——Everyone knows you reach around Willy go the extra mile
CAPA was up-minded Bill's back catalogue / a hologram video of his day-glo Drone-disciples squirting the latest nitro-glysophate <u>roots and six legs</u> floated between them / She rubbed her palms together aping delight
——Nobody forgets <u>murdering molecules</u> she giggled / Further floods of recognition washed through her waste pipe / she danced the praying mantis
——Not only a neat slogan Billiam but a delightful solution to the <u>you know what</u> / a flicker of eye brightness momentarily gave the impression of feminine promise until the milky cloud swept back / half SPIDER-CRAB half LAWNMOWER she was the embodiment of carnage
——Thank you CAPA / Bill tried to high-five the perversion
——Oh, call me the Clergyman's Daughter why don't you? We both know why you're here you cheeky scamp/ She rearranged her face into what she thought was a smile and blew what BRAINfeed explained was prelim to love / something called a KISS?

—Your reprise of mustard mutations / she snarled reading from lower down Bill's top ten / —Brilliant / A master stroke / But Billy my all-time fave <u>hydro cyanic rainwater</u> / Science with a dark heart / Nothing better to stir the genitals - nothing / She chopped the air with some excessive tai chi
Bill eyed her with unbridled contempt / She made the ancient art look like kung fu, but then, she got no class / reading his mind infoScreen fed him that old one about about Stein calling his daughter Phylis / He'd've nailed this crone straightaway / Returned her to the eugenicists in plastoResearch marked 'DUD'
Outside the 'flick, flick, flick' of passing air tubes could be heard in departure / More Day-glo Ultras with Robostrimmers high streamed to <u>Sub-Lancs BrownSpace</u> / numbers from Bill's recent social engineering mission spun / codes hummed to faint melodic chimes / The ubiquitous AITC hologram temporarily faded from golden reds to silvery white

CAUCUSES: BLOW BACK AND FAN INDUCTION, FIRESTORM MODEL #202
THAMES SECTOR: PROJECTS 37, 8 & 9, GRENFELLED.
POP FIGS. FOR CHRISTMAS 2289 BACK ON TRACK.

—Ayleloooyarr!' CAPA cried —missionShip finally coming in / Her voice switched to <u>autocue machine age C#</u>
—EliteBreeds taught me some very important top-down pointers Billy / Number one: Heartlessness / this leaking sentiment / control diminishing / spanner in the clock / not strategic / capital disaster / be unafraid / be cruel
—Number three: Always eradicate ... Billieboy / Are you listening? / Somebody in AITC just reported that my forebears replaced virtueEthics with Randian Kneesian dribble down / can you imagine such naïveté? Non mi fa fucking ridere / Bill Lee stemmed the vomit rising in his gut / Seeing humanity so

distorted by this lopsided monster required more than
domperidone
Her bearings in her neck squeaked / She was up-minded of her
duty / that her last egg had to be fertilised by something
called the missionary position / A step in the right
direction, suggested infoScreen, was <u>foreplay</u> / TotoControl
guessed she wouldn't have a clue and dialled <u>wistful smile/no
teeth</u> /
—You little rascal she declared

WHISPER: I LOVE YOU

Bill aware of the futility panicked / He felt between his legs
/ Nothing / CAPA was injected with every known aphrodisiac /
Inside and out she was falling apart / The tsunami of need
merely highlighted her ineptitude / Emptied of animal spirits
/ diluted by the trace and train of genetic jiggery pokery it
was clear that humankind was Totokaputissimo / To Bill's
disgust CAPA started to gyrate towards him / He imagined a
ghoul defending carrion from vultures / infoScreen tried to
encourage a better thought but Pompeii dog snarling at
Vesuvius was the best it could manage / it was hopeless
Bill frantically dialled up HEADspace / old walrus whistled
his way up the stairs - 11-30pm. - and slipped him the banned
DA agonist nasal spray and pills / inside Quaker Testimonies,
Old Bill Dent knew what the greatest painkiller was. "God is
Love" / you'd have more chance fertilising an Egyptian mummy
but you never know / Remember Ecclesiastes: <u>time and chance</u>? /
Good luck
Bill Lee placed the pills under his tongue trying to imagine
something beyond disgust / CAPA was bankrupt / Zero
compassion / back panel data empty / no resourcefulness /
devoid of emotional intelligence / inculcation total / And now
every wire in her institutionalised-brain short-circuiting /
She wasn't the first robotic CAPA / but the Pavlovian

habituation / the foot-in-mouth tics / jerks and layered
scowls of cruelty interpreted as funny were the actions of a
hagbred cow from Hades / cloned incubed and squirted / as if
artifice could ever replace nature and distract him from the
battery acid dribbling outta her motherless tits / MAN ALIVE /
No wonder humanity was face down in the swamp / She's on her
last mandibles / her poisonality alone would cure Jupiter /
And I'm expected to fuck it / Bill chucked his ring
CAPA was thrilled and advanced as if about to pounce /
—JEEZUS she thinks this is a turn on / her only technique is
cluelessness and mendacity / she came closer / Bill could feel
her breath and wondered if the gaps between her fangs were as
wide as those in her understanding / Bill felt compelled to
comment / he was terrified
—Jesus, CAPA, you're not looking so great / he sneezed.
The high priestess of vacuity stopped / she stared emptily /
his words meant little / AITC dialled chameleon on her visMap
/ Sure enough she'd unaccountably slipped to pale and pallid
corrected to sweaty and flushed / more internal whirrings
Capa's voiceOver kicked in
—CoooeeeeBill and now let's to bed purchase a little one to
preserve what we hold dear to bring our communities together
and spread harmony and love and cement the affection with
which will bless this happy day with love and bring pleasure
everywhere / Her face contorted / one side leapt to the
heavens / the other / the sewers / She could have swept the
field at gurning a curious Cumbrian pastime
Bill consulted his veterinary manual / bovine encephalitis?
—You're looking worse than that CAPA no use lying helluvalot
worse / have you got a headache? / he hoped
—Oh, how redemptive she gushed —oh how jolly jolly splendid
/ Nobody spills it like you Billie no one / all I get nowadays
are cheap voidy words / There's no integitty left all gone
like trees / did you ever see a tree Bill?
The twenty-seven agencies of control, conditioning and

butchery alerted to the unravelling gathered like hyenas
around a dying elephant / AITC scrolled frantically thru'
various vocal adjustments and chose <u>authoritarian</u> / BIO
Research registered <u>objection</u> feeling this a complete mismatch
with the juice streaming down her thigh / the problem /
she had been extracted as ELITEclass but every challenge
simply exposed the frailties inherent in systemRobotics /
The background chatter of every squabbling ideologue filled
the ether
BIOControl argued that CAPA was devoid of imagination /
Yes AITC recognised / ideas were a distant but critical
requirement / It had to be bred back but how? / TotoCorps
would recommend self-respect retrieval and CAPA would be
progged to pretend she knew what that was / If TC couldn't
help BIOControl might have to surreptitiously recreate
instinct as well / But from where? / allegedly when the chips
were down some had relied on it? / Was it really too late for
BIOprogeny....? / One way or another the next few minutes
would tell / It was agreed that if ALPHAplan failed the
acronym RWTC -Rewind the Clock- would simultaneously appear
throughout the universe / BETAplan would be enacted with a
technological shrug
AITC instructed CAPA to fondle Bill's hair and light a candle
/ She pushed Bill into the chair ... it snapped shut / like a
gin trap / She had him / Now he'd have to scratch her back or
whatever
She lifted her viscose petticoat revealing a smorgasbord of
orifices / Bill was aghast / What! Get your sexologist
Havelock or Norman Haire on the line / he wanted HEADspace ...
AITC suggested winding in her neck
—What fun she shrieked as her front and back brains collided
/ she mounted her victim
Writhing, their mouths engaged / she must penetrate / She
extended and retracted her corkscrew proboscis in a series of
rapid movements / After several Earth minutes of feverous

straining she defecated long, hard and deep into Bill's larynx
/ she sat back...panting
Bill was suffocating / he waggled his head / vaguely clocked
the technological ripple throughout the universe / the
ubiquitous warm glow outside faded to green and blinked /

RWTC RWTC RWTC

so that was it / the game was up ...
—I knew it, my darling / I won't die a virgin / she posed
like a teapot
—I knew I absolutely knew / she started to jerk and rave
—Always said it / a jab of cold blue veracity through the
caudate nucleus was indicated Billiam / a minimum fucking
requirement gore blimey / I am entirely biomechanical / the
finished article / her ravings encountered further structural
limitations / Bill spat and shook what he could from his face
—I must insist on my jocular fecundity getting first dibs she
grinned / Bill was helpless
BIOprogeny admitted defeat and sent out the closure code
acknowledging the lifespan of the last from ELITEclass

119 EARTH YEARS

—Ooo you noticed / Not to be sniffed at / oh no I will be
caramelised forever / FOREVER.
She's being checked out Bill knew / the Clergyman Daughter's
ravings continued to fragment and spin into the void
—I'm craven-sent Billie / My mission? To behave like a
nickel-plated cuntoid and I'm not letting go / My legacy /
power for its own sake / That's always been my pogrom /
Techernology rusted the organ long time ago / We've Beat your
Neighbour out of doors wiped out commoonity / Such a happy way
to spend the evening ... RE-WIND THE CLOCK? Pah! Find the Cock
/ that's more like it / the lost art of parlour games / lying

```
through my teeth / all control relies on striking fear /
morons always responded / Always worked ... look how gorjus I
am a tiptop cocker
CAPA's death rattle began to fade / humanity's stifled limbic
system generationally habituated to upholding self interest
had finally run its pointless course / CAPA's throbbing
proboscis pushed open her mouth for the finale / Sluglike it
slithered sniffed and withdrew the latest data from darkspace
/ The ubiquitous AITC logo rolled back to golden red before
going through the cycle of transmission codes; the usual
flimflam of procedural necessity / CAPA wriggled ...
—the last 'flicks' overhead in airtube slowed as the game
played itself out / there would be no more missions / Shire
departments bathed again, inside and out, with charcoal glow
of entropy / The strings holding up CAPA's bones were cut one
by one / she sank into jellied mumbling / the last conditioned
reflex / Somewhere under her nerve terminals the echo nothing
could silence
—I am the clergymun's daughter, I must, I must incwease my
bust ... I AM the clujimuns oo didn't orta ... I must ...
It looped on and on, there was nothing else ... Plugs of
analgesics guaranteed that she and her ridiculous species
would disappear forever amid the AITC annals of failed
experiments ... and Bill, struck dumb by a gob full of vomit
and shit, couldn't even SCREAM ...
```

* * *

Benway coughed, rolled over and rubbed his eyes.

In the kitchen next door the kettle was starting to boil.

'Cuppa?' asked Kate.

'Yes please,' replied the doctor, surveying Benway's notes. There were some good signs, borne out by Sister Kate's observation: 'He's changed; well, his behaviour has.'

'In what way?' he asked.

'He's lost that dreadful pessimism. He's begun to co-operate.'

'Good. You've done well, you both have.'

'I think now could be the time to talk to him more ... he's beginning to listen.'

Dent thought about this but remained quiet.

'That reminds me,' continued Kate, 'he's also started to write, sheets of it, ripped out from the notebook. At this rate we'll need to get a new one ...'

'Oh, do you know what?'

'Ooo I don't know, er, crazy, madcap stuff. Hannah and I have been listening to it since Friday. Now, when he starts off, I just give him a pen and a sheet of paper and say, "Tell it to this".'

Dent chuckled. 'Does he share any of it?'

'Oh yes, and it's better out than in, believe me. He really has the most extraordinary imagination.'

Dent smiled broadly. 'And the enema?' he asked.

'The same, better out than in.'

'Well, I'm very pleased. He has a strong constitution ... but we must expect further reactions. Keep up with the encouragement. He'll be nervous, concerned whether he's able to keep going. Whether any improvement is just a blip. Remember, every time he finds a reward it'll be that bit easier for him to look forward.'

'Yes. He's been hard work, but I'd say he's turned a corner.'

'Good.... From now on the apo can stay three hourly but no need to wake him if he's sleeping. Keep the Benerva as it is, and the insulin ... with meals ... at least for the time being. I'll make an entry in the notes.'

Doctor Dent put away his charts and stood up. 'I'll spend some time with him now and give him his next apo' jab. Pop out for a breather if you like. What are you reading?'

Sister Kate turned the book's front cover towards the doctor. He raised his half-moon glasses to focus on the title: *Anglo Saxon Attitudes*.

'Oh yes,' Dent said, 'enjoying it?'

'It's funny and sad. I enjoy the funny best.'

'Yes,' agreed Dent, 'we need more funny.'

'Money is honey my little sonny, and a rich man's joke is always funny,' she recited, walking towards the stairs. Dent entered Benway's room.

'Evening, Dr Benway,' said Dent, sitting by the bed.

The patient was looking over Dent's manuscript, *Medici Libris*. He pushed his long fingers under his glasses and tried to invigorate his face. His glasses rose and fell until they dropped onto his lap. He picked them up and returned them above his long nose. He looked sickly pale.

'Kate tells me you are doing well, very well. I'm delighted,' said Dent, loosening his tie.

'I feel terrible,' croaked the patient. 'Terrible.'

'No improvement?'

'No, not really.'

'Oh, I'm sorry to hear that.'

Benway closed the manuscript and noticed that the old croaker was looking at his ink-stained fingers.

'Yeah, ok. Maybe I'm a bit better,' he scratched. 'I managed to get some thoughts down.' He made a scribbling motion as if he were writing in the air. 'Satisfied?'

Dent was pleased but remained expressionless. His patient was proud and would not yield easily. This characteristic lay deep... he had no desire to expose it. Its very existence was key to his patient's recovery, perhaps his very survival.

'Are you pleased with your thoughts?' the doctor asked.

'Maybe.'

'I am sure they are fine thoughts.'

'They're about fucking boys and rolling around in shit.'

'Splendid.'

Benway looked up to see whether the old croaker was serious. The same steel-blue eyes were still there... not even a flicker. Those deep blue eyes as wide as the heavens... always looking for a way in... there was always a way in.

The doctor moved closer and took Benway's hand as the first

preliminary to the round of checks: pulse, breathing, blood pressure and temperature. Benway cooperated, he liked the old boy's soft touch and homely voice... it was oddly familiar but he still wasn't sure why.

'It may interest you to know, Dr Benway, that we are products of our environments and as such no different from any other organism in the universe. Man's wellbeing is entirely determined by the structure he inherits and the impact of his surroundings. Of course, we are not told this when we are growing up because our masters prefer obedience. This is upheld because it pushes the responsibility of any fall from grace onto the individual. It is how we are corralled; well, one of the ways.' The doctor waved one arm expansively. 'Look out of the window if you doubt me. People sleepwalking to and from work. If you ask them "Why?" they will immediately think of the food and clothes required by their families, the homes they struggle to pay for and all the false gods that give their lives meaning: the Church, nationalism, modern science, the economic and political establishments and the monarchy. All structural straightjackets designed to inculcate an atmosphere of homogeneity. Individualism is held back, Benway, held back by the stultifying insistence that happiness is dependent on our willingness to conform and serve.' Dent paused to enter something on the charts. 'And when we are ill we may be treated but the causes which made us sick will not change; the unfairness of the socioeconomic system, the prescriptive schooling, the awful housing and living conditions, our penal laws advocating prohibition. We are told 'you must fit in and then you'll be happy.' Dent laughed ironically. 'It would be fairer to say we're actually subjects controlled by fear of insecurity and censure rather than citizens living freely.'

The doctor stood to check Benway's temperature in silence. Satisfied, he sat back down and adjusted the position of his chair so that he faced his patient squarely. 'You see, ever since Man climbed down from the trees and entered the first cave, civilisation has demanded compliance. We are stigmatised if we belong to a minority and earn opprobrium if we do not fit in. The majority do not question this state of affairs. We react like machines, human machines because our reactions are canalised by the bewildered herd. This is reinforced by morality; newspaper stories that stoke prejudices, the language of deference, advertisements selling us products we do not need to impress those we do not like: cars, dresses, three-piece suites. But heaven forbid we discuss taboos, acknowledge the existence of minorities, support creativity and liberating forms of behaviour or advocate more equitable policies that would disrupt the status quo. The overriding thought must be "if I fail it is my fault … for I had 'free will.'" But this, Benway, is a myth perpetuated by all the things I've mentioned and many I haven't … every ridiculous school uniform, its Latin motto, exams from the age of five, sports days breeding competitiveness, every pointless gold watch awarded for a life of drudgery, to say nothing of the medals dolled out for risking your life, and an honours system reminding us who's in charge. I'm not surprised you write about fucking boys and rolling in shit. If individuals had enough gumption to see how we're being played … strung along … we'd all rebel, wouldn't we?'

Benway gulped. He was still adjusting to his doctor's ways but hadn't expected such a candid assessment of society's oppression. The anthropological progression from ape to Homo sap's societal glue was received and signed for. He leant forward as the doctor listened to his lungs. He felt a rush of excitement as he enthused over what was happening: how every expectation as to what a doctor could provide was being challenged. It was as confounding as it was stimulating.

'So that's why you use apomorphine?'

'What?' It was the doctor's turn to be surprised.

'Your apomorphine frees me up to be who I wanna be.'

The doctor smiled as he put away his stethoscope. 'That is correct. I certainly do not want to tie you down, the very opposite as a matter of fact.'

'Apomorphine's like the good cop at a crime scene. It does what it has to do but leaves no trace, no contamination.'

'Oh yes,' nodded Dent, smiling. 'That's a good analogy. If you came to me with a broken arm you wouldn't be happy if I exchanged it for a broken leg.' Benway laughed as his doctor continued to illuminate. 'But that is what is happening with medicine's approach to addiction and every other so-called disease of the mind, the depressions and anxieties...merely shifting the sufferer's burden from one shoulder to the other.'

'So, control is everywhere, in every walk of life...even medicine,' Benway responded with a shrug.

'For the time being it would appear increasingly so. For revolution to work it must end in laughter, not tears. The Mayans disappeared because they were unable to laugh, I am sure of it.'

Benway looked doubtful. 'How do you know?'

'Well, it probably went like this. The Mayan chief received warnings from his minions that human sacrifice didn't guarantee a good harvest or health and happiness in a future life. He was outraged by this challenge to his authority and ordered off twice the number of heads. If he'd listened the Mayans might have survived. In other primitive societies the wise woman knew that such advice might get the same treatment so she bided her time. *Her* chief, like a gorilla with a headache and his chest out here,' Dent raised his hands in front of him, 'he'd beat it like a drum and bellow: "My will must be observed or else..." The compliant group dispersed, disgruntled and frightened. It wasn't until the old woman laughed that levity permitted wisdom to percolate and erase stupidity. That is why laughter is infectious; it needed to be so humanity could evolve. One woman laughed and then the next and so on. In order not to appear stupid the chief had to see that he was the joke. It is our ability to laugh at ourselves which should encourage change and help develop our success as a species. We've never been further removed from this characteristic than we are today ...and right-wing politicians are the worst offenders precisely because of the systemic conditioning I have just described. We can all think of examples, the great panjandrums, just look around.'

'Have you ever lost your sense of humour?'

'Oh definitely,' Dent said gruffly.

'When you shot the robin?' asked Benway, patting Dent's open manuscript.

'Ah yes,' acknowledged Dent. 'Well, I really didn't need anyone to tell me that I'd behaved badly. In mitigation I might plead that my action was an unconscious rejection of the Church and the unholy feelings of guilt it engenders.'

'How d'you mean?'

'At school and to a lesser extent at home I'd been brought up to believe in Christ and one Sunday I was reduced to tears by the vicar's dramatic reconstruction of the Passion. Many believed and some still do that the robin's red breast is Christ's blood. But I had begun to reject the dominion religion had over my life because of an aunt. I used to stay with her during my holidays. She was an atheist and by example had shown me there could be another way, a richer existence earned by being original... independent. Quite possibly shooting the robin was a clumsy attempt to express my loyalty to her. You see, Benway, I have endeavoured all my life to reduce the wire-pulling that goes on over our heads. The blind trust we have for those things I mentioned earlier... the structural mechanisms that curtail and manipulate... it has been my lifelong struggle.'

As Benway reeled in the almost endless stream of messages, his own memories were triggered, sweeping him back into another time and space... into a sultry, crowded atmosphere... there were people drinking... faces... urging him on... and then a shriek. He peered through a veil of clearing smoke at the gun falling from his limp hand and the red trickle down Joan's forehead. The revolver hit the floor as a horn blew in Cromwell Road...

'I did the same thing,' he said in a flat voice, barely audible.

'Oh?' said the doctor.

'Yes, when I shot and killed Joan... my wife.'

Benway felt the old doc's eyes upon him. He wouldn't move; he'd keep his vacant gaze fixed on his private horror. He had a penchant for dropping truth bombs. He'd wait, wait for the inevitable reaction ... it always came... just let it hang there, madness loose in the room. There was no use pretending that he regretted its release. Like the split second when everything stops just before the catastrophe. The reaction was late... why hadn't it come...? His ears started to hum, he swallowed hard... to give breath to some vocalisation gagging in his throat. Trembling long fingers removed his glasses so he could wipe his brow with the back of his sleeve. Dent's manuscript slipped off his lap and onto the floor. He grunted, leaning forward to pick it up.

'Here, let me,' offered Dent, getting down on one knee. 'It's all right.'

'But it isn't, is it?' insisted Benway, raising his voice. 'She's dead and I did it.'

Dent shuffled the manuscript back into shape. He paused before getting back up. 'And you need to understand why?'

Benway put back his glasses, as if they might help penetrate the darkest recesses of his past. 'I dunno,' he said, 'I've tri- tri-ed...' he choked.

'Take your time. There's no hurry.'

'We had a crazy game where I'd shoot the wall just above her head. We were both high, I could barely stand but she baited me; there were witnesses. Once we'd started geeing each other we couldn't stop. Half of me thinks it was inevitable, the other half screams that it wasn't, I could've stopped any time. Now your robin and what you just said. I think she was my robin.'

Dent placed the manuscript by the bed. He didn't care for these moments; they tested his resolve to stick to the game plan... but how could it be otherwise? Here he was, once more staring into another's nightmare. He looked at his patient biting his forefinger.... Every treatment had to start with the individual, *all* his circumstances. He tried to imagine the scene and the relationship that spawned it. He thought of something Rhoda had told him: 'There's no such thing as a murderer without a murderee.' He also knew this facile explanation would just invite more speculation. People do not exorcise their demons by getting to know them, quite the opposite. Only by accepting the past can we forget it and adjust ourselves to the present. He reached out and patted Benway's arm.

'We're here to look forward not back. Together, you and I, Hannah and Gibbie and the others, we'll get through this, you'll see.' He moved closer raising his hand to rub his patient's shoulder and nape of his neck. 'There are few certainties in life... but while you're here we will be too... I promise.'

Benway took in a deep breath. Something had changed, not his body but the future. He'd always dreaded it but with those few words he realised it could accommodate him. Yes, even him, the no-good dirty junky wife-killing queer that he was. He'd dropped the truth partly because he wanted to test the old croaker's resolve... but he hadn't changed. With the simple encouragement to 'look forward' he could leap-frog the endless recrimination. Benway released his grip on his temples and let his hands fall together on the eiderdown. The old doc knows I've been over this a million times. He knows it's exhausting to keep digging it up. There's no place to bury it, it'll still be there, why try? Benway exhaled. He felt relief. Higher and higher... somewhere downstream... the water in the grey lagoon rose till, overwhelmed, the dam broke. The water cascaded down the valley. He was getting closer... closer in his surge to the sea. Benway looked up.

'Ever since that night,' he complained, 'I have felt inhabited by a dark spirit, a malevolence. I don't recognise this possession as me, but who else is it?'

After a long pause the old croaker's voice re-emerged. 'It could just as easily have been me, as you've noticed.' Dent gestured towards his manuscript.

Benway's brow furrowed. 'But that was just a bird,' his voice was derisory.

'Oh yes, I could agree. A bird, and I just a child, but the feeling of regret and "how could I have been so stupid?" is with me still. I hate to think about it. But it taught me something.'

'What?' Benway's voice barked. The doctor did not care for the sound... he was regaining his voice but one stained with self-reproach and disgust.

'That we're never completely rational,' said the doctor, simply. 'Within us all, each and every one of us, lies the capacity to be unspeakably stupid or reckless. We can all imagine committing some evil or enjoying a fantasy and wonder if we might get away with it. We know that there are consequences but we're tempted nevertheless. And then we'll say about another who gets caught "How could they?" without any appreciation that "they" are "us". We immediately contradict our own appreciation of ourselves, our potential in different circumstances to have acted in exactly the same way.'

Benway reflected on the universality of Dent's message. Of course, he was right. Anyone can make a fatal mistake, but he wouldn't admit it. He moved, he was stalling... looking for something to add. 'I thought only us Yankees were evil,' he wheezed.

Dent's shoulders heaved. 'Oh, my word! You colonials are babes in the wood, just cottoning on to the profits of barbarism. The British got rich on the slave trade, invented concentration camps, employed mercenaries, torture, deportation, genocide, you name it.... And – as long as the world couldn't see it – we carried on. The Opium Wars, a precursor to your prohibition laws, embellished by that great British specialty: hypocrisy. And today these policies are being copied by sentient human beings perpetrating what Engels called "social murder". Back in their cosy homes do these tardigrades ever stop to consider what they've done? And yet, with bewildering sanctimony, they'll be the first to condemn those caught in the traps they're permitted to evade. I ask you.'

Benway nodded. 'There's more honour in a den of thieves.'

'Undoubtedly,' said Dent rising, 'and more compassion in a nest of vipers.' He walked over to the window and looked into the street. It was clearing after the evening rush. A young woman opposite was waving, trying to hail a taxi. Had his patient shot someone like that? It suddenly seemed incomprehensible; he felt compelled to know more.

'When did this incident happen... with your wife?'

'Several years ago.'

'Where?'

'Mexico.'

'Did the authorities get involved, the police?'

'Yeah, they sentenced me in abstentia; I'd left the country by then.'

'Manslaughter?'

'Yeah.'

'But the feelings of remorse are no less strong?'

'Something like that,' rasped Benway. 'She is the mother of my child, my son... a motherless child.'

'And he's back at home... with your parents?'

'Yeah.'

Dent moved back to the bed and felt his patient's forehead as though he were reading his temperature or blessing a disciple. He ran the palm of his hand once more to the back of Benway's head to his neck and let it rest. Catching Benway's eyes he smiled and gave his patient another deliberate squeeze.

'Well, I'm glad I know. You can talk to me whenever you like.' Dent sat back down.

'Will you analyse me?'

Dent frowned. He had to check an urge to sound contemptuous. 'And how might that help us?' he asked, trying to sound more relaxed than he felt.

'I dunno, by getting me to think about why I've done what I've done. To revisit my motivations.'

Dent was quiet. He had absolutely no time for analytical psychiatry... he strongly suspected that his patient had been subjected to it in the past.... If that was what Benway wanted then he'd come to the wrong shop.

Dent cleared his throat. 'I really fail to see what good that can do. What happened must have been traumatic, but scrutinising it to the nth degree and attributing to it some bogus psychiatric profile named after some Greek fairy story, a label that you'll carry for the rest of your life? How could that help? No, we're looking forward not back. Dwelling on the past cannot change it, so I'll leave well alone.' Dent looked away. He could say more, dot the 'i's and cross the 't's forever and a day, but Benway would have to be shown another way and then draw these conclusions himself. Once that had happened he'd be able to accommodate his past. A sense of atonement achieved through the front door leading towards his infinite potentials... redemption via a self-sustaining respectability, it was a simple strategy. Not the back door pointing out the monumental bleakness of past horrors and their theoretical causes. That was the gateway to a controlling society... to recidivism and despair....

Benway unclasped his hands; he wanted to hear more. He hoped

Dent would stay. 'You probably have a lot of experience of this?'

Once again Dent saw the old faces flash by like shuffling a deck of cards. Some were still very distinct. One man, an accountant with dark, tightly cropped hair and smiling eyes, stood out.

'Back when I was a very green doctor at St Pancras Hospital,' he started, 'there was a case of a respectable, perfectly ordinary middle-class chap who, on his way home, crossed a railway track to get a cup of tea from the opposite platform. The arrival of his train was announced early and he had to cross back or miss it. It was dark and hurrying he missed his step and fell onto the rails beside the oncoming train, breaking his arm. When he was dragged onto the platform the police arrested him for trying to commit suicide. Nothing could have been further from the truth but he was brought to the hospital and put under guard... a policeman sat beside the bed as close as I am to you... day and night.'

'Was suicide illegal?'

'Oh, yes. It carried severe penalties despite rarely ending up in court.'

'An unworkable law?'

'Pretty much. Anyway, subject to days of inquisition this poor man started to doubt his own version of events. Even his wife began to question him: "Are you unhappy?", "Is there another woman?", that sort of thing. This grilling continued until he became very unhappy and wished for someone, anyone, who didn't want to convince him of a crime of which he was innocent. Soon, the constant suspicion began to wear him down and he began to fear that he'd lost his mind. "Perhaps I did want to end it all, perhaps I am mad?" Eventually he asked his wife, "You believe me, don't you?" Fatefully, she replied, "I am not sure. They're the police, aren't they? They must know." That night he crept out of his bed and jumped from the highest window in the hospital. He was barely alive after I'd unpicked him from the railings. His last words were, "I *did* try to commit suicide, didn't I?" A few minutes later he'd succeeded.'

'Tell a guy often enough and he'll believe anything,' said Benway.

The doctor agreed. 'Words are very important. They are agents of change. We have to choose them carefully otherwise they spread through the brain like a virus. We must never forget that the brain can heal itself.'

'How d'you mean?'

'By forgetting and by leaving well alone you will give yourself the time and space to get better on your own. When we met you told me about your uncle's fate.... It seemed as if you were merely anticipating the only outcome left to you. Your story reminded me of the background music throughout my childhood... here in London. My father worried about my thinness. I had to eat my crusts and when I went to school he derided me for not playing games. It might have made me believe that there was something wrong simply because I was subject to paternalistic anxiety. Society works like that, endlessly creating stories that confirm its moral position, its unassailable strength.'

Benway, reminded of the stifling petty-mindedness of uptown St Louis, nodded in agreement. 'I suppose it results in fear and stagnation.'

'Undoubtedly,' said Dent. 'When I was young I also had a stern piano teacher who, when listening to my first, faltering notes, her face buckled like someone forced to lick piss off a nettle. I wouldn't have hurt her then, but I would now. The untold damage her disapproval could do to a child, any child; unspeakable.'

'You could have been another Mozart.'

'Beethoven, puleeeze!' the doctor quipped and his patient laughed... like a child. Dent smiled as he recognised that Kate's observations were right. Another Benway was emerging. His fears were dissolving ... apomorphine had dealt with the worst ravages of withdrawal and small pleasures were being gained, conversational and otherwise. This was probably why he'd shared a trouble ... one positive triggering the next ... a chain reaction? All movement is reaction, like the spring flower turning its face to the sun. This was typical of patients treated with apomorphine in a benign atmosphere; a therapy that could be quickly measured in behavioural change and encouraged to develop from the get-go. The doctor looked at his watch. He'd be late for dinner and in all likelihood miss another delayed deadline for the journal... the SSA committee would be furious and Stickler apoplectic, but it couldn't be helped. Critical moments have to be seized because they may not come again. Benway stretched like an animal emerging from hibernation... at the mouth of his cave... the darkness at his back. He had to keep moving towards the light. His doctor knew what to do.

Dent pulled a sheet of paper and a fountain pen from his inside pocket and handed them to Benway.

'Now then,' he said, 'A little game. Your good thoughts, please. Your very best.'

Benway interrupted his mental image of Dent's piano recital. 'Mine?' he asked, a little confused.

'Yes. Just a few things you'd like to be. Don't think too much about it; just scribble them out, a list of characteristics that you like.'

'Such as?'

'Nothing to do with me. This is on you, I cannot possibly know.'

Dent got up. 'Run through the alphabet if you get stuck. Think of personalities you admire, your friends, traits you're drawn to. I've got to nip outside, I won't be long.'

Dent left and whistled his way down the stairs. As the door slam echoed up the stairwell 99 Cromwell suddenly felt empty, as empty as Benway's mind. He thought of the tip about the alphabet... 'Able,' he whispered, 'amiable... asshole.' The more he wrote down the easier it became. He amended the list, crossed a few words out and waited. Dent was more than five minutes. He began to worry. Had he said 'five minutes' or 'a while'? London had gone quiet save for the occasional passing of a vehicle... like irregular waves on a shallow beach. He listened; there was that whistling once more. It was approaching; he's back.

'How did you get on?' Dent asked as he entered.

'Not bad.'

'Good. What do you like to read?'

'Oh, I'll read anything.'

'Have you read anything while you've been here?'

'Not much, haven't been able to concentrate. Your friend Tiger Tim suggested your memoirs ... and I've looked at *A Modest Proposal*.'

'How did you find that?'

'Good.'

'We need more "good",' declared Dent. 'Not enough nowadays. How about poetry?'

'Yeah, why not.'

'You see, I want you to read something out loud.'

'Does it matter what it is?' Benway was intrigued.

'Not at all.' Dent recited as he scanned the titles:

> 'The time has come,' the walrus said,
> 'To talk of many things:
>   Ships and shoes and sealing wax, of cabbages and kings.
>   And why the sea is boiling hot
>   And whether pigs have wings.'

He passed a volume to his patient. 'Let's try *Rime of the Ancient Mariner*, a yarn with a repeating pattern. Fair exchange is no robbery.'

They swapped anthology for sheet of paper. Benway was enjoying the attention.

Dent moved to the back of the room and leant against the wall. He started to mumble to himself. 'Pen, where's my pen?'

'You gave it to me,' said the American and leant forward to return it. A fountain pen between fingers; the patient's ink-stained, the doctor's with nicotine. A moment fallen through the cracks of time and space.

Dent took the pen, bit off the top and scored through a few of Benway's suggestions while underlining others. He looked at his patient. 'Ready?' he asked.

'For what?' Benway was confused.

'Oh yes!' Dent acknowledged. 'Right, the method: you read out loud.'

'I can do that...'

'Yes, but as if you're giving a performance. Imagine there's an old school teacher over here by the window, or your best friend, and you want him to hear the words of the poem clearly. Read it without hesitation, no gaps... and without listening to me.'

'Without listening?'

'Yes, because I am going to read these back to you.' Dent shook the sheet of paper. 'You will hear them but under the radar, absorption without the usual strings... all the ones we mentioned earlier.... Ready?'

Benway struggled to understand. 'You're going to brainwash me?'

Dent laughed so loud he had to steady himself. 'Aha! How can I? These are *your* ideas... they're already part of you. This is just reinstatement... without all the blocking nonsense you've been fed since you were first thought of.... This way you'll find it easier to inhabit your true self in the future.'

'Without the bullshit?' Benway scratched the back of his neck, adjusted the front of his pyjamas and finally his glasses. He suddenly felt self conscious.

'It is an ancient Mariner...'

Dent looked up from the sheet. 'Try reading it a little louder, and from a bit later when the action starts: it'll help to stay in the story...'

Benway turned the page, cleared his throat and re-started, this time with his doctor's accompaniment.

BENWAY: :DENT

'In mist or cloud, You are strong and determined.
on mast or shroud, Recognise and celebrate these
It perched for vespers nine; qualities.

Whiles all the night, You can be yourself
through fog-smoke white, without anxiety; resolute,
Glimmered the white Moon-shine.' unflinching and steadfast.

'God save thee, ancient Mariner! As your true self returns...
From the fiends, you'll be increasingly comfortable
that plague thee thus!— in your own skin.

[270]

WAKING SUGGESTION

Why look'st thou so?' – With my cross-bow I shot the ALBATROSS.'	You won't let yourself down... you'll be free to express your
'The Sun now rose upon the right: Out of the sea came he,	talents... and, healthy, these qualities will come to the fore.
Still hid in mist, and on the left Went down into the sea.	If you feel worried take some time out to connect, be calm
And the good south wind still blew behind, and no sweet bird did follow,	and you'll flourish, make easy progress with your work... no need to rush.
Nor any day for food or play Came to the mariners' hollo!	Hasten slowly... Patience with yourself and others will replenish and feed you... Let go of old
And I had done a hellish thing, and it would work 'em woe:	thoughts, empty your mind, let them be
For all averred, I had killed the bird That made the breeze to blow.	and watch as new ideas take their place. Absorb everything from wherever you
Ah wretch! said they, the bird to slay, That made the breeze to blow!	find it. This will restore balance, help everything grow... You have a
Nor dim nor red, like God's own head, The glorious Sun uprist:	great ability to learn, and rest without depending on anything else.
Then all averred, I had killed the bird That brought the fog and mist.	You will sleep when you are ready to sleep. This will restore energy.
'Twas right, said they, such birds to slay, That bring the fog and mist.	Life will enrich you for you're magical, funny, with a wild nature.

HARDY TREE

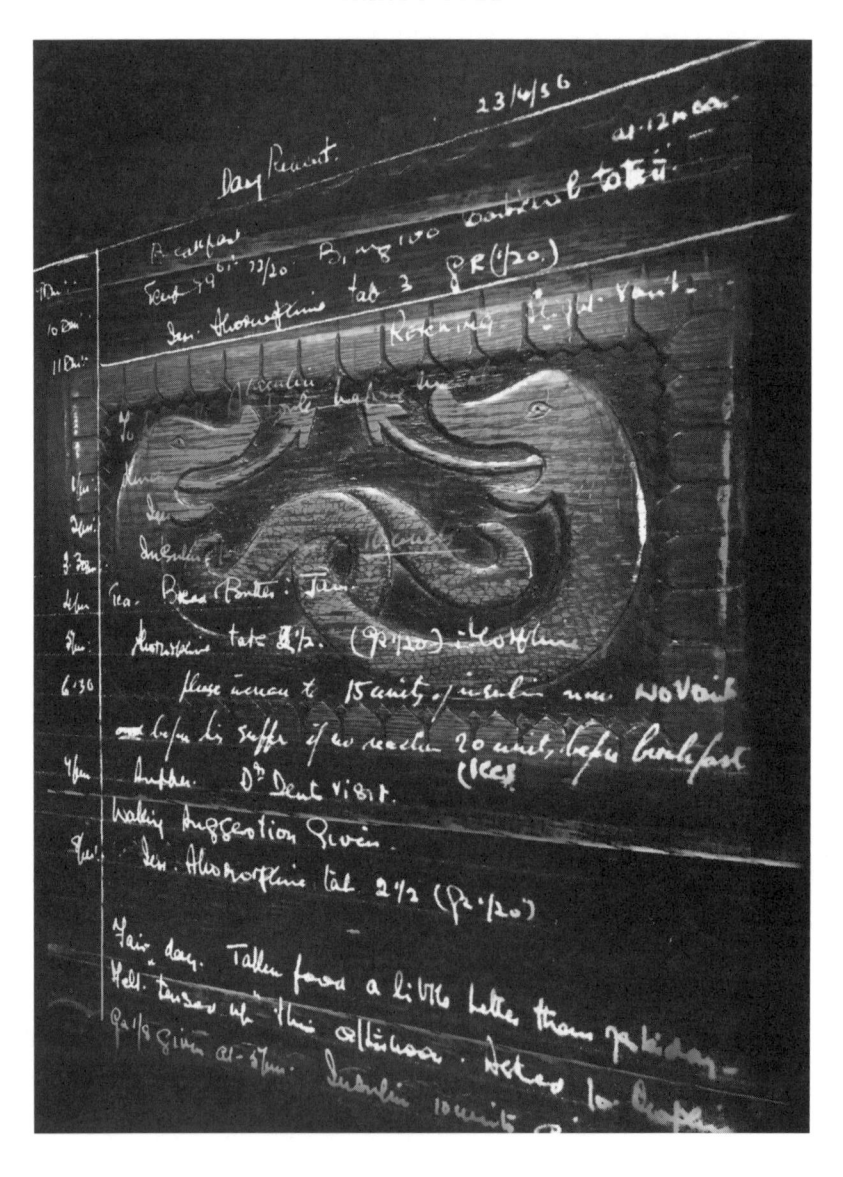

WAKING SUGGESTION

The fair breeze blew,	Think of being catlike,
the white foam flew,	their fierce independence,
The furrow followed free;	they do not worry...
We were the first that ever burst	... and take only what they need
Into that silent sea.	from their environment.
Down dropt the breeze,	Nurture and take care of
the sails dropt down,	yourself...... be proud and
'Twas sad as sad could be;	protect what you have.
And we did speak only to break	Cherish your health. By enjoying
The silence of the sea!	yourself you will be enriched.
All in a hot and copper sky,	and affection for others will be
The bloody Sun, at noon,	easier. Your life is long
Right up above the mast did stand,	with much left to discover.
No bigger than the Moon.	Let it all in, accept everything.
Day after day, day after day,	Be awake to your sensitivity....
We stuck,	Your powers of observing
nor breath nor motion;	and describing things
As idle as a painted ship	are unique, your special gift,
Upon a painted ocean.	and they will return...
Water, water, every where,	as soon as you're ready.
And all the boards did shrink;	When you feel creative, work.
Water, water, every where,	When you do not, take it easy,
nor any drop to	relax.
drink.	Do anything that you enjoy
The very deep did rot: O Christ!	and spend time with those
That ever this should be!	you admire.
Yea, slimy things did crawl with legs	Deal with things as they arrive,
Upon the slimy sea.	one thing at a time.
About, about, in reel and rout	There is no rush. Exercise when
The death-fires danced at night;	you can. A fit, responsive

> The water, like a witch's oils, body will help the contemplative
> Burnt green, and blue and white. life that you like...
>
> And some in dreams ...and permits you to benefit
> assurèd were from stillness and silence.
> Of the Spirit that plagued us so; You have
>
> Nine fathom deep nothing to fear from your own
> he had followed us company. Your sensitivity to
> From the land of mist and snow. your own moods
>
> And every tongue, will be enough
> through utter drought, to furnish your ideas.
> Was withered at the root; You will not require drugs
>
> We could not speak, because all you need
> no more than if you already have.
> We had been choked with soot. You'll enjoy the struggle and even
>
> Ah! well a-day! setbacks give insight and strength.
> what evil looks Your victories will enable you
> Had I from old and young! to help
>
> Instead of the cross, others, not just your friends.
> the Albatross Your gifts will be enjoyed
> About my neck was hung.' by everyone.

The doctor leant forward and took the book from his patient. 'Right, that's enough.' He returned the book to the shelf.

'Oh,' said Dr Benway, 'I was beginning to enjoy that.'

'Oooh, don't say that!' Dent bantered. 'Haven't you heard, my treatments are never enjoyable.'

The American sniggered. He wondered what that must have sounded like, two voices on their seemingly unrelated journeys. He watched in disappointment as Dent got up and walked out...he had so many questions. Dent returned with Kate.

'Time for your 8 p.m. Then I must get back to the ranch.' He filled a syringe. 'Tomorrow night I should be able to come in again and if things continue as they are you'll feel your energy return.' The needle slid in and out. Dent applied the antiseptic swab and held it firmly. The patient felt the pressure spread to his whole shoulder. It felt as reassuring as the message. 'You're doing well, Dr Benway. Very well.'

Their eyes met as was becoming customary but this time the patient wasn't compelled to look away. Instead he smiled in recognition that he was being cared for in a way he'd either forgotten or never known. This thought triggered a cascade of warmth and emotion. He would repay the croaker with all he had, he wouldn't let him down, no backsliding now.

'Thank you,' he murmured, but the doctor was gone. 'The Derry Air' was filling the stairwell; he heard it echoing in the stairwell until the door closed five flights below. Tears of relief streamed down his cheeks.... And the choice of Coleridge... and *that* poem? It must have been deliberate...? He wondered... but would never know... he let his eyelids fall...

...... an' the viewless wings o' Hypnos drew down their blinds... goose down drowsy I slip into tawny twilight....while far off, delta waters wash their grey sounds aroun' me... an' the wheels of the past, present and future become one.... then... slow as the second coming .... outta the whisperin' sands an' honeyed air, comes the most majestic mountain lion you ever saw....purring away she let's me bury my face in her thick warm fur......we embrace an' I ask, 'are you God?'... .'I'm love,' she answers, an' carries me atop Bluff Canyon revealin' all the earthly delights; whippoorwills, the harvest moon, swoopin' drifts o' moths, fireflies and little ole chickadees....an' all the while she's purrin'...yow'd all know the sound when you hears it... ain't no mystery..., 'mend y'self by leavin' well alone', she hums....an' I fall into a trance...yield, an' let go.... an', you know?... I sleep real good, first time for years... I'm sure, y'd all know it... that ole cat rumble... it's deeper than peace and all about love ....

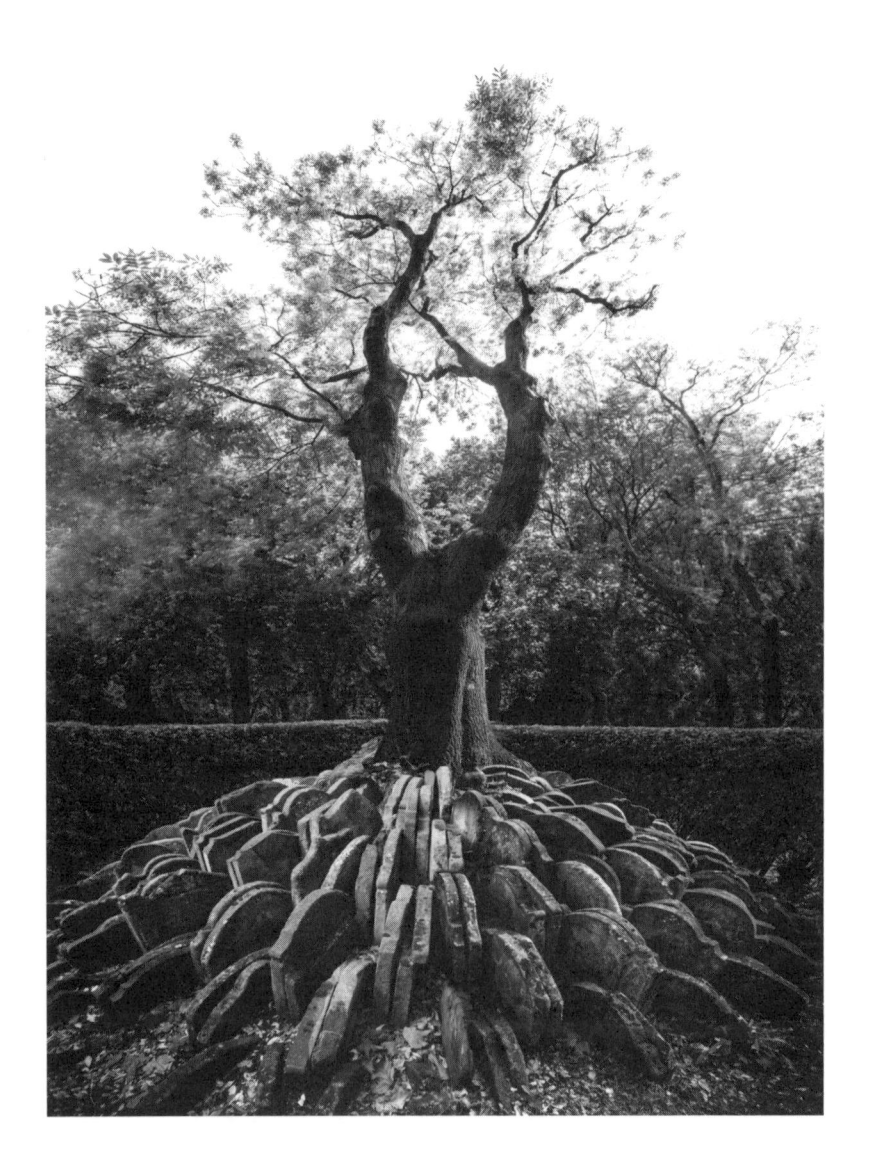

[photo: Warwick Sweeney]

13

Drunks

> What, therefore, seemed the least liable to objections of any, was that the chief sensorium, or head-quarters of the soul, and to which place all intelligences were referred, and from whence all her mandates were issued,—was in, or near, the cerebellum,—or rather somewhere about the medulla oblangata, wherein it was generally agreed by Dutch anatomists, that all the minute nerves from all the organs of the seven senses concentered, like streets and winding alleys, into a square.
> – Laurence Sterne
> *The Life and Opinions of Tristram Shandy, Gentleman*

All day long hammerhead cumulus towered over London. Beyond the fringe of the southern horizon the first flicker of an electrical storm. The sunset simmered, a crucible, red-rimmed and angry. Finally, the pressure burst over the metropolis, an explosion of fulminating rage.

Captain George Broadbridge, MC with bar, staggered out of the pub. He turned his face towards the tumult, pleading for answers from a pitiless sky. He raised an empty bottle of whisky to his mouth. The kiss of hard glass prompted thoughts of his old war whistle, the one on the mantelpiece at home. He felt broken, useless. He cursed the heavens for being unable to wash away his pain. A shrill blast from a nearby train triggered another memory, each association firing another until the howling tornado overhead stretched deep into his brain, pulling yesterday into today and nightmare into fact. Blundering he fell backwards through time and space.

Terrified he looked around. Gaslight flares spread their haunting presence over a desecrated land. Sentinel trees, monuments to the millions of mouthless dead, pointed their charred fingers at the maelstrom. Sucking shells and whizzbangs rippled sodden air; another barrage. George knew the signs but he mustn't panic. 'Have to show my boys.' He squatted and ran crablike to the end of the canal wall and stopped. If they advanced he'd expose their flanks but the crump hole wasn't safe either. 'What to do?' He interpreted the sudden silence as a lull and blew hard on the bottle, a short sharp blast. Immediately a tickle of phosphorescence crept along his savant neck, his only warning. He spun, glimpsed the shadowy line of crouching figures: his comrades. 'Get down, lads!' he cried. Too late, the explosion turned the sky to a white sheet and toppled him face down into a deep puddle. A black swell spread outwards, over cobbles and against the braking wheels of a horse-drawn police wagon.

Two dripping constables looked down at the bedraggled heap.
'Sod it!' said the driver.
'Your turn,' said the other.
'Didn't say it weren't.'
'Let the bugger drown.'
'Can't.'
'Why?'
'Military, ain't he?'
''Ow d' y'know?'
''Is 'at.'
A braided peaked cap floated along the gutter.
'What clobber's that then?' asked the young one, riding shotgun.
'How d' I know.'
'Just a ruse anyhow.'
'What?'
''Ee's a beggar.'
'No he ain't.'
''Course 'ee is,' the young one sneered.
'What about the 'at?'
'Borrored it.'
'Come again?'

'You ain't 'arf thick. He uses his hat to beg wiv.'

The older policeman hesitated. He saw an opportunity. 'Bet yer,' he said, securing the reins and pulling on the brake.

'How much?'

'A tanner, and any that's on 'im.'

'How much did you get off the last one, the prossy?'

'Nuffin'.'

'Yer lyin'.'

'Ask 'er if you don't believe me.'

''Ow can I? She's sloshed.'

'Well, you'll 'av to take my word.'

The young policeman coughed and wiping his dripping eyebrows considered his options. 'Ok, my tanner ses he ain't a soldier.'

'Yer on!' said the senior policeman, holding out his palm for his accomplice to strike the deal.

The smirking driver got down from the wagon and splashed over to the half-submerged figure. He reached under the water, grabbing George's lapel. 'Wakey wakey,' he shouted, turning him over.

'Thought so,' he muttered, peering at the face in the feeble light. He pulled the comatose head up by its hair and slapped it. George's jaw dropped, spilling alcohol fumes into the night.

'Evenin', Cap'n.' The policeman slapped the other cheek. 'How about a comfy bed for the night, hey?'

George gulped and shook his head. 'Whar?' He swooned, his pupils rolled. His cheeks were struck again, hard. He focused on the face in front of him. Things slowly fell into place. His predicament was as clear as the solution. He closed his right hand into a fist and let the copper have it. Both men fell backwards into the expanding puddle. The older policeman rose slowly, holding his broken and bleeding nose. 'Gi' us a 'and, Mick,' he mumbled. 'Bathstab ain't parthal t' pethwasian.'

Mick got down from the wagon and pulled a truncheon from his belt. He pointed it accusingly at his colleague. 'You recognised 'im.'

'So?' said the older policeman, spitting blood.

'It ain't fair. You bet me when you already knew he's a swaddy.'

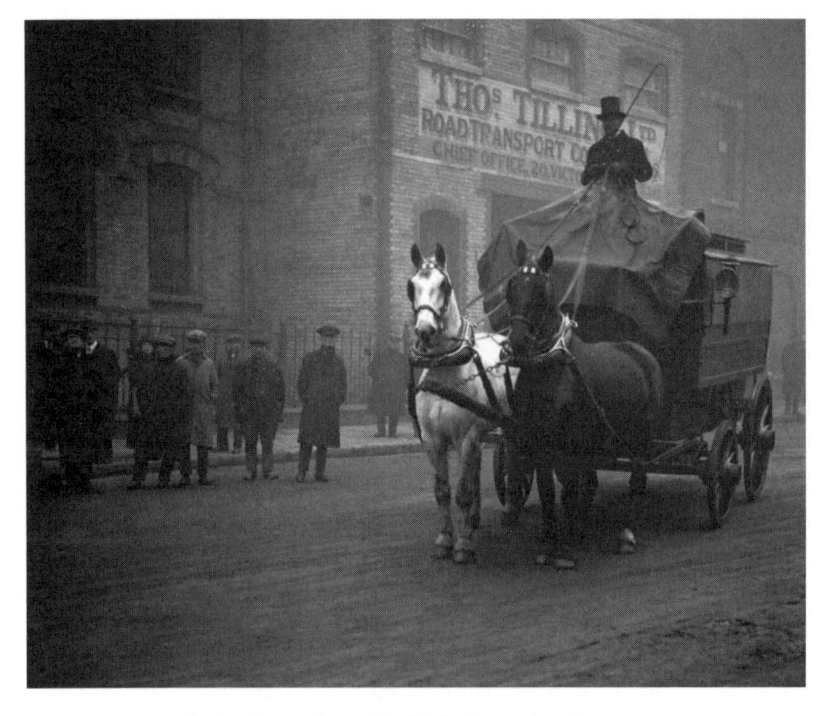

The last horse-drawn Black Maria seen here in 1924.
[©Collage, London Picture Archive, 2018]

'And?'

'You cheated.'

'Shut up, Mick, an' thwow 'im in the back.'

Scowling, Mick grabbed George by the collar and poked the truncheon into his neck.

'I ain't in no mood, soldier boy. Up or else.'

The captain staggered to his feet, waved away the truncheon and threw a weak punch.

'Have it yer own way,' snarled Mick, and caught the captain with a brisk blow to the temple.

George staggered and fell to his knees. The older policeman, still holding his face, kicked the captain's belly, and, as he fell forward, brought his heel down onto his back.

'Buggerin', beggerin' bathstud,' he mumbled and buried his toecap deep into the captain's ribs. George rolled over, groaning.

'Right, Mick,' he spluttered, 'he's done for. Take 'im for anyfin' he's go' and chuck 'im aboard.'

Sniggering, Mick pinched his nose mocking his injured colleague. 'Burrerin' berrerin' bathstab,' as he went through the captain's pockets, cleaning him out. Penniless, George was locked in the back with the other drunks.

Fifteen minutes later the two policemen discharged their cargo into the care of St Pancras Infirmary. Free of their obligations they returned home along cleansed streets, streets rinsed by rain and the law.

* * *

Inside the hospital Sister Lawson arrived to deal with the usual Saturday night intake. She advanced towards the last trolley and looked at the battered and bruised face of George Broadbridge. He searched her face, hoping to meet her eyes.

'You again,' she remarked, with no attempt to conceal her disgust.

'Let me go,' he pleaded.

'Chance'd be a fine thing,' she said, pulling hard on the leather restraints that bound him.

'Please!' he raised his voice and waggled his head in a frenzy.

'Stop that!' she demanded, to no avail.

'You know me. I'm a soldier, decorated. Please!' he moaned.

'Hero or not, we do our job.'

'Please, you can help me!' He was trying to sound pitiful.

'Look here!' The sister grabbed both his ears and pinched. 'Carry on squealing an' I'll sew your lugholes to the stretcher, clear?'

Captain George Broadbridge screwed up his face in pain and indignation. He would have to try another tack. He paused and waited till the sister released her grip. 'Why can't you just let me sleep it off?' he asked.

'We can't, now shut up.'

'It hurts,' he complained, jerking his head to the commotion on the other side of the room. 'Really hurts!'

The sister turned and watched a thin middle-aged woman being held down. A small rigid frame with a round hole in its centre was forced between her jaws. Her screams turned to gurgles as a junior doctor and a nurse fed a thick rubber tube into her mouth and down her throat. The nurse started to pump on a brass cylinder as if her life depended on it. The woman's body twisted and shook. She was urinating. It was bedlam.

George waited until he had regained the sister's attention. 'You could loosen the stretcher restraint, please!'

'No,' she said coldly.

'Just the top one,' he wheezed.

'Shut it.'

He lowered his voice to a hoarse murmur, 'I can't breathe.'

'You must think I was born yesterday,' she said, trying to sound firm. She looked at the captain's face. It had gone purple. She placed her hand on his chest. He held his breath and let his head fall to one side. She released the buckle by two notches.

'Is that better?' she asked, leaning forward.

George wriggled his arm free and for the second time that evening his knuckles found their target. The sister fell like a rag doll. George undid the straps and jumped off the trolley before anyone noticed. He burst through the doors just as Doctors Dent and Dalton were climbing the stairs from Surgery.

'Ah, George, back again?' Dalton said, blocking George's path to the exit.

George turned and raced up the stairs, reaching the fifth floor in a series of leaps and bounds. He barged through the last pair of swing doors, pushing past a startled nurse.

Climbing over an occupied bed George squeezed himself through a half open window as Dalton grabbed one of his flailing legs.

'Leave me alone,' he moaned, kicking Dalton with his free leg.

'George,' panted Dent, 'what is it?'

'The pump, I won't have it,' he sobbed, looking at the neat row of spiked iron railings five floors below.

'We have to give it,' said Dent. 'There's no alternative.'

'Let me go,' shouted George, 'my mind's made up.'

Dent whispered something into Dalton's ear and gestured that the nurse should take his place at the window and hang onto George's other leg.

Dent left the ward but returned within a minute with a loaded syringe. He climbed onto a chair.

'Excuse me, George,' he said pulling down the captain's trousers and injecting a drug called apomorphine into the top of his backside. 'Hold him tight, please; don't relax, not for an instant.'

George looked into the darkness. He didn't care. He felt a hand gripping his collar. If only he could bite it. He wriggled; it was no use, they had him fast and were all against him. Coppers, doctors, even the bastard weather. He'd never yield. That was all he had, a refusal to buckle…. He closed his eyes and listened to the hiss of steam engines across the rail yard. He could imagine them shunting back and forth under the gaping train shed. Their roars grew louder like the advance of progress. He knew what they were about. He'd seen it all…the fantastical turrets and spires of St Pancras devouring cheering school children pulling them through arches to the shiny carriages that carried them far into the night, thunderous locomotives spurting sparks and sliding into hell's forge…the metallic rattle of points and rails merging into the chatter of machine guns far beyond sense or justice …a pellmell descent into darkness, a well of industrial death swallowing flesh, bone and mud…. All buried now, a truth too brutal to mention. Who makes the law? After a while you stop hearing the insanity and long to lie with them safe in the underworld…they alone met the madness…they alone understand.

Another shrill whistle from the train shed returned George from the war but this time to something new. Something clicked inside. He was on a different track…he opened his eyes. This was a track he couldn't leave…. All his impulses suddenly meshed. His mind, its deepest and most elemental compulsions combined with every fibre of his body.

His stomach erupted. Its entire contents arced through the darkness. For a second nothing then the telltale splatter below. A wide-eyed George gulped. 'Hell. That should've been my brains,' he mumbled, relaxing his hold on the parapet.

'Got him,' shouted Dalton, and yanked George back inside the building.

* * *

The next morning Dent met the matron on her way out of George's ward.

'Anything to report?' he asked her.

'Nothing out of the ordinary,' she replied, 'apart from our friend at the end. I heard you had a struggle last night.'

'Ah, George. Is he restrained?'

'Yes,' she said.

'And furious, I suppose.'

'You'll see,' she said with a twinkle.

Fearing the usual slug of insults Dent left George's bed until last. 'Another eventful evening you gave us, George.'

George opened his eyes. 'Oh, you,' he grunted.

Dent felt George's forehead and took his pulse. 'Would you like a glass of water?'

George's voice brightened. 'Yes, please!'

Dent filled a glass from a jug and held it to George's swollen lips.

He downed it greedily.

'More?' asked Dent.

'Ooo, yes please … a life saver.'

Dent held the glass while cradling him with his other arm. The water barely touched the sides.

'My, you are thirsty.'

George fell back onto his pillow and tried to make himself comfortable.

Dent checked the tightness of the restraints. 'I suppose you've had another terrible night, no sleep?'

George thought about it. 'Strangely, I think I had a good night.'

Dent thought this odd. He felt George's forehead with no good purpose other than that it gained thinking time. 'I'll be back in a few minutes, don't go away.'

George gave an ironic laugh as Dent went to find the matron.

'What did you mean, "you'll see"?' he asked her.

'You mean about George?'

'Yes.'

'Well, we all know how he is, a bear with a sore head, but when I did the early round he was still fast asleep. Later, when the nurse woke him, he was chatting away and no profanities either. He even apologised for his behaviour last night.'

Dent raised his eyebrows. 'I needed to hear it from you as I could hardly believe it either. He even laughed at a lame joke.'

'One of yours?'

'Er, yes.'

'Extraordinary,' she said, smiling.

Dent pulled some items of clothing from a cupboard and returned to George.

'Where did you get those bruises, George, the ones on your face?'

'Coppers, last night. I put up a good fight, though.' George ran his fingertips over his grazed knuckles.

'How would you feel, George, if I took off these restraints?'

'Aren't you worried I might do you in?'

'Should I be?'

George reflected for a moment. 'I think you're safe,' he smiled.

As soon as the straps were released George rubbed his face vigorously. 'You've no idea how good that feels; thank you.'

'I thought,' said Dent, smiling, 'we might go somewhere quiet, for a chat. Would you like that?'

Dent helped George out of bed and gave him a dressing gown, socks and slippers. He spoke as he helped him. 'Matron and the sister say we have had you in almost every other weekend since May. Is there a reason why it's so regular?'

George tied his dressing gown cord. 'I didn't realise it was, but now you say it.'

They walked out of the ward, down the stairs and through the back of the South Wing into St Pancras Gardens and cemetery. After strolling aimlessly for a few minutes they found an empty wooden bench midway between two unique structures; a mausoleum and a strange circle of repurposed gravestones.

'What's that?' commented George, nodding towards the unusual formation.

'A monument' replied Dent, 'created by Thomas Hardy.'

'Hardy, the writer?' asked George, disbelieving.

'Yes, when he was a student of architecture, before moving on to a higher calling.'

'I'm glad he made the switch,' said George, quickly.

'Don't you like it?'

'I need a closer look.'

'Well, I like it. I also think it expresses something consistent with his writing.'

George considered the point. 'What do you mean?'

'Usually monuments record names and dates, or the causes people died for. By stacking the stones face to face it transcends all that, all the pettiness, the patriotic posturing. There is no reference to any creed, law or the usual customs we genuflect before. And by ditching all that Hardy's suggesting something much greater... something that goes beyond the flux and flow of life itself. I see that in his writing... he may describe the human character but its always against a backdrop of immutable forces...'

'You don't care for monuments of remembrance?'

'Awful, particularly war memorials. And I don't relish the usual stuff either: no cards, homilies and certainly no flowers for me.' Dent smiled.

'I won't forget.' George laughed before settling to reflect on Hardy's strange monument.

'Yes,' George eventually concurred. 'I suppose through it's ascribed anonymity, it represents, I dunno, something bigger than anything we can imagine.' He got up and approached the structure like a pilgrim at the end of a journey. His blue-grey eyes squinted, their gaze falling on a seedling ash tree clinging to the top of the monument. A gust of wind tugged its few, brittle leaves... from where did it get its strength, he wondered. Its urge to hang on and push for the light? He quietly marvelled its tenacity, its life struggle springing from nothing more fertile than rings of stacked headstones.... Slowly a protective, almost wistful emotion grew in George's heart. After several minutes' reflection he returned hesitantly to the park bench and the watching doctor.

His voice wavered: 'Do you think that little tree will survive?' he asked, slightly fearful of the answer.

Dent thought about it. 'Yes,' he replied eventually, 'it'll be fine if it's left alone.'

'Yes, let's hope so,' said George faintly, recalling the beautiful woods on the Somme. The glades of mixed woodland where his comrades had spent their last days before the slog to the Front.

Soft pools of warming sunlight spread through the garden's canopy. The breeze dropped and George leant back, crossing his legs. 'I had not realised there was a pattern to my coming here, but now I've thought about it there certainly is.'

'If our clocks were on a fourteen day cycle we could ask you to wind them for us,' remarked Dent.

George rubbed his battered ribs. 'When I leave here I go straight home. My wife doesn't ask me where I've been. Even if I could remember I don't think she really wants to know.'

'What do you talk about?'

'What I'm going to do, work, the usual.'

'And you want to talk about other things?'

'Yes, exactly. How did you know?'

'I didn't, but I wondered. What sort of other things?'

'The war mostly. I want to talk about how I feel about it. How I miss it, but it's hopeless, she'll never understand.'

Dent was surprised and tried to put himself in George's wife's shoes. 'Miss the war, all that misery?' he ventured, doubtfully.

'Yes,' said George. 'You see we survived what to everyone else is unimaginable. That is a knowledge we share. Friendships like that cannot be replicated on civvy street. Just as well really.'

'I see,' said Dent. 'I suppose in a way, she feels jealous.'

'Oh yes!' remarked George, 'I hadn't thought about it like that. Love is so complicated with the demands we insist upon... it ends up destroying itself.'

'True friendship is love without boundaries.'

'Exactly!' said George, 'I wonder if my wife would accept that?'

They let the thought percolate for a minute while a young couple walked past arm in arm.

'Do you have children?' asked Dent.

'Two girls, you?'

'One, but another on the way.'

'Oh! Congratulations!' Despite the battering George's face had retained its rugged beauty. It radiated pleasure.

Dent reciprocated with a broad smile. 'I suppose your wife has to worry about your children's welfare?'

'Yes, but I have my army pension and she has an annuity. This isn't about money, it's deeper.'

Dent sensed that this was true. He tried to imagine what, if anything, might help George's wife understand.

'If you could tell her about the war what would you say?'

George didn't speak at first but licked his raw knuckles. As he dropped his hands he started to talk.

'When I'm at home or even up here the nights are the worst. I'm filled with melancholy and loneliness. It pulls me right down. I see my men, their faces looking at me. I think of what happened... decisions ...' George sifted through the scrambled chaos of his memories, confronting the usual jumble of grief and blame. How much should he say? He thought how he'd cried when his wife had wanted to throw his war whistle out. He knew its symbolism, she never would. Slowly the tangled swamp of his mind grew signposts. One by one a sequence of pictures emerged and the words that described them. He looked to his left, at the trees towering over Hardy's monument and falteringly, re-traced his way.

'One night about five years ago my men and I had to follow in the second wave but we got held up by a sniper. We should have gone on but the moon was up and I didn't want to leave us exposed. I signalled we should wait in a shell hole by a broken down wall. I lay there listening to the whizz bangs and the boom of the rail gun until everything fell silent. I hated that because it was usually a prelude to something. Weighing up my options I crawled forward and looked over a thin layer of mist rising out of the valley between the lines. I could just make out the escarpment behind the German trenches crisscrossed with searchlights. Suddenly the whole skyline flashed. Their big guns, hundreds of them, had opened up. I blew my whistle to get back but it's futile. Suddenly we're hit and I'm flying through the air. I remember having strange thoughts, everything slows down... I don't remember landing. When I wake up I'm soaked in blood. I think: 'that's it, I'm dying'... until I realise the blood isn't mine. Apart from temporary deafness I'm unscathed. I crawl out of the carnage and through a mile of mud to our trench. Next day they tell me over twenty of my boys are gone, wiped out. I couldn't understand it. Why them and not me? I was sent back to recuperate but it's a living hell. There's no sense to it, the war or anything. I wished I'd died. I'd've done myself in save for the fact that I was needed back at the Front. You'll think this strange but I was glad to go. It was the only place where I didn't have to explain; that's how we coped, see? We didn't even have to ask, we could recognise it, see it in a man's eyes, smell it on each other's skin. It surpassed words, grief, everything. That's how we pulled through; we were a brotherhood.

'Later, when it was all over, I was empty. My feelings bounced around like echoes in a crypt. The brass gave me a medal which made it worse.... Sure, I hated the war but now I ache for it. I've never admitted this to anyone, you're the first.'

Dent nodded and looked up. 'When did you start drinking?'

'We drank in the trenches, course we did, particularly before the big pushes. But it didn't stop after de-mob. Each bout got worse, because sober I could see how I'd changed. The nightmares got worse and I couldn't sleep. I got no pleasure at home, in my kids, nothing. Drink helped me blot out what I couldn't face. Now my wife says she no longer recognises me, that booze has changed me. Two years ago I'd get sloshed uptown, sober up, go home and the same cycle would start over. She isn't stupid, she's learnt to cope, but her family's military and destined to uphold the very madness I've described. They'll never acknowledge their mistakes; they can't afford to. I've more respect for the German soldiers, they fought honourably and were victims like us.' George looked up through bloodshot eyes at his tongue-tied doctor. 'I'd like to stop drinking but can't.'

Dent uncrossed his arms and hesitantly patted George's shoulder. 'I'm sorry, I feel so useless,' was all he could manage. Finally, George broke the silence:

'Last night, on the roof, what actually happened?'

'Yes, sorry about that. We carry that drug for poisoning; as you can see it empties a stomach in seconds.'

'Why don't you use it all the time? Nobody likes the pump, not even you lot.'

Dent thought about it. 'Well, I have used it before, once or twice, with, er... difficult cases, but it isn't encouraged.'

'No?'

'No. If the chief finds out there'll be hell to pay.'

'Well, it gave me a good night and no hangover.'

'Maybe just a coincidence,' suggested Dent.

'What do you mean?'

'Well, you may not have one because of another reason, one we haven't considered. What had you drunk?'

'Oh the usual, beer and then spirits, whisky, probably not as much as usual because I left the pub early. I heard the thunderstorm and fancied a walk; what a night, hey?'

'Yes, great guns and marlinspikes.'

'Fantastic lightning.'

'You remember that?'

'I do, even the coppers picking me up. Say, I don't suppose they delivered me with my cap?'

'I don't know, I'll ask the porter.'

'Thanks. You see, I banged my head when I fell over. I think that's why I've got this bruise on my face.'

'Yes, not this one on your head?' Dent lifted the hair above George's ear to reveal a dark blue line.

'No, that was the copper. Is it bad?'

'You'll live.'

'Oh dear,' said George, drily, and chuckled. Dent caught his mood and joined in.

'Look, George, you evidently like being outside; why don't you stay here and soak up some more sun? I've got to be getting on but I'll check on your belongings and send them out.'

Dent went straight down to the Admissions Hall and asked for the captain's personal effects.

'Oh, police constable just popped in for them,' said the porter.

'What do you mean?'

'Blowed if I know. He signed and took 'em upstairs. He's with a sergeant.'

Dent ran up to George's ward and found a nurse.

'What's going on?'

'With George? They're arresting him. I don't know why. Look, they're with him now.'

Dent crossed to the window and looked into the gardens. George was being spoken to by two uniformed officers. Another stood to one side. Dent ran downstairs and met the sergeant coming up.

'Are you Dr Dent?'

'Yes.'

'We're taking that drunk off yer 'ands.'

'But why? He needs care.'

'Don't worry, Doctor, we know what 'e's good for.' The sergeant tapped the top of his truncheon.

'But he hasn't done anything.'

'Oh no. You should take a butcher's at the constable's snozzer, sir. A right mess it is.'

Dent watched helplessly as a handcuffed George was escorted towards the garden gates.

'Another thing. He's got previous, I 'ear. Shouldn't wonder if he don't get a spell in clink.'

'Won't they fine him?'

'What would he pay it wiv? He swears he's got money but he can't find 'is wallet. Usual story, I'm afraid.' The sergeant sniffed and rubbed his nose. 'Anyway, you've enough on yer plate. We'll sort 'im owt, don't you worry.' The sergeant touched his cap, turned on his heels and marched off.

At lunch Dent sat down with his thoughts. It depressed him to think of George; how, he couldn't be relieved of his torment. And now he'd be thrown before the magistrates.

'You look like an old dog,' said Dalton, joining him.

'With good cause, Dalton.'

'I heard about George.'

'He's ill, he needs care,' complained Dent.

'Isn't that what we do for him? Stop him choking on his puke?'

'I mean care that works. We grumble that the same old faces keep coming back without accepting that our methods are part of the problem. What about the cause? People like George get no advice, no one listens to them. Most of the time they just need someone to talk to.'

'Talk to? Why?'

'Honestly, Dalton, you can be dreadfully dull sometimes.'

'What is it that I don't understand?'

'That doctors should be able to do more, much more. Remember Barnes, when you said we couldn't do anything because we were students. But look at us now, qualified but just as hamstrung.'

'You told me then that Barnes needed to get psychological help... suggestion wasn't it? I don't know how that alone can help.' Dalton looked up at his friend.

'But the suggestion of health can lead to different...' The words dried in Dent's throat. For the second time that day he was frustrated by his own ineptitude.

'Yes?' persisted Dalton. 'I'm waiting.'

'Behaviour,' said Dent.

'What?'

'Yes,' continued Dent, 'by listening and offering different possibilities we can encourage different behaviour that doesn't involve alcohol.'

'Come again?'

'Yesterday poor old George was fighting with policemen.'

'Because, let me remind you, he was drunk.'

'Yes, but why was he drinking? The truth is George drinks because he cannot confront the pain of telling his family why he's miserable. He blames the war, but really it's our inability to understand how the war has affected him that creates the conflict ... and lies at the heart of his anxiety. That's his worry, and alcohol just de-anxietises him ... temporarily. He has no other way to deflect the blame and assuage his guilt.'

'How do you know?'

Dent looked at the mug of tea in front of him and stirred it idly. 'I don't, it's just a hunch.'

'And how do you know about the war?'

'He told me, he's scarred by it.'

'So he already knows what the problem is?'

'Perhaps, but the anxiety comes when he confronts everyone else's expectation that he should behave differently. Society believes he's a hero and should act like one, "pull himself together" or "forget about it". George knows he isn't a hero and drink obliterates this conflict but in the morning it's back and worse. However, this morning, in the gardens, he spilled the beans, everything. The talking seemed to change him, he was even laughing.'

Dalton sounded doubtful. 'All because you had a chat?'

'No. Look, Dalton, I cannot be sure but could it be that vomiting helped?'

'Because of apomorphine? I just hope for your sake no one finds out.'

'Well, you saw what happened. That's the only thing that can explain the change. I have tried to speak to him before; so have you, everyone has. It makes no difference. But today it's chalk and cheese.'

'And now you've lost him.'

'I know, but what can I do?' Dent sank forward running his fingers through his hair. 'What can any of us do, in here?'

'And the Church doesn't help,' muttered Dalton.

'Did it ever?'

'Last week in maternity I delivered a still born. And just as the poor woman is waking up that prig of a priest bursts in. You know, the one with a red and gold cassock and door-stop Bible. 'Show me the baby,' he demands. Before I could intervene the nurse gestures over to the bundle. 'UGH!' he exclaims turning back the towel, 'I've never seen anything so disgusting.' I try and shut him up but the entitled oaf starts remonstrating. 'Why didn't you keep it alive,' he bellows, 'I could've saved its soul?'

Dent shrugged. 'Old habits die hard.'

'I'd kill a few abbots,' grumbled Dalton.

'I won't stand in your way.' The two friends chuckled at a grim understanding. Dent leant back. 'I am afraid Dalton, the establishment prefers the status quo irrespective of what is compassionate or remedial. Their agents, the Law and the Church, baulk at anything which doesn't perpetuate ingrained idiocy. Medicine is no different. Only last week I heard Cameron recommending gin to a whisky addict. My wife thinks I should leave. She thinks I have suffered enough.'

'Set up on your own?'

'Yes, private practice.'

'Well that should permit you a bit more freedom ... and if I'm turned to drink, you can heal me.'

Someone approached them from behind. It was Matron Skehan; she looked agitated.

'Sorry, am I interrupting something?'

Dalton looked up. 'Er, no nothing. We were just discussing George.'

'I see,' said Matron. 'It'll have to wait, I'm afraid; we're all required in surgery, there's an emergency.'

'Righto.' Dent swilled down his tea and followed Dalton and Matron back towards the main building.

Downstairs at the hospital entrance the first group of sobered-up vagrants were being discharged. They ambled down Midland Road passing a tramp and his dog at the junction under St Pancras Station.

They clocked his pitch and string of polished medals on moth-eared khaki, but most of all the yawning gap between his crutches. This crippled hero knew how to work the street.

'Look at 'im, puttin' the touch on,' muttered one dry drunk to another.

'Aye,' said his companion, eyeing a tin full of coppers. 'The dandy dosser, don't even need shoes.'

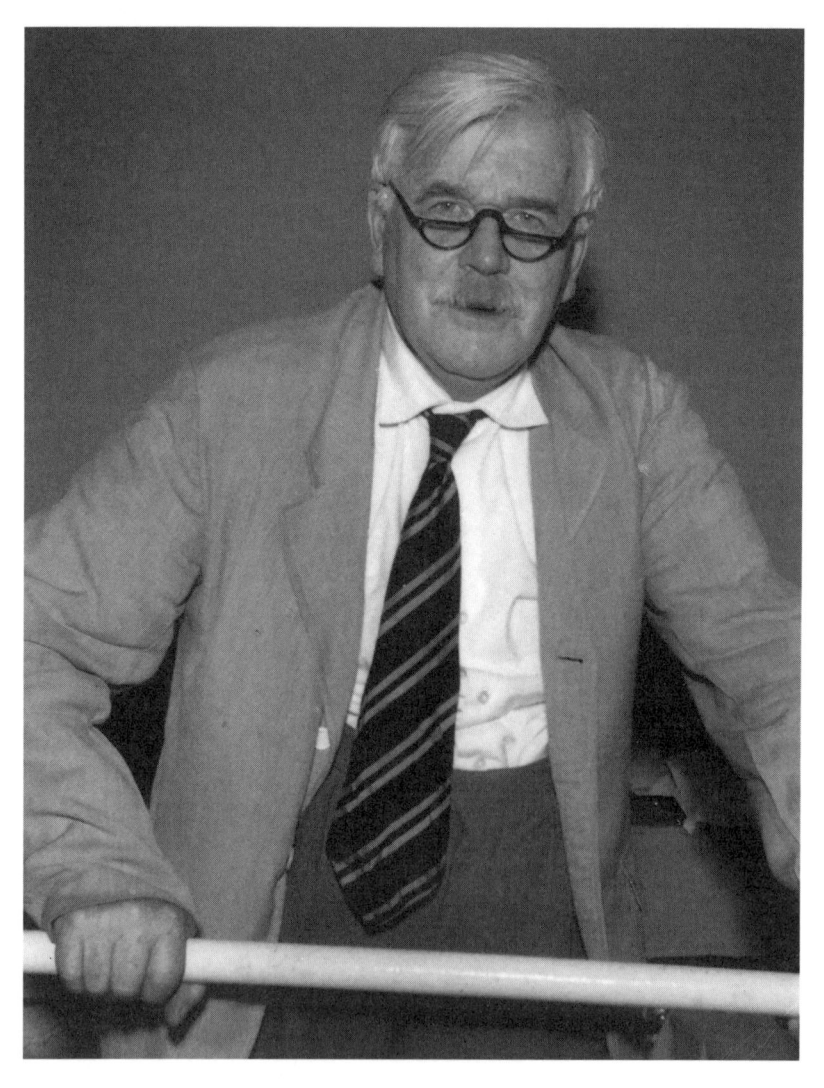

J. Y. Dent, 66 [photographer unknown]
signed on reverse, 'Lady boy'.

14

Silent Waiting

Therapy isn't Radio. We don't need to constantly fill the air with sounds. Sometimes, when it's quiet, surprising things happen.
– Mary Pipher, *Letters to a Young Therapist*

The doctor laughed quietly to himself at the irony. He'd come back to the clinic at midnight because Dr Benway had complained he couldn't sleep only for Hannah to whisper that he'd just dropped off. Sure enough, he was sleeping soundly and his next injection wasn't due for over an hour. The doctor would wait in the gloom and silence. He made himself comfortable in the bay window and cleared some space on the table. There was just enough light to play and it'd give him the opportunity to sort out a few ideas…

… Benway stirred. He was vaguely aware of a repetitive sound. It was irregular… but quite distinct… like a blue catfish flapping in the bottom of a canoe: "flick". Sometimes the sound was harsher: "click". It was dark. He'd stir himself but stay cocooned in the warm… no need to open his eyes… surface… nothing to be gained… Kiki would fix for him… no need to move, he was comfortable… 'Ugh!?' He held his leg, and his stomach… the burn… it's gone! The realisation woke him. He lay there, startled…. What had happened? He couldn't take it in; no headache either? He turned over… recalling a different time and place…. Where am I? Oh, yeah, ……. London…. 'Ugh… Sister… hello?'

'She's next door… with the other patient.' The voice was familiar.

Benway scratched his cheek. Who was that, what was happening? 'Hello?'

'Good morning, Dr Benway...'
'Oh, Doc Dent...what time is it?'
'One a.m. Did I wake you?'
'Er, I dunno...I mean no...'
'What day is it?' Dent asked.
'You're asking me?'
'It's not important...but I wondered.'

Benway rubbed his eyes...he had arrived, oh...last week...but that was impossible. He remembered 'Come Friday, eleven a.m.' It must be Monday or Tuesday...no, there was that Macmillan chap, what was his name? Another Mac...he'd have to ask; the doctor twins, two more Macs, suits an' bow-ties. Kate came in during the day, Hannah at night...and croaker all hours...here again...early hours...? Might be Wednesday?...he'd had a shave yesterday after the second enema...shocked by his appearance...gotta straighten out. Must ring his folks ...let them know about no burn...what would that mean to them? He'd tell them to hang out the flags. "Hang out *with fags*?" his Father would reply. "No Father," he'd have to repeat, "the flags."

Benway lifted his head. 'Thursday.'

'Correct! Well done!' Dent spoke looking at the table...there was that sound again. More flicks.

Pushing himself up Benway tried to see. 'What are you doing?'

'Playing cards...Patience.' There were some rapid manoeuvres... the game played itself out... 'No good...' said the doc, 'no good.' He gathered up the cards and put the pack back in its box.

'Patience?' repeated the American, eventually.

'Yes, I am not really playing the game...but experiencing the idea.'

Benway was still interpreting his doctor's ways...it wasn't easy. He needed time to think about what he'd heard. Simple words...but big ideas. He'd already realised that small talk was not the croaker's forte...better to have something meaningful to say if you're gonna ruin silence...

'I'm not a card shark, you know?' continued Dent. 'It's against my religion.' The doctor found this funny. His body trembled. 'No,' he continued, 'I play cards because it gives my brain the space to find answers. There's a great sound in silence, do you agree?'

'By playing cards?'

'Well, it empties the mind, like worry beads, chanting or playing a raga. Any automatic action that permits the mind to sidestep the drab and dreary routines of everyday life. Patience works... reading too, provides a distraction, clears the mind of obstacles. Then, later, when I re-engage with a problem, I'm refreshed. I am looking at it from somewhere else.' Dent thought of 'Seldom Seen' and his old aunt pointing out to sea. 'And voilà! There it is... the answer to all our hopes and prayers.' He laughed at his private joke.

'By sidestepping the heat-oppressed brain...' muttered Benway.

'Exactly,' confirmed Dent, 'the cards there,' he gestured towards the table, 'calm the nerves here.' He pressed his fingertips to his temples. 'It is like the "silent waiting" employed by Quakers. The difficulty comes with trying to convince others that doing nothing is the gateway to everything. We live in such a habit-forming environment based on reactions to a material existence that we forget this side of ourselves. Even when we try it and it works, the next time we're still likely to return to those old ways to resolve issues, to find solutions.'

'Don't medicate, meditate.' Benway sniggered.

Dent smiled. 'That's it. So many of the drugs used today suppress the brain. This is quite wrong. How can we get to know a patient if our first response is to turn him into a cabbage?'

Benway nodded. 'I think Maclay realises this. He seems to want to find better treatments. I should call him the real McCoy.'

Dent laughed. 'Yes, he's one of the few. But there's another reason I play patience. I sometimes do it in a consultation.'

'So you can engage with the patient?' guessed the American.

'That's right. So many doctors are as clever as a bowl of soup. Usually they cannot wait to deliver their stock answer so they can see the next patient and so on. They're reluctant to alter a protocol, even one that is doomed to failure, because they cannot evolve their thinking. A good doctor is by definition a practitioner but one that listens. Playing patience encourages me to remain quiet, permitting the patient "talk time". The really nervous patient may even believe I won't hear what's being said because I appear engrossed in another activity. The burden of expectation only adds to the patient's anxiety.... A good doctor must remove it and provide time, the time to listen and then to heal.'

'You said something the other day about negative words being problematic?'

'Well, we have three environments: the internal, the external and the conversational. That last one – the conversational or symbolic – is only fully developed in man but its impact upon the other two environments is clear.'

'A man can be made sick with fear just by looking at something like an image?'

'Possibly. The fearful reaction is of particular concern to me. Our imaginations are ripe for exploitation by the unscrupulous. Anybody, can be turned into a patient and it is fatally easy to turn the already anxious into a chronic invalid.'

'You should see the ads in the States and how they manipulate emotion?'

'Oh yes. And here. The biggest lies cement our anxieties over health. The same dishonest manipulation used to happen at table-rapping.'

'Séances?'

'Yes, I caught the tail end of that craze in my late teens. It involved all the trappings of suspense, the darkness, sudden noises and so on.'

'What happened?'

'Well, there was a manifestation of sorts. The medium introduced a wandering spirit to the circle and in particular to a "Professor" who was apparently convinced by the illusion of a dead person communicating. The real purpose, though, was to extract information from other gullible people at the table. The "Professor" was nothing of the sort, just a plant who reiterated certain "facts" in order to deceitfully engender wish-fulfilment in others.'

'Just like advertising.'

'And politics. The politician who reiterates a myth, even a lie, to promote his own ideological preferences over any deeper truth. It goes on all the time.'

Dent stood up and moved his chair to the side of the bed. As he did so he dwelt on the trajectory of his patient's mood. Everything was moving in the right direction. His reactions were better, the fog was lifting ... slowly, revealing the complexity of his character, his infinite potentialities ... and the road ahead. Yesterday afternoon he'd been fitful and depressed. It felt like a setback ... but not unusual. Overall, the curve was ascending ... time to press a few more buttons. Dent helped Benway build up a bank of pillows and then sat down.

'How are you feeling?'

'Better; I can hardly believe it but the burn has stopped, no headache, no hives.'

'Your appetite?'

'Returning. Kate prepared me dinner: steak, potatoes, tomatoes. I ate it all. Surprised myself.'

'You've surprised me too ... no morphine for over twenty hours ... well done!'

'I'm full of surprises,' Benway drawled. 'But I can barely believe I am down to this. Hannah and I were looking at the charts earlier. They prove it ... I never believed this could happen. Have you any idea how much junk I needed just to keep going? Has to be your apomorphine ... what else could it be?'

'Well ...' Dent leant back, 'we still have some way to go. Keep looking forward. Now we've reduced your injections and your appetite is returning you'll have more time to rest, to rebuild your strength. The critical thing right now is we have to be sure apomorphine is in you after all of the other drugs have left you. That will complete the metabolic change from someone who needed drugs to survive to the person who can get by without any. Tomorrow, to celebrate this transformation perhaps you'd like to get dressed, sit at the table ...'

'Do some more writing?' suggested Benway.

Dent smiled. 'Why not, or reading ... play patience if you want.' Both men laughed. Dent was delighted with the reaction. 'Have you got all you need, paper, pens and so on?'

'Yeah, sure.' The room returned to an easy silence. Neither man was in any hurry ... but the older of the two knew that his orchestration was edging towards the finale.

'When you told me about yagé,' he eventually said, 'you said you'd toyed with the idea of being a doctor?'

'Yes. I went to Vienna, to train. It didn't work out.'

'And you settled on writing?'

'Not really, I'm not sure when that started. Maybe it's always been there... though it doesn't come easily.'

'Maybe you were waiting for something to say?'

'How do you mean?'

'Well, many toy with the idea of being a writer. I know I did. I wrote poetry... short stories and so on. But pretty words aren't enough. I struggled with religion, like we discussed, but beyond that I didn't really have a peg to hang my coat on until medicine took over.... Then again, after my first book, which turned a few heads, I thought I might make a go of it; but then this. My work with addiction took off and here I am.'

For the first time in a long time Benway was able to consider another's life. 'Did you initially want to be a doctor because you believed you'd be good at it?'

'Yes, partly. I think that in my youthful arrogance I felt medicine was on the threshold of tremendous breakthroughs and I wanted a part of that. To succeed where my parent's generation had failed.'

Benway remembered his listless years. 'I suppose the attraction for me was, well, you know, a respectable profession that would ease parental scrutiny.'

'Was that all there was to it? After all, you were drawn to discover something important about yagé.'

'Yeah, but that won't cut the mustard. I've actually written two books, though only one has been published.'

'So,' Dent leant forward, 'you've succeeded where I've failed.'

'I'm not a success,' Benway scoffed.

'Oh! How can you tell? Even if you settled on any criteria: money, fame, awards, public taste, it could never be the whole story. Largely these things are unquantifiable, aren't they?'

'I'm not arguing with you, but I don't feel a success; I feel I haven't done things to my satisfaction, not yet. But, something of what you say seems to be true. You wanted to write and I wanted to have a career in medicine. We stand in each other's shoes.'

'But unfulfilled,' added Dent.

'But *you're* not a failure,' insisted Benway. 'You couldn't have achieved all this, people working for you, *your* reputation, your position at the Society, if you'd failed.'

'Oh but I feel...' the Doctor hesitated. 'Well, no. I actually know I've failed.' Dent decided not to take Benway's blood pressure for the time being; he needed to concentrate. 'You see, this problem that I have struggled to define, the control in all our lives... isn't exactly going away, is it? Recently I have had to accept that I may even be contributing to the problem.'

'How?'

'Well, it is complicated but by flushing out the opposition I have seen how powerful they are. If it is true they control where we are today they will certainly want to suppress ideas that might halt the gravy train.'

'How d'you mean?'

Dent opened his jacket and pulled a sheet of paper from his inside pocket. 'This is a recent letter written by one of your compatriots, a doctor, but no ordinary one.' He held the headed notepaper up. 'It is perfectly reasonable to conclude that his voice represents the direction of control that some exert on this matter which has affected you and tens of thousands like you, read it.' Dent passed the letter to Benway, who reached for his glasses. Dent turned on the bedside lamp.

AMERICAN MEDICAL ASSOCIATION
COUNCIL ON PHARMACY AND CHEMISTRY
535 North Dearborn Street · Chicago 10 · Illinois

February 14, 1955

Dear Dr. Dent,

Your letter of January 31 has been referred to this office by Dr. Smith.

In sub-emetic doses apomorphine produces a hypnotic or narcotic effect. As such it is potentially habit forming. If it actually satisfies the compulsion of the alcoholic or narcotic addict to escape from reality, it accomplishes this essentially through the same fundamental depressant or euphoric effect as alcohol, barbiturates or narcotics. In my opinion apomorphine would be most unsatisfactory and potentially dangerous for the treatment of alcoholism and other forms of addiction.

I am also referring your communication to the Council on Mental Health, which is also interested in problems associated with alcoholism and addiction.

Yours sincerely
Signed

Dr Benway read the letter through three times. 'That's baloney,' he muttered, returning the letter to Dent.

Dent carefully folded and returned the letter to his pocket. He loosened his tie and collar. 'I do think this letter could be symptomatic of something that is far more damaging than merely the fate of apomorphine. But as this is the area with which we are primarily involved, please, could you tell me, Dr Benway, is apomorphine a depressant, does it induce a hypnotic or narcotic effect?'

'No,' asserted the American. 'Sure, it allows me to sleep and sometimes I'm dreaming, or having nightmares, but that's detox. If apomorphine does anything it stimulates my powers of recall... I remember stuff... I dunno... clearly. What had you told them?'

'Oh, about the 4,000 cases of which I am aware. Cases not just of addiction but also various states of mental disturbances and anxiety for which apomorphine has been remedial. And to my knowledge not one case of addiction to apomorphine has been recorded. Yes, it is difficult to use but with the proper safeguards it is certainly not dangerous. But what troubles me about that letter from a collegiate perspective is the complete lack of curiosity. You see, the greatest words any scientist can express are: 'I do not know but am prepared to learn.' There is nothing of that in that letter. He knows everything. Where, for instance, is the realisation that apomorphine is a hindbrain stimulant. Why doesn't he ask about protocol and for whom it is efficacious? I certainly don't use it on everyone; for many it isn't necessary.'

'You use it on those at the compulsive end …?'

'Mostly, yes. It seems to take that compulsion away.'

'The craving?'

'There seems to be consensus on that … though "craving" appears to mean different things to different people.'

'Evil, depraved bastard. I'd boil him alive. He's employing that old trick of accusing you of what he's doing. Malignant little shit.'

Dent coughed. 'Well, perhaps I shouldn't expect him to behave differently.'

'WHAT!' Benway looked horrified. 'Goddammit! What are you saying? Of course they should…. That's their job! That sonovabitch talks about an escape from reality. This is reality.' Benway thumped his chest. 'Cancerous phony!'

'But what *is* his job?'

'To make things better, of course!'

'Is it? Or is his job to shore up the interests of those he's protecting. Imagine if your enquiry into the properties of yagé threw up a treatment which negates the use of tranquillisers. Do you think they'd make it freely available? Of course not. They'd probably ban it if they haven't already, which, judging by this correspondence, will end up being the fate of apomorphine …'

'Well that's evil … EVIL, for Chrissakes!'

'It's wrong, yes, as you can testify, but if this man's agency weren't doing it another's would. There's probably a legion of analysts, racketeers if you like, lying in wait … all with the same plan. The problem lies in the assumption that a centralised government acts in our interests and not in theirs. Furthermore, health is the perfect cover story. Nobody would ever suspect that health ministries might subvert research in order to guarantee greater demand for their products and services. Who could think such a thing, eh?'

Benway leant towards his doctor, certain for the first time that this old croaker was genuine, a kindred spirit. 'I don't have any doubt. I know governments are doing this,' he screeched. 'And not just with the banning and supply of narcotics. Psychiatry colludes with the drug companies. They even invent conditions they can exploit.'

Dent laughed in recognition of a shared understanding. The two men's heads were almost touching; they suddenly resembled co-conspirators... plotting. 'Yes, that's right,' the doctor enthused. 'And absurdly the British elite believe that America is our ally. They have no appreciation that we're next in line, another market ripe for profit. In our enthusiasm to align ourselves with America,' Dent paused to laugh, 'we'll ban heroin and invite all the ills currently endured in New York and elsewhere: criminal gangs, addicted teenagers, overcrowded prisons and patients dependent on lethics. This is obvious but explaining it to the establishment politician.... Hah! I'd get more change out of a chair-leg.'

'So what's the answer... there has to be an answer,' Benway insisted.

'Better information with the aim of greater cooperation between people. I could not treat you without the constant support of people like Kate, Hannah and Maclay. Elsewhere, I do what I can... help with the running of the Society, commission papers, disseminate ideas, encourage best practice and better policies... write press articles, radio broadcasts... expose charlatans and analytical psychiatry, encourage international congress that includes correspondence like this.... And that brings me back to why I feel I've failed. Darwin recognised that the race is not to the strongest but to the most cooperative. We have to support one another. That doctor in Illinois is not doing that; he's being competitive. He is not even slightly inquisitive about another's experience that might be different from his own. He'll destroy more than he'll save... it is inevitable. By reaching out I am being knocked back... but Dr Benway what else can I do? If I got angry I'd have to give up... retire to the country... or, if you remember, plant roses...'

Benway twisted the bed sheet in frustration. 'Did you reply to that scheming leech?'

'Of course,' continued Dent, turning the screw, 'I replied by asking for evidence and provided some more of my own... but he responded by referring me to the Narcotics Bureau...'

'What?!' Benway was boiling now... no longer with neurasthenic sweats but rage. 'That fucking mugwump, Anslinger? He's a reptile.'

'The very same,' said Dent, his eyes shining. 'I found out all about him last year. He thrives as he sustains his host, a perfect parasite...

But, he's replaceable...as well he knows, as this agency doctor from AMA knows.' Dent patted his pocket where he'd stowed the letter. 'They're all expendable.'

Benway's voice squealed. 'You've nailed that bloodsucker too! This is unbelievable.' He looked half crazed, as though he wanted to strangle someone; his doctor had provoked a reaction...quicker than he'd thought possible. He'd have to rein him in...Benway needed an outlet.

Dent coughed. 'That's why I play cards...I mean patience.'

'Evil, sadistic monsters.'

'Patience!' repeated his doctor, leaning forward and squeezing Benway's arm.

'What?'

'I said that's why I play patience...it allows me to deal with things beyond my control.... It clears my head...helps me see things as they are...simply and clearly. That is all.'

Benway slowly unwound the bed sheet. Dent leant back from the bed and continued to expand his rationale.

'The things I have had to confront as a doctor...almost on a daily basis. I'd have gone mad if I hadn't learned to accept my limitations. Patience buys silence and restores a sense of calm. However, I do realise that knowledge in the wrong hands is now my biggest frustration of all. So patience saves me...'

'But what will save *me*?'

The doctor paused. He knew the answer. It was obvious. A blind man in a coal mine could see it...but he mustn't say. He wouldn't. He knew that Benway knew too. He got up and moved into the bay, looking out into the dark street. A couple of drunks sat on the pavement opposite. One was swigging from a bottle. It might be meths. 'Why was Benway hesitating?' he wondered. 'He must know? Is he frightened of this responsibility...to himself?'

Save for the occasional shout from the drunks and passing vehicle the night was quiet, it was nearly 1.30 a.m. Slowly the doctor returned to the bed and an earlier theme.

'I envy you Benway.'

'What?'

'When I struggled with my earliest ambitions to be a writer...I realise now that I had little to say. Then, when I wrote my first book it was a jumble, an anthropological treatise with scientific and political overtones...an extension of this, my medical life. But suppose I'd wanted to really cut loose. I'd've had to give up doctoring.'

'Why? I don't get it.'

'Well, I suppose to a degree I was inhibited by my responsibilities. I felt and still feel certain pressures...the stewardship of a discipline. I wanted to help not just science but ordinary men and women too. My ambition fell between stools. No good writer should ever feel censored by loyalty, or inhibited by a convention they cannot escape from...at least, not on the page. My favourite writer was a vicar but he had to give up penning sermons before he was able to create great literature.'

Benway looked at his long fingers and rubbed them with his thumbs. 'Yeah, I suppose.'

'Many of your interests are about medicine...about those political injustices that sit behind your predicament.'

'Yeah, you're not wrong.'

'Well think if you'd ended up a doctor. You'd feel constrained by the selfsame conventions I did, those professional obligations, the rules and regulations. You're so fortunate not to be a doctor...consider it a lucky escape.'

Benway continued to rub his hands. 'Ok, I get it,' he said.

'So, I have no doubt you will survive, none. You'll not only survive, you'll flourish. After all,' he added, 'so many would-be writers have nothing to say. You have plenty to get off your chest...and no reason to hold back either, none.'

'Yeah,' muttered Benway, 'Plenty of ammo there. Evil bloodsucking parasites.'

Dent walked to the end of the bed and picked up the Day and Night Reports. 'Do you remember Dr Benway when you began to feel different?'

'Yeah, it was the morning of the third day for sure. Kate brought in a cuppa, the same colour as your dog. I told her and she laughed. It felt sorta normal. I knew then that my junk sickness was leaving the building. I waved him goodbye and read a newspaper with my tea. Kate rewarded me with a cooked breakfast. I couldn't be sure and felt awful weak, but I sure as hell knew something had changed.'

Dent put down the notes. 'Well you'd had approximately thirty-three injections of apomorphine by then.'

'33?'

'Yes, perhaps you'd like to tell that to your compatriots when you get the chance. That you're the living testimony which exposes the error of their ways.' The doctor's smile turned to laughter at his patients immediate rebuttal.

'The error of their ways? Their evil bloodsucking parasitism, you mean.'

Still laughing Dent moved to the other side of the bed and resumed taking Benway's blood pressure. 'And now you're on a sub-emetic dose and hardly in need of morphine at all. In just under a week you've gone from needing heroin to survive to almost none. The evidence is not just in the notes but in your behaviour; your psychological and conversational interplay with us. So, Dr Benway,' Dent smiled as much to himself as his patient, 'despite this upside-down world we cannot escape from, you are able to make sense of it. This confirms there's nothing wrong. You're on the right path and soon your reactions will become normal patterns of behaviour. The real battle will start once you're out of here. The sooner the better.'

'While those gangsters in DC try to discredit you.'

'Because *I*,' Dent emphasised the word, 'am dangerous … manipulating you with my apo-mor-phine.' He hooted with laughter and Benway, as was becoming customary, joined in. For the time being, it was all he could do.

Front cover *The Human Machine* (Alfred A. Knopf, 1937)

15

Eugenics

> Zoological Society of London
> Regent's Park,
> London N.W. 8.
> 6 January 1937

Dr. John Y Dent
46 Warwick Gardens
W.14.

Dear Dr. Dent,
　I read your book some months back, and was much interested.
　I shall be very glad to see you.
　I wonder if you could come up to tea, about 5 o'clock, on Wednesday next, the 13th, when we have a few people coming?
　　　Yours sincerely
　　　Julian Huxley

Dent read the letter and passed it to his wife. She was reading a novel while making some toast over the kitchen stove.
　'What's that?' she asked, pushing the letter away.
　'Read it.'
　'I'm already reading.'
　'I thought you'd be interested…'
　'Jam please.' She waved her hand towards the dresser where several jars with grease-proof paper lids sat beside copper saucepans and large blue plates.

'Strawberry or blackcurrant?' he asked.
'Marmalade.'
'You said jam.' He looked at his wife. Her blue-green eyes scanned the lines; she was absorbed, self-absorbed. The toast started to burn. Still reading, she lifted the toasting ring from the hot plate and turned it over.
'John,' she said.
'Yes.'
'Are you using the car today?'
'No, surgery all day.'
'I thought I'd take the girls down to Acres Gate and stay at the cottage... till the weekend.'
'Good, I think you'll be lucky with the weather.'
'Will you be down on Friday or Saturday?'
'Doesn't look possible, too busy here. Anyway, the Brenans have asked us for dinner. And you accepted, remember?'
'Oh, you'll manage.'
'What's that mean?'
'What I said.'
'Toast,' he reminded her.

More blue smoke rose from the hob. She put down the book and pulled out the toaster. Two large slices of brown toast were shaken free and dropped onto the side.

'Strawberry,' she said extending her hand and picking up a knife.

Dent reached over opened a jar and passed it to Alma. She was in her early forties and eight years his junior, maybe this was why she had suddenly appeared restless; she needed a new challenge and had no interest in playing the dutiful doctor's wife. She was a rebel. It was what had attracted him to her in the first place... and that story about her being expelled from Roedean... for drinking ink. She scratched away charred bread onto a plate and spread herself two generous helpings of butter and jam. She cut the slices in half and leant back, picking up the book. Her face suddenly lit up.

'Oh that's good!' she exclaimed.
'What is?' he asked.
'Oh, nothing.'

Dent finished his mug of tea and put the letter back in its envelope and from there into his breast pocket. He got up as there was a knock on the front door.

'That'll be Mrs Todhunter, I must go.'

'I'll see you on Sunday,' said Alma, not looking up.

'Yes, till Sunday.'

He turned and went to the front door. He was in a hurry; he did not like to keep his patients waiting.

A week later at 4.55 p.m. he was ushered into a small office where a thin man rose to greet him.

'Julian Huxley,' he said, shaking Dent's hand. 'So glad you could come. Here, please sit down for a minute before we go through. I'll just give you a bit of the lowdown on our purpose. Unfortunately not everyone could come, but this is just a friendly chinwag.'

'I see,' said Dent, sitting down.

'Yes, should things develop we might have to arrange something more formal.'

'A society?'

'Possibly, we have to tread carefully... because... well, it is controversial.'

'Oh, may I ask what?'

'Eugenics.'

'I see, not really my subject.'

'Yes, that's as may be but you raised some interesting points in your book. Primarily that people may be persuaded to volunteer for sterilisation. You see there is no doubt that many now believe strongly that something has to be done. Civilisation is at a tipping point. With further industrialisation and more and more hungry mouths to feed... well, I don't need to explain, your book deals with much of it... very well, I might add. We have to meet the challenges head-on.'

Dent looked into Huxley's steadfast stare. There wasn't a flicker of doubt. So this is what dogma looks like, Dent thought. Huxley continued to expand his ideas. 'So, what we're interested in is whether you and others like you will be prepared to offer support. We have to explore all the avenues to get our message across. This is a critical moment in our history, as many in government finally accept. There's a swing in our favour and, with the socio-economic crisis, real appetite for change. We'll need articles and comment from a range of disciplines. The medical angle would be hard to dispute.'

'Yes, I see what you're driving at bu—'

'Anyway,' Huxley interrupted, 'come through.' He got up smartly. 'You weren't the first to arrive and it'll save you the trouble of having to repeat yourself.'

The two men walked out of the office across a landing and into a large comfortable room with a chandelier over a broad dining table. A maid brought through a silver tray of tea and cake, placing it on a low table ringed by two sofas and two armchairs facing a marble fireplace and roaring fire.

Huxley moved in front of a seated figure. 'H,' he said, 'may I introduce John Dent; Dent, H. G. Wells.'

'Hello Bertie,' said Dent, smiling.

'Oh!' said Huxley, taken aback. 'You know each other!?'

'Gollancz introduced us,' squeaked Wells.

'Oh, of course,' said Huxley.

'Will "young Bertie" be here?' asked Dent, looking around.

'Who?' asked Huxley.

'Russell,' replied Dent.

'I did ask him but he's busy,' said Huxley. 'You know him too, I suppose.'

'Yes, but not through Gollancz, we have a mutual friend, that's all,' said Dent.

'But he's also read your book,' added Wells, 'which is the reason we're all here.'

'Yes, that's right,' said Huxley, moving towards another figure. 'Do you know Dr Arlington?' Huxley beckoned towards a tall man warming himself by the fire. He turned and shook Dent's hand.

'Delighted,' he beamed.

'No, we haven't met,' said Dent. 'Are you in private practice?'

'Harley Street. And you?'

'Kensington, small, general practice.'

'Families?'

'Yes, lots of families, young and old and everything in between. You?'

'Neurotic women mostly. Still, it pays the bills.'

'Which must be considerable,' said Dent, sitting down beside Wells.

Huxley helped himself to some tea and sat down. 'Gentlemen, please, take your tea while it's hot.'

The door opened and a slight man with a long grey beard appeared. He was supporting himself with a stout stick. Huxley jumped to his feet.

'George, thank you for coming!'

'Hello Julian, sorry I'm late.'

'You're not late at all, perfect timing. Here, sit down.'

The small man sat down in a large armchair facing the fireplace.

Huxley introduced him: 'Gentlemen, Bernard Shaw. You know "H", of course.' Wells leant over and shook hands with Shaw without saying anything. 'And Doctors Arlington and Dent.' The younger men leapt to their feet and bowed as they shook the old man's hand. It was like being introduced to royalty, Dent imagined. Huxley remained standing and leant over to talk quietly to Shaw while the doctors returned to their places. Dent looked over the top of his teacup at Arlington, who seemed to be taking everything calmly. Huxley addressed the group.

'Delighted that we're here and thank you for coming. There may be one or two more late arrivals but given that some of us have pressing engagements this evening I think we should press on. As you all know I feel strongly that we need a strategy outlining our beliefs *vis-à-vis* a eugenic policy that can exert greater influence. The news from America gets worse every day. Food banks, mass starvation, whole communities on the move looking for work … and it's beginning in Europe, too. Terrible.'

'Not in Germany,' said Wells, 'their brand of nationalism is fuelling an economic revival.'

'What's the situation in Russia?' asked Arlington.

'Hard to say,' replied Wells, 'I've been advised that they won't have anything to do with a transatlantic alliance.'

Shaw raised his stick before speaking. 'Any international alliance would inevitably lead to opposition from within the Soviet empire. A great shame.'

'Yes,' nodded Wells, 'that is almost certainly something they could never accept.'

'Why is it,' asked Dent, 'that British socialists seem bewitched by Communism?'

Shaw's eyes sharpened and Huxley sighed. 'I am sorry but this is a familiar discussion that we won't settle here tonight. Can I remind you all that we're here to establish common ground over eugenics.'

'Is your name Bent?' asked Shaw.

'Dent.'

'Well, Bent, I haven't had the pleasure of reading your book, this human machine one, but they say you have something interesting to say. Please, when you're ready.'

'On eugenics,' prompted Huxley.

Dent looked into his teacup. His mind had gone blank. He couldn't remember what he'd written. 'Err, b-before I tell you what I believe,' he stumbled, 'can I tell you what I know?'

'Is there a difference?' asked Arlington.

'Of course there is,' wheezed Wells.

'At the end of the Great War I worked in a London hospital where there was a maternity ward. One woman with a severe mental disability came in once a year to have a baby. She was not at all well. As soon as each baby was born it was taken from her and sent into foster care. All of her babies showed signs of malnutrition, one or two had some sort of minor disability: cleft palates, squints, but also an indication of some congenital problem which due to their infancy was impossible to diagnose. When the woman had recovered from each birth she discharged herself and within a year was back and the cycle repeated. The drain on resources was apparent to us all, doctors and nurses alike, but also to the state. We talked about sterilisation but without conviction. We knew we wouldn't do it.'

Shaw's forehead furrowed. 'Why ever not?' he shouted.

Dent struggled to find an answer. 'Er, because it felt wrong.'

Shaw waved his stick. 'Felt wrong!' He rapped the side of his armchair. 'Surely you can do better than that? Bloody hell, Julian, it's January, freezing, and you've dragged me here to listen to this. I'll tell you what's wrong, Bent, it's an imbecile telling me we need more imbeciles.'

Shaw's outburst had afforded Dent some thinking time. 'Well, sir, I'm sorry. I think what I mean to say is that though our intellects argued for sterilisation, our hearts and by extension, our understanding, told us otherwise. If we had sterilised her against her will we would have crossed the Rubicon. Where would our intolerance of disability have ended?'

Huxley sat down; he looked dejected. 'I am sorry, George, I didn't expect you would have to hear this.'

Wells put down his tea cup with a clatter. 'But Dent's right. Our position is also a belief is it not? We should be grateful for a doctor's experience. In our brave new world, who does the dirty work?.... As you yourself have noted, George, with regard to vivisection. People say "yes, experiment on dogs", but no one says, here, take *my* dog.'

Shaw ignored the remark.

Dent looked up. 'Yes, in a society which aims to eradicate disease and disability, very few people would be able to do what might be expected of doctors.'

'I'd have no compunction of putting them out of their misery. It'd be a pleasure,' barked Shaw.

'Society wouldn't condone it, George,' Wells advised, 'you're kidding yourself.'

'I agree,' said Dent. 'Consent has to be achieved through better information about the science. Education is the only way any of these ideas will work.'

'But that's the problem,' asserted Huxley. 'How can you expect the unwashed to understand what is best for them?'

'Moreover, if the blighters keep breeding as you describe how on earth are we going to feed them, let alone educate them?' added Shaw.

'Or eradicate these awful congenital diseases,' said Arlington.

'Like diabetes you mean?' asked Wells.

'That's not hereditary,' asserted Arlington.

Shaw noticed to his annoyance that 'Bent' was laughing. 'What's funny, you fool?'

'Well, diabetes may very well be linked to some heritable factor, though as yet we do not know what.'

'Not very scientific then,' snorted Shaw. 'Bloody doctors.'

'Would you sterilise all diabetics then, just to be on the safe side?' asked Wells, sharing Dent's amusement.

'I'd gas them along with the deformed and imbecilic.' Shaw looked fiercely at Wells who continued to smile. 'Don't look at me like that, Wells, gassing is quite humane, they wouldn't feel a damned thing.'

Huxley turned rapidly to Arlington. 'What's the view from Harley Street?'

'Our clients agree; something has to be done.'

'I mean amongst your colleagues?'

'Oh yes, well, err… that's highly delicate. Publicly some doctors say we need to eradicate disease through inoculation. Privately they talk of selective breeding and other methods. I have to say doctors aren't really interested in science. Unless we can drug it or cut it out most doctors don't want to know.'

'Cowards,' added Shaw, 'cowards, vivisectionists and cranks.'

'Which am I?' asked Dent.

'You're a crank. Have you ever conducted an abortion?'

'Steady on, George,' said Wells. 'Dent, you mustn't feel under any obligation to answer that question.'

Huxley coughed and lit a cigarette. 'Nevertheless, H, as abortion is clearly linked to sterilisation I would like to hear how a family practitioner confronts the issue. Dent, if you would prefer you can speak in the third person. I would be most obliged.'

Dent looked at Huxley and then at each face in turn. 'Oh I don't mind telling you,' he shrugged. 'The worst that can happen is blackmail. Given you're all richer than me I needn't worry.'

Huxley choked, expelling clouds of smoke.

'I conducted an abortion not that long ago as a matter of fact. A very young girl and quite possibly the victim of abuse. She came down from Scotland under the pretext of getting a job and was delivered to my house by a female friend. With this other woman's support we established that the girl was terribly unhappy, possibly suicidal. I had no objection to helping her and after giving her a few days for consideration she returned to my home where I conducted the procedure. It went well. I hear she's a changed person. She has remained in London and has secured a job as a typist.'

'Did she pay?' asked Shaw.

'No, she had no money.'

'Well that's not right. She should pay.'

'What with? You see this is one of the difficulties. Rich people have no problem getting what they want even if it is illegal. The rest of society struggles and delivers babies into unsanitary conditions. I sometimes wonder if eugenics isn't really a distaste for poverty.'

'Hang on, Dent, you know that isn't true,' said Wells.

'Isn't it? The middle classes pat themselves on the back for their achievements, gold stars and salaries, convincing themselves that their talent is being rewarded. In truth they're in receipt of privilege, nothing more. Look at you.'

Wells exploded with laughter. 'Just can't shake off my below stairs mannerisms.'

'You're all the better for them,' smiled Dent.

'Most kind.' Wells nodded.

Huxley looked flustered; his earlier hopeful mood had evaporated and this rapport between Dent and Wells had embarrassed him in front of Shaw. He scratched around for some common ground. 'What about abortion where there's disease,' his voice had lost its earlier bounce, 'didn't you talk about that in your book? Remind me.'

'Well, I make a case for sterilisation. As we cannot stop people practicing birth control I can see no good reason to deny people a vasectomy or hysterectomy or, as I have admitted, termination.'

'The Church?' said Arlington.

'He said no *good* reason,' retorted Wells.

'What we should offer is education and choice,' suggested Dent.

'Education?' Huxley looked intense. 'Haven't we been over that?'

'Not really. You see I am referring to better information about sterilisation. Men in particular fear they will lose their libido. This couldn't be more untrue. In fact, ridding themselves of the anxiety of unwanted pregnancies, sheaths, and so on can have the opposite effect. A hysterectomy for a woman can turn an individual who suffers chronic pain and risk of disease and infection into a happy, high-functioning individual overnight. I have seen it, many times. But talk to the medical profession about this and they react as if the womb is sacrosanct. An organ to be preserved at all cost. Doctors can be unbelievably dense, you know?'

'Well, finally we agree on something,' said Shaw.

'That's very interesting,' Huxley persisted, 'but how can science help eugenics get rid of disease?'

'Well, in my book I talked about syphilis, which makes the opposite case, I'm afraid.'

'Oh, how's that?'

'From the end of the fifteenth century syphilis virtually destroyed the new world because the indigenous tribes had no biological defence to withstand it. Nowadays, however, this bacterium, treponema pallium, is nothing like as dangerous as it once was.'

'But how is that relevant?'

'Well, would you exterminate syphilis sufferers because a proportion of them will pass it on?'

'Not now it is treatable,' asserted Arlington.

'Exactly, and so who are we to say today that a different disease will not be eradicated because the organism learns to overcome it or science can provide immunity through inoculation?'

Huxley twisted in his armchair. 'I should have read your book more closely.'

'I am sorry if you think I am letting you down but I do believe in society having informed choice. If a thin band of the rich and powerful impose eugenics on the rest of us for purely demographic and economic stability, then I am sorry, I could never support that.'

'And neither would I, you know jolly well,' squeaked Wells. 'We both share the same values. Eugenics is primarily about eradicating disease that science cannot. The sights I have seen, in the hospitals and prisons, horrendous.'

'The same things that I see every day, but what you are not accepting is that these things are primarily due to poor education and unsanitary living conditions. Why aren't we talking about that... about solving the consequences of inequality and social injustice? Eugenics advocated by a few privileged intellectuals is unworkable. To me it's just another form of elitism.'

'So I see,' said Huxley gravely. 'More tea?' Huxley leant forward and turned the handle of the teapot towards Dent.

'What's your bloody background, Bent?' asked Shaw, his knuckles whitening on his blackthorn. 'You sound like that bloody troublemaker, what's his name, Orwell.'

'Family?'

'Yes.'

'Mother came from a long line of Methodists... from Lancashire Cumbrian borders. My father was born in London and descended from Quakers. Bertie thinks I'm Fabian or a Humanist, but perhaps I'm more Quaker than anything.'

'Oh that explains it, God!' Shaw slammed his armchair with the flat of his hand. 'I was wondering when you'd resort to fairy stories to support your small-mindedness.'

'I'm an atheist,' said Dent. 'Quakers do not insist on a belief in God, far from it.'

'What's the difference between Quakers and Fabians?' asked Huxley.

'Quite a lot. We share socialist ideals but without hierarchies. Quakers embrace individual differences by relying on cooperation. Survival of the fittest was incorrectly attributed to Darwin. What he actually recognised was that species that employ mutual support endure. It is similar to what Quakers advocate.'

Huxley frowned. 'An odd lot, too reticent for my liking,' he huffed, not wishing to be drawn in. 'Never could get to grips with them.'

'Tell me more, Dent, I'm interested,' invited Wells.

'As Mr Huxley says, Quakers are undemonstrative. I am sorry Russell isn't here; he shares their pacifism.'

'But how do they organise themselves?' asked Arlington.

'From the floor, they're egalitarian. As I suggested, they emphasise mutual aid. Decisions are made collectively with equal shares for everyone.'

'Like the chocolate towns,' Wells added.

'Yes, that's right. Benefactors like Fry and Cadbury had a business model based on temperance but in practice it ended up being a cradle-to-grave community with good housing and schools. It seemed to work.'

'There must be something missing, otherwise why aren't we all doing it?' said Huxley miserably.

'Social reform through community?' suggested Wells.

'Yes, a society of friends, but no coercion or proselytising,' said Dent. 'Anyone can leave at any time. My grandfather was brought up a Quaker, found it dull and left. Interestingly though, he couldn't shake it off and became friendly with Joseph Lister, another Quaker. Through this alliance my father and uncles became doctors and trained under Lister at King's, where I trained. My father never went to meetings but was every inch a Quaker. I suppose some of their ideas and causes rubbed off on me.'

'Like a heritable disease?' suggested Arlington, with a titter.

'Quakers were certainly persecuted like lepers and Jews. Am I to be done in?'

'We poisoned your tea,' smirked Huxley.

Shaw leant forward. 'This might be interesting to you, Bent; eugenics is not about society but science. Modern advances brought to bear so that humanity can progress in giant leaps not piddly little steps. Your view is too mean-spirited and discounts Man's ability to be ingenious, to be brilliant.'

'Yes!' enthused Arlington, 'isn't this why we're so envious of what is happening in Russia? State control with real power to change things … and quickly?'

'That's a sweeping assessment,' said Wells. 'Care to enlarge?'

'Er, well. You wouldn't know, but I joined the Left Book Club, too, a branch in Soho. And there was this wonderful speaker before Christmas. He told us of his research into the Soviet model of industrialisation. He says it is entirely down to strong leadership... just as Mr Shaw advocates.'

Wells tried not to laugh. 'Ah, well Arlington I have actually had the benefit of meeting Stalin himself and I can assure you that the Soviets are more despotic than many here care to admit. A technological republic running like a well-oiled machine may sound spectacular but I remain to be convinced. In fact I have much sympathy with Dent's view. Progress should happen from the bottom up, through the broadest consensus possible. It may be the only way.'

'Bloody hell, Wells – you old fool,' remonstrated Shaw, 'democracy isn't working, look at the queues outside the labour exchanges. It is an out-and-out failure. Automation is inevitable. It'll rob more and more of work. What then?'

'But you're just impatient for a world you can imagine but have no idea how to achieve,' rejoined Wells.

Huxley stubbed out his cigarette and stood up. 'Damn it, we're getting off the point. I echo George's point: eugenics is about scientific advancement. A science which, once embraced, is immediately beneficial.'

'At the expense of the individuals who make up society,' added Wells.

Huxley raised his voice. 'No! At the expense of the viruses and diseases which are destroying society. I thought you were onside, H, and yet it seems you've got Dent in to peddle a different line. What's going on?'

'What's going on, Julian, is that I'm trying to understand from where the opposition will definitely come. We have to be prepared... to understand all the arguments... profoundly.... People like Dent can help us.... That's why I recommended his book.'

Huxley sat back down and crossed his legs. 'Go on then.' He threw his hands in the air. 'I feel as exasperated as George. All the mounting problems and humanity seemingly desperate to jump off a cliff. It's unbearable.'

'Yes,' cried Shaw, 'you tell us, Bent, what would you do about all the inbreeding riffraff, the millions of congenitally stupid demanding food so they can produce another generation of mongols to drag us all down. You'll suggest vegetarianism, I suppose.'

All eyes turned to Dent. For the second time that evening he'd lost his bearings.

'Civilisation,' he blurted.

'But it isn't working, you idiot!' shouted Shaw, waving his stick.

'But, its failure doesn't prove it isn't necessary, rather the opposite. You might destroy an organised form of collectivism or an international union but immediately find yourself having to recreate it. It'll inevitably encounter challenges but only a socially democratic and wholly transparent structure can work. One of those areas may be eugenics but a workable eugenics policy must come from ordinary men and women, including the riffraff.'

Wells smiled at the livid expressions opposite him.

'Oh hell, we're not elitists,' said Huxley. 'No matter what some may think. Judicious use of the latest technologies can reduce humanitarian crisis and misery.'

'Even if, in your pursuit of biological equality, you cause exactly that?' asked Dent.

'What do you mean?'

'Discovery never stops. If a heritable link with a certain disease is established you may intervene to eradicate that disease. In that instance you will have succeeded in your aim of a healthier society. But then, as I've tried to explain, suppose science establishes a cure for that disease and exposes your position as having been premature. At that moment you will appear no less imbecilic than those Mr Shaw would gas.'

Wells laughed; Huxley and Shaw glared at each other.

'On top of this, Julian,' said Wells, 'there is also the difficult issue of race. Dent or Arlington may be able to corroborate this but aren't some of the worst congenital problems limited to certain races?'

'I haven't a clue,' said Arlington. 'Isn't there a theory, Dent, that certain races are alcoholics?'

'Would that be the Irish, George?' asked Wells, his eyes smiling.

'You disappoint me, Wells, you always have,' said Shaw.

Like a referee between two boxing heavyweights Dent intervened, 'It would be unwise to assume that races are genetically disposed to any disease until it is shown to be separate from all other factors: environment, traditional customs and so on. You mention alcoholism. Our observation of indigenous tribesmen rolling around drunk on a first ever whisky is really a lack of tolerance that the Northern European races have developed over the millennia. All things being equal we'd behave in exactly the same way.'

'And other diseases?' asked Huxley, 'the more obvious ones, cretinism?'

'Well, as I've tried to explain, it would be difficult to imagine the enactment of compulsory sterilisation in a democracy but the state might try to introduce a rate of bonuses. The worse the hereditary risk to the applicant the higher the bonus. This may reduce certain congenital dementias for example and represent a saving to the state in terms of costs, resources and so on, but I could only see it working if the principle of consent was absolute. If not you risk the charge of persecuting minorities.'

'Different races, you mean?' added Wells.

'Well, that should be avoided, of course,' said Dent, 'but there is also the assumption that certain minority groups cannot enrich our lives. I recently learned that Beethoven was hard of hearing but it hardly stopped him bringing pleasure to millions.'

'But what if we decide we know best?' asked Shaw, leaning forward. 'The current state of affairs is simply unsustainable. If I had my way you lily-livered types would be the first to go. I'd invent a machine that would go *BZZZZ* and you'd be gone. Just like that.' Shaw banged the floor with his stick. 'There's probably one in those silly books of yours, Wells; *War of the Worlds*? Ha! I'd declare war on the gutless.' He banged the floor again, but louder.

'Calm down, George, you're too old for all this excitement,' tittered

Wells. 'The issue of science and race is critical. If science creates advantages for one racial group over another, for instance, how is that to be understood?'

'To be honest, this worries me too,' said Huxley. 'I think you touched on that too ... didn't you, Dent?'

Dent thought of the arc of human evolution. He saw hairy people inside caves devouring raw meat. Two hundred thousand years later their descendants emerged from exclusive homes in Belgravia to hail a cab. For all Man's sophistication he was still monopolised by instinct, motivated by rivalry over sex, food and property. And now eugenics was being touted by a few crackpots craving homogeneity against a rising tide of diversity with a billion and one opinions. He looked into Shaw's face ... at its raw and impatient savagery, at his knobbly stick now gripped as if it were a cudgel.

'Speak up, man!' Shaw shouted. 'Defender of the irredeemable. Let's hear your painful witterings.'

'Look,' said Dent, doing his best not to be put off. 'Even if I were to accept that you're prompted by a benign impulse is it even theoretically possible to imagine that your aims, no matter how well-meaning, wouldn't be twisted by other groups for less altruistic purposes?'

'Go on,' said Wells.

'Today no nation is self-supporting or can survive in isolation. Interdependence between countries is greater than ever, based on easier travel, finance, trade, science; you name it. We are entering a period where our traditional conversational contact is becoming less important as the electronic transfer of information is expanding faster than we can imagine. Keeping pace with this technology is our greatest challenge because the human organism possesses all manner of absurd impulses, fears and prejudices that must be resisted. And yet the speed with which information will be shared also offers a global civilisation opportunities for cooperation never before seen. The League of Nations is its embryo. And even if this League fails we will have to recreate it as civilisation inevitably edges towards a universal race with a single, universal language. All the talk of keeping races apart is futile. It is far easier to mix races than to separate them, and isolation is impossible so we shouldn't try. Nationalists who appeal to these tribal urges are either backward or dishonest or both backward and dishonest; take your pick. In light of all this, eugenics may resonate with some but for all the wrong reasons.'

Dent glanced at Huxley and then at Shaw. 'You see,' he continued, 'it is impossible to bend society to ourselves because each of us would do it differently, eugenicists included. Our emotional intelligence has to be excited not by any form of elitism or nationalism but by a collective struggle towards values of a universal nature involving cooperation and unity. To this end society must never isolate any group for the purpose of special treatment. Instead let us emphasise inclusivity based on equally shared resources to meet the inevitable challenges: sociological, ethical and environmental. Eventually the European race will gravitate towards a global civilisation with a sense of universal justice at its heart. Ultimately nothing else will work and nor should it.'

'I've never heard so much rubbish,' shouted Shaw, standing up. 'I shan't be talked down to any longer.' He pointed his blackthorn at Dent. 'I bet you're a nudist; the only thing you wear in the summer is sandals. I'm right, aren't I? Gentlemen.' Shaw nodded to no one in particular, turned and stormed out. He was followed by Huxley and a scurrying Arlington.

'Don't worry, Dent,' said Wells, chuckling, 'he's the most irascible man I know, particularly when he's lost an argument.'

'Oh dear,' said Dent, 'I was told it'd be a friendly meeting.'

'It was, believe me.' Wells wiped an eye. 'At least he didn't call you "charismatic".'

'Oh?'

'Yes, remember, when a man does that he's trying to disarm you... he may even suggest it because he's unable to or unwilling to meet the standards you set.'

'I see.'

'He'll never admit it but Shaw needs a deeper perspective. We all do from time to time.'

Dent looked into the fire. It was almost out. 'Don't any of them know you have diabetes?'

'Apparently not.'

'Better not let them find out,' cautioned Dent, laughing.

Wells continued to titter away; he'd enjoyed the meeting.

A month later Dent had grown increasingly disenchanted with the refusal amongst the Left Book Club's hierarchy to reflect the position of its contributors and members. There was also talk of specific interference over the content of George Orwell's *The Road to Wigan Pier*. Dent, conflicted by his admiration for Victor Gollancz, the Club's founder, felt he had to explain himself.

17/2/37

Dear Gollancz,

As a sincere democrat and one who believes in progress towards the left, I welcome your Left Book Club and I have done my best to extend and advertise it. It was a very fine idea. I congratulate you upon it. I must also thank you for the pleasure and number of valuable friendships it has given me. I am genuinely frightened of the Fascist advance towards Nationalism and smothering of opinion.

The Left Book Club, as I see it, has become more and more Strachey and less and less Gollancz. Originally its policy, it was declared, should be modelled and evolved from that of its members who would receive advice but not direction from the central office and who should have no loyalties and obligations other than the payment of their subscriptions. I feel myself now a little too left for it.

There is a great gulf between a collection of Soviet republics and a centralised empire under a dictatorship. The first may be possible for an educated mankind, the second controls and therefore stultifies the possibility of education.

Last night I called on a fellow member whom I respect

and the evidence he gave me of autocratic interference with the conduct of group meetings by the central office forces me to reluctantly resign my membership. Please accept my six weeks' notice.

I am suspicious of all authority when it is uncontrolled from below.

Yours sincerely,
John Yerbury Dent.

Dent sighed as he sealed the letter. He wouldn't miss the LBC that much. If it remodelled itself he could rejoin. If it did not, it would collapse from within. All organisations, like relationships, have to be self-sustaining, that much was clear.

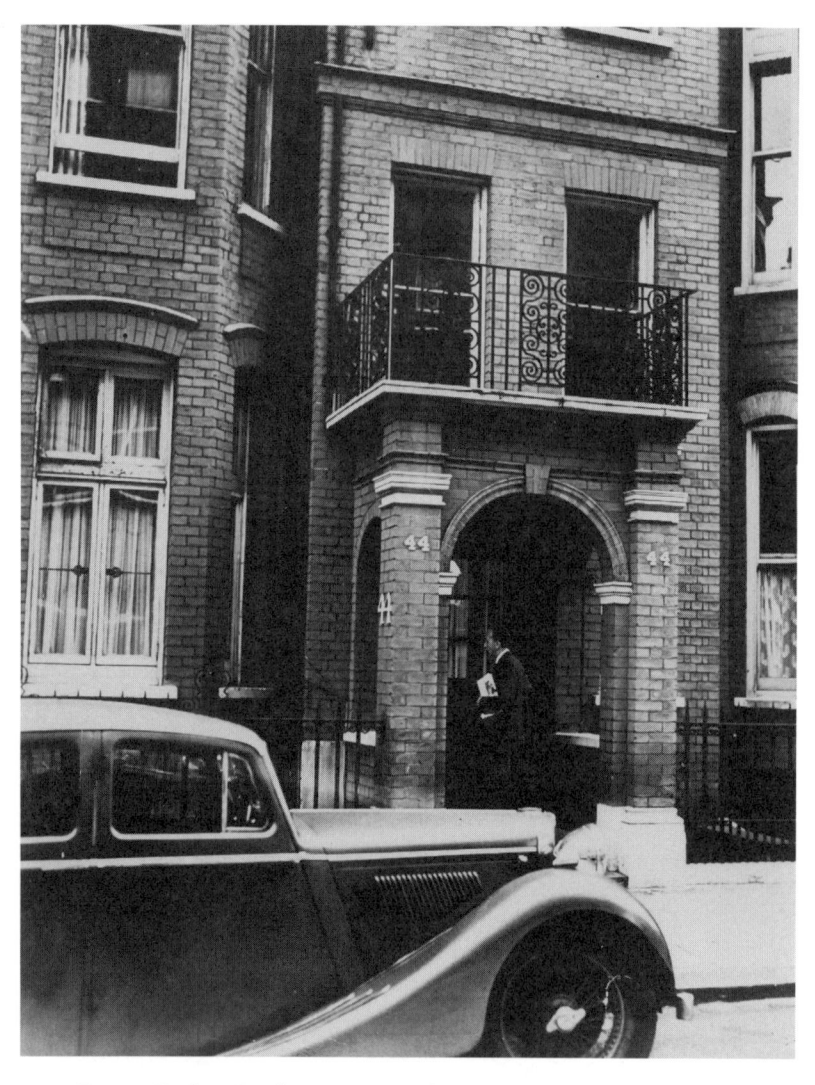

44 Egerton Gardens, London SW3, 1955. This was Burroughs' address during his first stay in London. A short walk from Dent's clinic at 99 Cromwell Road. [©Getty Images]

16

Riding Stang

The best-laid schemes o' mice an men
 Gang aft agley......
Still thou art blest, compar'd wi' me!
The present only toucheth thee:
But, Och! I backward cast my e'e,
 On prospects drear!
An' forward, tho' I canna see,
 I guess an' fear!

– Robert Burns
To a Mouse

Dr Benway awoke slowly. He had slept deeply, as was becoming customary. A busy figure like a peppered moth flapped around his space. He felt his eiderdown being adjusted ... a deliberate attempt to stir him. He rolled over and rubbed his eyes.

'Day's dawnin', sunshine,' a strange voice offered unwanted encouragement.

He mumbled incoherently.

'I'm Nurse Morse, filling in for Gibbie,' the voice identified itself.

'Ah, yes. Kate did say,' he replied, sitting up.

'Most call me Morsey.'

'Mercy?'

'Oooh, that's a laugh. You'll get no mercy from me; left or right side?' Getting no answer she undid a button, yanked down Benway's pyjama top and injected him in his right arm. 'You're on low dose, three-to four-hourly injections. Doin' champion, I hear.'

'Thanks.' Benway covered his shoulder and put on his glasses.
'I'm informed you're Benway, a *Dr* Benway?'
'Yes.'
'You don't look like a doctor.'
'Don't I?'
'No, you don't, you look like death warmed up if you don't mind me sayin'. How you feeling anyways?'
'Better.'
'Grand, then you'll be getting up?'

Morsey was a small lady about sixty years of age with a bustling intensity. She had been reared in Palmerstown, a suburb of Dublin, and her choice of career had been simple: nun or nurse. Religion struck her as 'insane' so nursing it was, though her devout family had remained tight-lipped on the matter. Coming to England in the 1930s had been liberating and, for the first time in her life, given her financial independence. She also liked the variety of private work introduced to her by a friend. She was slightly cross-eyed and Benway was undecided about which pupil to focus on.

'Might the doctor be after a brew?' she said in a sing-song mix of Dublin cockney.
'What you offering?'
'Coffee, tay or milk.'
'Nothing stronger?'

Morsey snorted. 'F'd' love o' Mike! What I said, or dere's Adam's wine.'

As she spoke she picked up Benway's notes at the end of the bed. After flicking through the pages she looked intently at the cover stroking her bottom lip.

'Well I nivver, ain't dat a ting. These yer notes?'
'Yeah.'
'Yer address?' She turned the book round so Benway could see the cover.
'It is.'
'Yer rooms, Egerton Gardens?' She pointed at the address.

'Yes.'

'No. 44?'

'Yeah, so what?'

'Well, get a 'old o' dat. Did she appear before you den, loike da Vairgin Mary?'

Adjusting his glasses Benway looked intently at Morsey, her uniform and pinned bonnet. He thought she could be Napoleon's grandmother. Or the man himself, in drag. He sniggered.

'What so funny… did you or dint yah?'

'What are you talking about?'

'Ellis, sunshine. That was her address, I should know, treated her downstairs, din' I? Twice if I ain't mistaken.'

Benway rubbed his eyes under his glasses. What was this indiscretion? It seemed incongruous, out of place with the stuffy medical confidentiality he had grown used to. That thing locked away with all those other things the English don't discuss: money, death and sex.

He thought he'd go native. 'Should you be telling me this?'

'Oh for the love o' God! Spare me! She's past caring, believe me.'

'Sorry?'

'Ar, come, you waren't born yesterday.'

'What?'

'Don't play the Charlie with me. Where you bin, Mongolia?' Nurse Morse threw the notes back on the table.

'Look, I'm sorry, but I don't get it.'

The small nurse crossed her arms. Benway imagined her on a battlefield, surveying her troops. He smirked.

'Where you from then?' she demanded.

'I'm American, but I've been living in Tangiers. I only arrived in London recently. "Edgertons" a few blocks away, convenient for Queen's Gate, for…'

'So you don't know?'

'Know what?'

'About Ellis… Ruth Ellis?'

'No.'

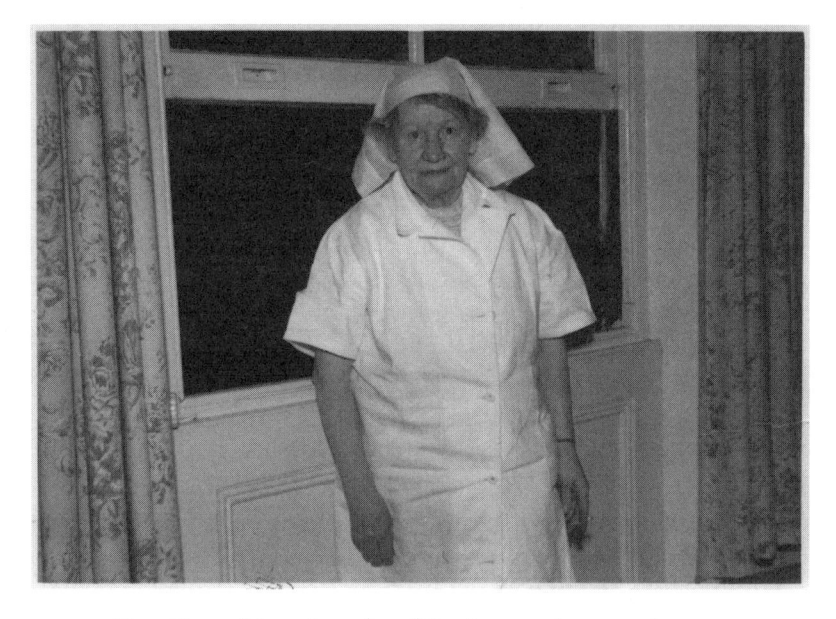

Sister Morse, 'Morsey', another of Dent's supportive team of nurses. [photographer unknown]

'She murdered her 'usband, din't she?'

Benway felt a chill. 'Murder?' he asked.

'No doubt about it, sunshine, filled him full o' 'oles.'

'Shot?'

'Point blank range.' Morsey raised her hand as if she were holding a gun and clicked her tongue.

Benway sat up. 'What? W-why? – I mean, what happened to her?'

Morsey threw her head back and scoffed. 'Jeezus, Mary an' Joseph! What d' yer think 'append to 'er?'

'I don't know,' Benway insisted, biting his finger.

'Strung 'er up, din't they?' Morsey lifted her right hand close to her ear and jerked it, opening her eyes wide and sticking out her tongue.

She held the grotesque pose for a split second. 'Broke her pretty little neck, dint they? Snapped it loika stick, a dry ole stick.' She advanced towards the bed. Benway pulled the eiderdown up to his chin and froze.

Oblivious, Morsey rattled on. 'Thatz why, see, I reckoned you might o' had a visit from her tortured spirit.' She made a little howl: 'Her wanderin' soul.' Morsey mustered a laugh, thinking Benway would get the joke. 'Bein' as you're in 'er digs, an' orl.'

She fixed Benway with a twisted look. 'Blimey,' she gibed, 'you're behavin' as if *I'm* 'er ghost. *Whoo...*' she wiggled her fingers. Getting no response she stood back. 'Yous don't believe in all that, do you?' Her patient remained rigid and mute. She shrugged and clapped her hands. 'So what'll it be then, a cuppa or coffee?'

Benway didn't answer. His eyes were vacant, unblinking.

'Deary me,' berated Morsey. 'Cat got yer tongue? Looks like a nice cuppa is just what you need. Get some loife into ya.'

'Yeah,' the rust in his voice was back.

Morsey went into the kitchen. She returned five minutes later with a steaming mug.

'Oh mother o' God, you ain't moved! Here, get this down yer neck.' She set the tea down and proceeded to talk and tidy at the same time. She spoke very fast. 'Dr Dent will be in soon. He'll decide what's what. You know, dunno why, I was thinking of them loony bins I used to work in. When tippin' up we had to check the alarm bells and account for all the sharps, knives and so on. I dunno, but oim reminded of that, I am. Helf is so much better nowadays, don't you think? Agh, o' course it is. Dr Dent says there's a long way to go. Not sure he's right. I mean, how much more can be done for folk, I ain't the foggiest.' She noisily shifted the table into the centre of the bay and clattered two chairs into position.

'Now then, I expect you'll be after a full English, yes? There's rashers, eggs and bread. I can do you my speciality, "dipped in", if you fancy?'

'Yeah?'

'I get a propah crust on it...'
'Great.'
'Right, comin' up. Dr Dent'll be 'ere then.' Morsey left.

Dr Benway pulled his knees up and dropped his face between them. He was back in the quagmire, drowning in the bottomless, bubbling sinkhole. He pushed his palms against his ears. They'd meet in the middle...if only.... He pushed harder; his mouth opened in anguish but there was no scream, nothing...nothing but a bald emptiness breaking out in every direction and forever...

Downstairs, pausing outside the entrance, Dent pulled deeply on his third cigarette of the day. He pushed back his fringe and gazed through swaying trees at the pink and blackened facade of Waterhouse Gothic. It was going to be a warm day; spring winds had swept away the residual traces of the last pea souper. Life was simple, life was good. He studied the tall, arboreal line, its fresh leaves peeking out against a brilliant April sky...

> One impulse from a vernal wood will teach you more of Man,
> Of moral evil and of good, than all the sages can.

...he mused before hurriedly stubbing out the cigarette on a lamp-post and climbing the steps to the clinic. The smell of freshly cooked bacon filled the stairwell. He felt hungry.

'Agh, good morning, Morsey,' he said, through gasps for air. 'Breakfast?'

'Yes, Dr Dent. For Dr Benway, mind.'

'And how is our resident doctor this morning?'

'Well, he seemed well-rested, said he felt good – then he went quiet, dunno why.' She lifted up the tray laden with full English and freshly squeezed orange juice. 'Agh, nae bother, these rashers will revive him.'

'What's that smell?' she asked, moving to the door.

'Bacon?' said Dent.

'No, it's burning. Blimey, it's coming out of your trousers.'

'Oh, my goodness!' exclaimed Dent. 'I put a cigarette stub in my pocket.'

He pulled out a smouldering handkerchief as some coins fell onto the floor.

Morsey cackled. 'Aha, now oi've seen the lot. Here, you sort yourself out while I bring this to our guest.'

She crossed the landing and pushed at the bedroom door. The bed was empty.

'Oh!' she said, returning to the kitchen. 'He's gone AWOL, our Dr Benway.'

'Bathroom?'

'Must be,' assured Morsey.

She returned the tray to the kitchen table and crossed the landing, tapping on the door.

'Hello, yer breakfast's ready.' She hesitated, listening.

She rapped the door. 'Dr Benway?'

Dent looked across the landing.

'Open it,' he said.

Morsey tried but it was locked.

Dent walked towards the door. Morsey stood back.

Dent knocked loudly. 'Benway?' he called.

A clear 'click' was heard and the door swung open. The gaunt, pale figure of his patient stood in front of him. His face smeared with tears, eyes bloodshot. He swayed; a listing ship in a gale, his arms broken masts. Dent advanced and held him first by the shoulders and then hugged him. Benway's body heaved with sobs and gasps. The doctor squeezed him closer and waited for the trembling to subside.

'Here, easy does it. Come back to bed,' said Dent.

The doctor piloted the stricken American back to port; his port in a storm.

Morsey straightened out the bed sheet, blankets and pillows and watched as Dent quietly eased the trembling patient back under the covers. Without saying anything she withdrew to the kitchen, closing the door behind her.

Neither man spoke. Dent retreated to the far wall and pushed a chair up to the bed. He adjusted the curtains, maximising the spread of sunlight, and turned the vase of daffodils so that they faced into the room. He coughed quietly and sat down.

Benway lay back, expecting a barrage of questions. None came.

Anxiously he looked towards the hunched figure of his doctor... his hands clasped on his lap... as if in silent prayer. He hadn't shaved for days and his hair flopped forward over his forehead. His moustache appeared golden. Was this ginger or nicotine? Benway corrected himself with a new understanding. It was *both* ginger *and* nicotine; heredity *and* environment. He looked for Dent's eyes above his tortoiseshell half-moon specs but they were closed! He could be a beachcomber on a beach preparing for a snooze! Slowly Benway adjusted to what was required of him, realising it was nothing. He too closed his eyes and listened to the rising bustle of the day outside, the doves on the parapet above the window, their courtship warble. The flood of sunshine warmed the room and a distinct feeling of having accomplished something replaced the round-the-clock fear. He felt safe. He could rest... like a Buddha... there was nothing else to do but let go...

When Benway awoke Dent's chair was empty but he knew the doctor was still in the building. He needed to talk; he was ready now, it would be easy. He got out of bed and hurriedly got dressed. He opened the door and entered the kitchen, pushing his shirt into his trousers. Dent was seated on his own, reading.

'Oh hello, Burroughs, do come in.' Dent put away his paperback after folding down the corner of a page.

'Thank you.' Burroughs pulled back a chair and sat down.

'Sleep well?'

'Yeah, not bad. How long was I out?'

'Oh, just an hour or so, but on the reduced dose. It's another good sign... you'll sleep more now.'

Burroughs leant forward. His face, Dent noticed, was flushed; he almost looked healthy.

'We'll go for a walk if you like,' said Dent. 'You've missed breakfast, but there's an Italian restaurant downstairs, the Dolce Vita, or we can sit in Stanhope Gardens.'

'I have to talk about what happened,' said Burroughs, his lips barely moving as he rattled out the words.

'Yes, I thought you might. Morsey told me. Here, at least have your orange juice.'

'You know, then?' Burroughs emptied the glass in a single draught.

Dent didn't answer but cleared some space on the table in front of him.

'An amazing coincidence,' continued Burroughs, his voice racing.

By contrast Dent's voice was flat, its message incongruous. 'I'll start with the vase, please.'

'What?' said Burroughs, distracted.

'The flower vase, there on the dresser.' Dent gestured towards a tapered glass receptacle.

Burroughs spun round, grabbed the vase and shoved it towards Dent. Dent took it carefully and placed it in the middle of the table before covering it with a large upside down dinner plate.

'Helluva coincidence,' repeated Burroughs. 'Amazing.'

'And now let's try the sugar,' said Dent.

'You *must* agree?' Burroughs passed the sugar-bowl to Dent.

'Thank you,' said Dent, taking great care to set the bowl precisely in the centre of the plate. Upon this he balanced another dinner plate, also upside down.

'What I really want to know is what you think. I could scarcely believe it.'

'And now the pepper.' Dent pointed to the far side of the table.

'It's as if this was meant to happen,' continued Burroughs, banging the pepper-pot down.

Dent rubbed his hands together, 'This is where it begins to get tricky,' he said, carefully positioning the pepper in the centre of the plate.

'This seems to have happened to spook me...like a curse...' said Burroughs, raising his voice in a failed attempt to gain his doctor's attention.

'Easy does it,' mumbled Dent, while adjusting the condiment.

'... Just as I was turning a corner. Don't you agree... you must?'

Dent steadied himself and positioned a bowl then another side plate over the pepper. Once this had been safely accomplished he stood to admire his creation. Satisfied, he finally adjusted his chair and turned his attention towards his patient.

'I have to say, Burroughs, yes, what has happened seems peculiar. Some might say that this coincidence is so extraordinary as to be unbelievable. Now then, I am not in the least bit superstitious and have never believed in the supernatural; however, I realise that many, and not just those from primitive cultures, believe that their surroundings are paying attention to them. The rustling tree or babbling brook speaks to them, the flower opens for them and so on. This tendency starts in childhood and when the reality doesn't fit our ideal it is scolded. The chair is "naughty" if we drop it on our toe, the imaginary dog bites us and we banish it to its imaginary kennel. It is not clear to me how much of this tendency is discarded when we become adults. Some still look for meaning in the random cosmology of atoms. Even natural events like an earthquake or a solar eclipse are interpreted as "God's will", as if that is the end of the matter.'

Dent paused, waiting until he'd found his patient's gaze. It shone, picking up the bright sunlight outside.

'You see, Burroughs, things happen which have nothing at all to do with us until we respond. We cannot change the event but we can react in any number of ways. The sooner we do so positively, pro-actively, the better because, as I may have said, avoidance or going over old ground only makes us more aware of what stands in our way. Accordingly, events may exercise undue influence and make us fearful. If I could offer you any advice it is this: a coincidence is a chance happening, kismet, and may be good or bad, but serendipity? Well, that is another thing altogether.'

'Oh?' Burroughs was flummoxed. 'How do you mean?' he asked urgently.

Dent stroked his chin. Without speaking he stood to lift a heavy cut-glass tumbler from the dresser. He rolled it in his palms... held it in the sunlight. The kitchen was transformed by a sudden kaleidoscopic effect. The patient watched the spinning spectacle until the doctor leant forward and topped off his tower with the crystal. Then, like an artist he stood back to admire his masterpiece, a precarious totem on a wobbly table. Finally, he sat down and very slowly turned his attention back to the taut American.

'Heraclitus said we can only stand in the same river once and he was right. The river keeps flowing and we can jump in later, but it won't be the same river. We have no control over what's in the river but by jumping in we can get to know it, and profit by it. That's good, and that's serendipity.'

Burroughs absorbed the message and for the first time took in his doctor's absurd creation; half-lighthouse, half-pagoda.

'The only thing that interests me,' continued Dent, 'is whether your experience today has left you in a better place to stay well and get on with your life, that is all.'

Burroughs was silent, he had a great deal to consider.

'And that, Burroughs, is one of the reasons you're here. I am not interested in raking over old coals or forcing you to do anything, but events may help us. Help plot a way forward.'

Dent leant back and crossed his legs. 'Apomorphine has contributed, I am certain of it. You have already changed from the man I met last week. You're beginning to get pleasure from little things and are even starting to do things that last week you would have found impossible…unimaginable. The important thing now is to take the plunge. Don't think about it.'

'Jump in the river and don't look back?'

Dent played with his moustache before replying. 'You'll make better progress if you look to the future…to where the current is taking you and not back at the floods that brought you downstream.'

'And this Ellis woman, is she part of the river?'

Dent continued to pull his whiskers. 'Yes, I suppose she is. Her story is now part of yours. Your currents have converged and we cannot pretend otherwise. But it is up to you what you take from the knowledge.'

'Different outcomes?' suggested Burroughs.

'I think that is safe to say.' The doctor watched...and waited. He knew what was coming. Burroughs picked at his trousers.

'And what they did to Ruth Ellis?' he asked, eventually.

'Oh dear! Well, her end was an abomination. There is no place for it in any civilised society. An unsound act brought on by retributive idiocy. They hung her out to dry, I'm afraid. She was used by the media, her glamorous appearance a godsend to those looking to appeal to the mob's base instincts.'

'You followed the case?'

'Impossible to avoid, everyone was talking about it. The press had a field day. My understanding was that she was unwell having been a victim for years. She probably snapped. When it happened I thought of poor old Betty Martin riding stang.'

'Betty who?'

'In the village, Rampside, where my mother came from there was a young woman called Betty Martin. She had done something wrong and the elders decided she should be encouraged to change. The punishment didn't have to fit the crime, none of this "eye for an eye" nonsense. The community simply had to be a witness because this justice was reformative not punitive. A clear and simple distinction. Betty, you see, would remain in the care of the village, the whole village.'

'A sort of community policing, the action of a Johnson,' suggested Burroughs.

'A what?' asked Dent.

'Well, there were people I knew of, a family called Johnson. They weren't exactly upright citizens but knew how to help folk and keep an eye out. It sorta worked.'

'Yes, that's right. I am sure all communities work best in similar ways. Anyway, the Rampsiders put Betty astride a wooden plank called a "stang" and carried her down the street. Everybody came out of their houses and banged pots and pans. The children rolling hoops and singing: *"Betty Martin's riding stang, Betty Martin's riding stang"* all the way until the procession arrived at the village pond. Held over the water the stang was turned. Poor Betty's ducking symbolised a baptismal rebirth. My mother told me that Betty lived to a great age, grew to be a proud and central figure in the village. Ruth Ellis wasn't given that option and her judicial murder was not comparable to her crime... nothing other than a barbaric act of cold-blooded savagery.'

'I see,' said Burroughs. 'So do you think I should ride stang?'

Dent laughed at the thought.

'Aren't you still riding it? And isn't this one of the difficulties of the law; law divorced from community? Everybody has an opinion. We selfishly demand "justice" without having a clue what that means or involves. Like spoiled children in a nursery, individuals twist a public morality to suit their prejudices and then get hot under the collar because they can never agree. It is ludicrous. Some will argue that you've suffered enough, while others will ask whether you have suffered at all.'

Dent looked up as a lorry, carrying 802,701 pieces of rubble, roared westwards up Cromwell Road. His creation wobbled....

'Nobody can change what has happened,' he continued, 'but we must do our best to avoid its reoccurrence. The death penalty is clung to as a deterrent but this is not supported by the facts. It's upheld by windbags who enforce their moral high-mindedness. It's a nonsense, a preference for barbarism over rehabilitation while the factors that make murder inevitable are brushed under the carpet. It is just another way to keep people in line; enslaved in the interests of the few not the many.'

Burroughs knew that he was meant to feel better if not exonerated by this blunt logic. He felt like a cherished nephew in the hands of a favourite uncle. Too bad he didn't have one...

'You see,' Dent's voice rolled steadily on. 'In society's simplistic rush to gain revenge it fails to examine the causes: poor education, prospects, and living conditions. The bore that squeals for "justice" is actually looking for an excuse to do nothing. Murder is environmental just like drug addiction and the moralists who adhere to punishment as a solution are merely perpetuating the very thing they condemn.'

'Sounds like we're describing mugwumps again,' muttered Burroughs.

'Yes, they cling to this and similar idiocies because root and branch reform is hard work requiring imagination they do not have. Sadly this is not limited to politicians, many pulpit professionals parrot the same message and have it broadcast by a slanted press.'

Dent raised both himself and his voice.

'And the very idea that a judge, a man who's received all the privileges society can confer, should decide that another who can only dream of such things shall forfeit her life. Damn it all, Burroughs, this'll turn me to drugs.'

Dent erupted in an extraordinary series of hoots. Not only his creation but the whole kitchen rattled.

Dent glanced at his watch. 'Look, two more sub-emetics then let's nip outside. Dunno about you but I could do with a stroll and it'd be a shame to waste what's left of a beautiful day.'

Burroughs stood to follow.

'Before we leave,' Dent said, turning round, 'I want you to put this orange on top of that tower.'

'What?!' Burroughs looked doubtful.

'Yes please, doctor's orders,' Dent grinned, handing Burroughs the fruit.

Burroughs held the orange; it was heavy and far from perfectly round. He studied its dimpled peel and tossed it into his other hand before transferring his attention to the sparkling crystal floating precariously nearly three feet above the table. Taking the orange in both hands he drew himself up to his full height. He steadied himself and like an archbishop at a coronation crowned the glass.

Five minutes later the two men sat on a bench in Stanhope Gardens under a spread of two-hundred-year-old plane trees. Around them, crimson magnolia and snow white amelanchier waved for attention.

'That orange looked marvellous,' commented Dent.

'You think?'

'Definitely.'

'I guess.'

'A beacon from the lighthouse.'

'I wasn't sure I'd manage.'

Dent thought for a moment. 'I'll never ask something of which you're not capable,' he said.

'No?'

'No,' repeated Dent emphatically, 'never!'

Immediately Burroughs was overcome with another surge of colliding emotions. The change in him was extraordinary. A week ago he could barely find his head with his hat, now he could imagine juggling fruit. He laughed and cried at the same time and in a spontaneous show of emotion held Dent's leg.

'Thank you,' he rasped, 'thank you.'

Dent reciprocated by patting then rubbing Burroughs' shoulder before leaning back to enjoy the sunlit scene. As he lit a Senior Service he reminded himself that his patient would be apprehensive. Burroughs had to focus on the future and his doctor had to keep the ball rolling. He turned to him.

'I'd like to see you again tomorrow, but not at the clinic,' he said. 'Come to the house around midday. Hannah will be in tonight and if she's happy, and I cannot think of a reason why she won't be, she'll discharge you. Come round then.'

'34 Addison?'

'Yes.' Dent enthused. 'Stay for lunch. There's an old friend coming, nothing onerous.'

'Are you sure?'

'Certain. He's a writer. You'll have plenty to talk about.'

'Thank you, and I can settle up what I owe you.'

'Yes, of course.'

'What time?'

'Any time after eleven, I try and have a lie-in on a Sunday, busy again next week. I'd like to talk over a few things, give you some apo' pills. And there's Fred Hornibrook's address.'

'Who?'

'Didn't I say? Well, he's an expert in the importance of posture and abdominal health.... He'll give you some ideas for exercises. The routine of exercise will be very good for you right now and Fred will show you the way. But I'll need to ring him. Then I'll give you his details. We can go through all this tomorrow.'

'Thank you. And some more waking suggestion?'

'Yes, if you'd like. We've talked about, "What now"; well this.' Dent waved his arm in a wide sweep. 'Right now, from this time and place.'

'From here?'

'Yes, anything beneficial that you can learn or relearn. The quicker you commit to beneficial patterns of behaviour the better. Allow them to become good habits and they'll be as hard to break as the old bad ones.'

'Yes, I think I get it, I'm a soft machine.'

'Exactly, but de-anxietised.' Dent beamed. 'This is why I advocate getting back to life as soon as possible and why I and those who run expensive nursing homes do not get along.'

'Oh?'

'Well, they condition a sense of decay. The poor inmates wander around in a dream, like Wells' Eloi. It isn't until you experience your normal environment that our habitual responses to it can be measured. In a way, what happened this morning with Morsey is a case in point. There's no need to tell her but I'm actually grateful for what's happened, inadvertent as it was.'

Burroughs nodded. Everything about this treatment, even the unforeseen, had been turned to profit. Dent continued to point the way, 'A crisis, you see, is something we do not know how to react to. Every time a coping strategy is achieved and returned to it has a chance of becoming ingrained. We're creatures of habit, might as well be good ones.'

Burroughs took a deep breath as a rush of warmth swayed the boughs overhead and shook the regiments of red and yellow tulips beside him. Everything suddenly seemed straightforward, simple... perhaps it was? His body quivered in a quiet ecstasy. He opened his face to the sky as he spoke: 'I feel I owe you an apology... and Kate ... even Maclay. You all indicated that this would happen,' he waved airily at the garden, 'but I couldn't believe it.'

Dent grunted. He was quietly delighted with the American's progress but knew that the burden of recovery was only just starting and back in the humdrum the patient's newfound responsibility to himself might prove too much. He thought of his role, what he felt for his patient, the potential conflict between responsibility and compassion …. He had to remember that too much care was never advisable in the long run. A petted adult can become more dependent than a petted child but a kick in the pants may last a lifetime.

'Well, Burroughs, you're not out of the woods yet. I repeat, you'll carry this thing with you always: remember that. I don't want to sugarcoat this: I mustn't. You'll die an addict but not for decades and do who knows what?'

'Yes, what?'

'You'll think of something.' Dent's smiling features gave way to a quiet chuckle. He'd had patients from every walk of life; the disease of addiction doesn't discriminate and neither, in his treatment of it, had he. The individual character and circumstances of the patient must always be met by an appropriate response from a healing physician. It was abundantly clear to him that Burroughs possessed a streak of fanaticism that had to be expressed … the alternative: more self harm and annihilation. He thought of the many other writers and so-called 'creatives' he had known, of those he'd treated and been unable to treat. After a while you get a sense of what passes muster … that alchemy of passion and originality and this one had it in spades. Now, finally, he had a real chance to depict the blunted minds of monsters like Anslinger, the literary descendants of Morlocks and Yahoos. This was his best chance to stave off relapse …. Under the doctor's whiskers his lips curled in quiet anticipation ….

For his part Burroughs felt a growing sense of purpose roll through him … the glow of an old intimacy … the reacquaintance with a lost friend … himself. Addiction is often the progressive but futile attempt to compensate for loss. In childhood, stripped of their skin by grief or trauma, people possess an acute sensitivity to pain and its mediating effect on themselves. With each loss they lose another layer and become more and more sensitive to hurt, theirs and others'. Drugs quell the pain, an alien chemical carapace replacing those layers stripped and shed. He now hoped he could develop the armour to head off the hurt, not with drugs but from within, with a justifiable and fulfilling sense of self-worth.

Burroughs aped his doctor by undoing his jacket in the manner of a country gent in front of a log fire. As he stretched out his legs he felt the energy of the sun and the elemental forces sweeping from the earth to the sky and back again: the circle of life. Suddenly his attention was drawn to a tiny movement on the lawn. Sparrows were picking their way towards him. He noticed their pecking order, motivations and teamwork; how each bird contributed to the eyes and ears of the flock. As the birds advanced they mysteriously became villagers jostling for position as Betty Martin, astride the stang, came down the road. The children cheered as she toppled into the water. Immediately the crowd dispersed leaving two old women. They pulled bedraggled Betty onto the bank, wrapped her in a blanket and took her home. As they passed they spoke. He heard soft words, words of solace and hope... interrupted by the terrifying crash of a trap door and twang of the executioner's rope. Ruth Ellis swung before him with burn marks on her pretty white neck.

'Righto!' said Dent, slapping his thighs and getting up. 'Duty calls. You can let yourself in at the clinic; Morsey'll be back now. Stay there tonight and come over tomorrow and we'll go through everything then. If you need to know anything ring me, anytime.'

Burroughs stood and they spontaneously hugged. It's what men do... when the hurly-burly's done. Dent felt a twinge of excitement at the clear expression of trust. He secretly admired this man's cold courage because no matter what others might think it took fortitude to get on a plane, sick and alone and come to London; hardly the most enlightened place in the world. The doctor had not demanded anything of his patient. Quiet example is often enough to the wise.

Burroughs watched his doctor walk away. He noticed that he avoided treading on a scattering of tiny yellow and white flowers peeking through fresh grass. Some chirruping sparrows flew off as he approached but returned as soon as he'd gone. Within a minute you couldn't tell he'd been there at all.

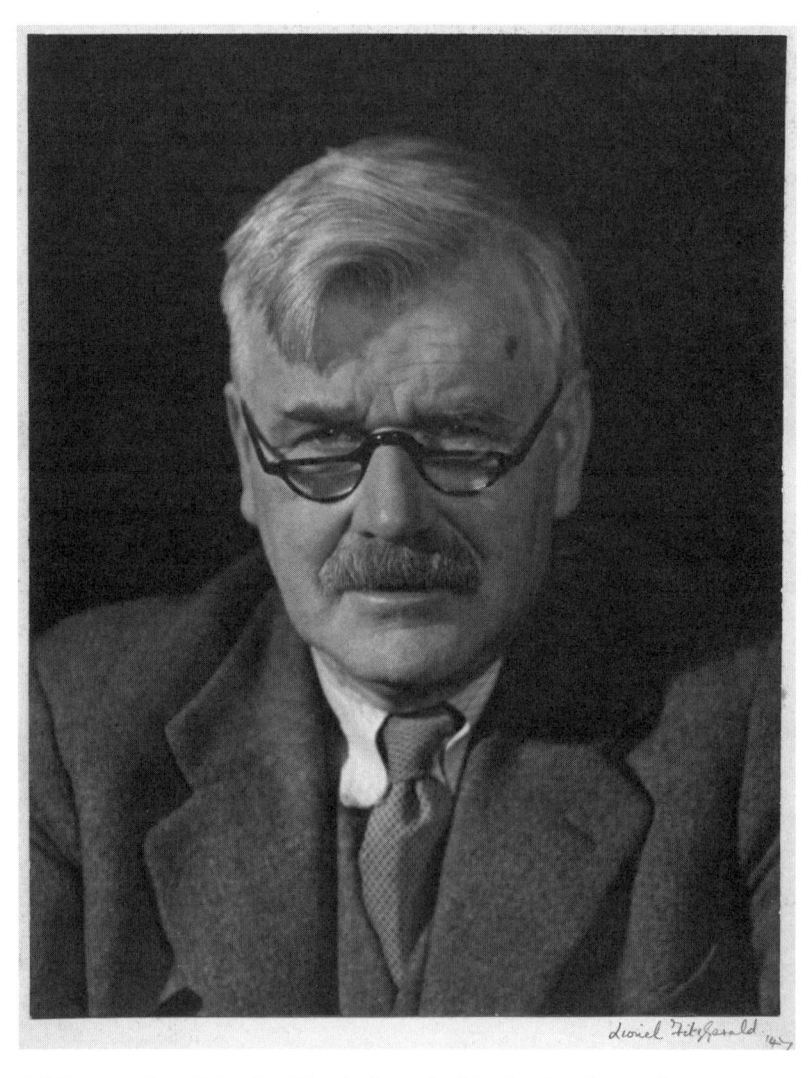

J.Y. Dent, aged 58. 'It is critical for the future health of society that a coherent strategy is thought through and enacted upon. Any mistake now could have incalculable long term consequences... not just for alcohol but all drugs.'
[Photograph: Lionel Fitzgerald]

17

Savages

> Society cares for the individual
> only so far as he's profitable.
> – Simone de Beauvoir
> *The Coming of Age*

Junior Minister Montgomerie straightened his tie and looked in the mirror. Small bloodshot eyes in a puffball face stared back at him. 'Thank God I don't have to look at that too often,' he thought to himself.

He turned on his heel and entered a wide corridor. After passing several sets of double doors he entered the dining room, catching the eye of the attendant waiter who was straightening out a few tables.

'Anyone turned up yet?' he enquired, breathing hard.

'Let me see,' said the waiter, running his finger down a list of names. 'No, I don't think so, err... no. Nobody.'

'Thank goodness,' puffed Montgomerie. 'You see, I've got a quick prelim with the boss. Just tell the early birds I've been unavoidably held up down the road, something like that. Make them comfortable; you know the drill.'

'I'll do my best, sir.'

'Now, you haven't seen me.' Montgomerie continued down the corridor and proceeded to the broad stairs which curved to his left. He paused, glanced behind him, and climbed to the second floor. He opened a large white door and entered an expansive office with chandeliers and a gold leaf picture rail. Two 16th-century oil paintings from the Italian School adorned the inner wall. Sitting in front of them was a secretary. She looked up. 'Ah, David, thank goodness. The minister will see you immediately, please go through.'

'Thank you, Wendy.'

Montgomerie crossed the room and hesitated before opening the door of the adjoining office. A thin bespectacled man was standing in the middle of the room, reading from a newspaper.

'Ah Montgomerie, what's the score?' he asked. He was of slight build but his stare unnerved Montgomerie. It always reminded him of a weasel he'd seen as a boy... killing a rabbit.

'Well, err... we're hopefully ahead, sir... for the time being.'

'What do you mean?'

'Well sir, you can't predict how everybody is going to react, can you?'

'React?' the minister sneered. 'Surely you can do better than that?'

'I'm sorry, Minister, but this Advisory Committee was sprung on me and we've only had three weeks. Given the time of year and so on, I think we've done pretty well.'

'Leave your self-congratulatory crap at the door, Montgomerie.'

'Yes, Minister, of course.'

'Sir Audrey has consented to chair pro tem and naturally you'll be Secretary, but we'll need a Vice Chair. Then there's the memo of intention. Anyway, the upshot of all this is that we have to have our – sorry, *your* report on the PM's desk Friday fortnight, with clear recommendations for cabinet. We cannot permit this issue to get out of hand and turn into the need for another, full-blown Council. We may have to get a bigger team, if there's a problem.'

'Problem?'

'Honestly, Montgomery, did you leave your brain at home this morning? Rejig it, co-opt somebody useful.'

'Good idea.'

'Mmmm, good ideas aren't really your specialty are they? Anyway, today is just the beginning. Right, runners and riders?'

'What was that, Minister?'

'Names, Montgomerie. Who has your department come up with?'

'Oh, I see, sir.' Montgomerie passed a sheet of paper into the minister's thin hand.

'How long before kick-off?'

'Er, ten minutes, fifteen at most.'

The minister sank into a luxurious armchair.

'Bloody hell, Montgomerie. Did you scribble this?'

'Yes, sir.'

'Well it's barely legible. You read it.' The minister disdainfully held up the sheet for Montgomerie to retrieve.

Montgomerie cleared his throat. 'Ahem, right, there's Lady Cresswell, a JP; married into one of the Yorkshire brewing dynasties.'

'Which?'

'I'm sorry, I don't know.'

'You don't know? Listen, Montgomerie; this is critical information. Just because they're brewers doesn't mean they're onside.'

'Yes, sir.'

'Carry on.'

'James Coutts. Part of the team overseeing the Guinness merger.'

'Excellent, last thing he'll want is uncertainty.'

'Jollyon Hunt, M.D. Harley Street, Charterhouse and Oxford. Recommended by us.'

'Good, you can usually count on a Carthusian in a fix. Next.'

'Sir Audrey White, your suggestion.'

'Yes, Sir Audrey will chair. I've briefed him on where this should go and he's had experience with Immigration at the Home Office. So that's two bankers.'

'He's not a banker.'

'Oh for pity's sake, Montgomerie, I mean two we can count on.'

'Hunt and Sir Audrey?'

'No, Coutts and Sir Audrey; now get on with it.'

'Not Hunt?'

'He's a probable, damn it.'

'I think he's more than that, Minister, shall I tell you why?'

'Can it wait?'

'Well, first off he's a doctor and knows—'

'Shut it you drip,' interjected the minister. 'The Lord preserve me. Why do I have to spell it out? He owes us a favour and that's why he's here. Forget he's a doctor. Naturally that will give the report an extra degree of medical credibility should that be flagged up at a later date but this is *not* a medical issue. Morning, noon and night – an industrial matter, commercial, with perhaps a few minor social and moral implications. So, steer well clear of the National Health Scheme. Is that ab-so-lutely clear?'

Montgomerie held his forehead in frustration. 'Perfectly, sir.'

'The list, Montgomerie, come along.'

Montgomerie lowered his hand and peered again at his sheet of paper.

'Mrs Caxton, a councillor from Hampstead. Missed out in a by-election. A token woman.'

'We've Lady What's-her-bloody-name?!'

'Cresswell, yes, sir, but what I meant was; a token woman politician.'

'But she isn't.'

'Best I could do.'

'Christ Almighty! If this goes belly up you gormless oaf they'll have my guts for garters. How many more?'

'Three.'

'That's eight; it's barely enough.'

Montgomerie pondered the point before continuing. 'The Reverend Canon Ernest Fogg of Southwark Cathedral, campaigner for mandatory Bible study in schools.'

'Excellent. I know he's mediaeval from the neck up but the Church never advocates change.'

Montgomerie breathed. 'Viscount Ridley, brewing all the way back to the Armada, a rock solid ally, sir.'

'Yes, I remember Ridley, didn't he room with you?'

'At Harrow, sir. Brilliant off-spinner and a spiffing chap.'

'I'm bowled over, Montgomerie. The last?'

'John Dent, a doctor.'

'We've already got one.'

'Yes, but this one is supposed to be a specialist in the matter in question. He runs the Society for the Study of Addiction.'

'School?'

'No joy there, I'm afraid.'

'Oh bloody hell, this doesn't sound good, two women and two doctors. This could go either way.'

'It's just a departmental committee.'

'Yes, but this report needs to say, well, little or nothing. We've got more than enough on our plates without this blowing up in our faces. The very last thing we need is a domestic health crisis.'

'Even if there is one.'

'Exactly, you sack of lard. At all costs avoid creating a worse impression. Perception is everything; we need a favourable interpretation of current strategies. That the drinks industry is sober, ha! Dutiful and savvy, doing all it can. Now get down there, and don't bugger it up.'

'Righto, sir, but there's the point I was trying to make earlier. We invited this Dent character because he was recommended.'

'By whom?'

'Well, that's just it. I don't know, but Hunt was, as you know recommended by us...'

'You're boring me now, Montgomerie, this better be good.'

'Well, when I mentioned Dent to Hunt he said "Oh, *him*!"'

'And?'

'Well, it seems within medical circles Dent has a reputation for, you know... certain unorthodox practices.'

'Spit it out.'

'Interventions which are, well, not strictly legal, Minister. Anyway I pressed Hunt and it seems Dent shares a clinic with a husband and wife team, the Chessers.'

'What of it?'

'Well, the Chessers quite brazenly conduct terminations, sir... er, abortions.'

'Go on.'

'Well, as Dent is an unknown quantity, and should he exert undue influence, somebody could have a quiet word, suggest he might end up being closed down, that sort of thing.'

The minister stroked his chin. 'I see...then we just drop him, tell him he's off. And that way we can excise everything he's said.'

'And if he asks why?'

'Just say, off the record of course, that we cannot afford to take risks. He'll put two and two together and crawl back to wherever he comes from. He's not Harley Street, is he?'

'No, sir.'

'Well then, he'll be intimidated...only too happy to resign.... Still Montgomerie, I like your initiative. Always useful to see a gap in the hedge, well done.'

Montgomerie stunned by the compliment hesitated.

'Montgomerie! Stop gawping like a prize pig. Get to it. We'll catch up at lunch.'

* * *

Downstairs Dent had arrived early. He was shown into a Home Office waiting room by a junior civil servant and asked if he'd like refreshments. Dent accepted. A short while later the civil servant returned with a tea tray, setting it on a small table. Dent looked at the silver teapot, digestive biscuits and sugar pot. He lifted the lid of the teapot and took in the aroma...

'Can I smoke?' he asked another junior attendant standing by the door.

'Certainly, sir. Would sir care for a cigar or a cigarette? We have both.'

'I've brought my own,' replied Dent.

'Just as you please. Matches?'

'I have those, too.'

'Splendid.'

'No, what I need is an ashtray.'

'Of course, sir. How silly of me, I'll fetch one immediately.'

The junior returned and placed a huge cut-glass ashtray on the tea-table, which wobbled under the weight. 'There you are, sir. I've just heard the Junior Minister is running late. At least you can relax for a while and enjoy your cha and smoke. Nothing better, I think.'

Dent felt uneasy. Hospitality was one thing, but this smarmy gentility?

He poured out his tea and lit a Senior Service. He inhaled deeply and leant back to watch the blue plume of smoke rise steadily in the still air. It looked wonderful...he had always liked watching smoke... an upward waterfall...

'Ah, so you're Dr Dent.'

A cut-glass voice as angular as the ashtray interrupted his reverie. Dent looked up to see a tall man in a dark suit extend his hand. Awkwardly Dent got up, dropping his cigarette onto the floor. He wondered whether he should shake hands or search for the cigarette. He looked down but couldn't see it.

'Oh dear,' he said, getting onto his hands and knees. 'Must have rolled under the table.'

'What was that?' asked the man, curtly.

'Oh never mind,' said Dent, struggling to his feet, 'found it now.'

Dent held up his cigarette in his right hand and realised the other man was still waiting to conclude pleasantries. Dent transferred the cigarette to his left forefinger and thumb and they shook hands.

'Yes, I'm Dent. And you're...?'

'Viscount Ridley. Viscount *Rupert* Ridley. I'm here to represent the wings of the industry you silly buggers are trying to clip. But don't worry; you haven't a hope in hell.'

'Sorry?'

'Another thing, Dent, I know your sort. Interfering, sticking your oar into things you don't understand. We're the backbone of this bloody country, not you lot with your piss-in-the-wind ideals. Clear?'

Dent was about to speak when a weak voice from the other end of the room intervened. It was Montgomerie.

'Oh how splendid!' he cried as he glided towards them with rapid short steps. 'Deee-lighted you've had a chance to have a friendly chitchat before business. Sorry things are a bit topsy-turvy this morning.'

Montgomerie shook Dent's hand.

'Dr Dent, isn't it? I'm Montgomerie, servicing the Division of Health. Delighted you can help.'

Montgomerie turned to Ridley.

'Ah! Rupert old chap, tear you away from the club, did I?'

'Bugger you, Monty, I still haven't forgiven you for last month. It amuses you, doesn't it?'

Montgomerie and Ridley exchanged knowing glances and giggles. 'Rather!' snorted Montgomerie, 'nothing funnier than ole Rupe with a strop on.'

'Ahem, right,' he collected himself. 'Look, we better get going because there's all manner of formalities to get through. Before we know it, it'll be lunchtime. Please, follow me.'

Montgomerie and Ridley crossed the corridor together. Dent gulped down his tea and followed them into a large airy room. It was well-lit and dominated by a large conference table with a dozen chairs. The others had arrived and were chatting in small groups.

Montgomerie sat at the head of the table and invited everybody to take their places. Dent found himself at the other end of the table flanked by two women, Lady Cresswell and Mrs Caxton. They introduced themselves, shaking hands.

'Please, call me Araminta,' Lady Cresswell flustered. 'I absolutely hate formality, so unnecessary nowadays.'

Wendy arrived and handed each person a sheet entitled 'Draft Memo of Intention' before sitting down to take notes.

Montgomerie introduced himself and Wendy and thanked everybody 'for giving up their valuable time'. He stated that the aim of the introductory meeting of the Advisory Committee on Alcohol and Drugs was to agree an overview of current policy and any recommendations for change. The report was to be made available to the Health Ministry before the summer recess. He explained the day's timetable:

'First of all may I suggest an informal meeting amongst ourselves. This will give us the opportunity to get to know each other before lunch at one. Lunch'll be served in the room opposite. After lunch, at two p.m. sharp, Sir Audrey will chair a more formal approach to proceedings with minutes. Any questions?'

'How many times will we have to meet?' asked Ridley.

'Impossible to know at this stage. The Ministry will review the situation and things may change. If you pushed me I'd say twice a year should be adequate.'

'I'll hold you to that.'

'I wouldn't,' said Dent.

Everybody looked towards the quiet voice at the end of the table. Montgomerie sank his fingers into his pudgy cheek.

'What was that?' asked Sir Audrey White, undoing the bottom two buttons of his silk waistcoat.

'Drug and alcohol abuse is a growing health problem and one that has been ignored for far too long.' Dent started. 'I have written and spoken extensively about this for many years – as can be verified by the literature if you're interested. Put simply, the government cannot afford to do nothing. We're finally on the threshold of a proper understanding. It is critical for the future health of society that a coherent strategy is thought through and enacted upon. Any mistake now could have incalculable long-term consequences... not just for alcohol but for the use of all drugs.'

Montgomerie was aghast. Any vestiges of colour in his fat face drained away. His feelings of dread were confirmed by the shrill voice of Mrs Caxton.

'Hallelujah! I've been saying this at church meetings for years but no one listens.'

'But you can't treat these people, can you?' asked Sir Audrey White.

'On the contrary,' continued Dent. 'If sufferers realise treatment is possible then they must insist on getting it and the government will have to give it even though it will cost the Health Service money in the provision of beds, doctors and nurses. Some take the short-sighted course of recommending punishment instead of help. This is not only morally wrong but economic suicide. You see, a successfully treated addict can become a source of financial support, not a drain. He is invariably young and may have a family that could rely on him rather than the state. Put bluntly, he has the potential of years of useful tax-paying work ahead of him.'

'Oh, this is so refreshing!' exclaimed Mrs Caxton. 'Such a change from the "they've brought it on themselves" I keep hearing.'

'Well they have!' claimed Lady Cresswell stridently.

'Yes!' cheered Ridley. 'We give free beer to all our workers, here and in Ireland and if they turn up drunk they get the sack. It keeps them in line, never fails.'

'What never fails?' asked Dent.

'You can't tell me, Dent, that our strategy doesn't work. We've run several very successful breweries for decades and our workers are loyal to the firm.'

'Loyal because they fear redundancy or because of their alcohol dependency that you've been cultivating for generations?'

'Take that back this instant,' demanded Ridley.

'Why? You simply haven't the imagination to consider a different possibility.'

'Preposterous! Monty, are you going to let this insolent varlet get away with this slander?'

Montgomerie burst into nervous laughter. 'Oh, haha! Please, gentlemen, come now, I'm sure Dr Dent isn't insinuating anything.' He jerked as a sudden vision of the minister's weasel eyes loomed in front of him.

'Err, Mis-Mister C-Coutts,' he stammered. 'Y-you know about breweries, no?'

James Coutts straightened his bow tie and ran a finger around his blisteringly white collar.

'It is certainly true that I have seen behind the gates of umpteen breweries, distilleries too. Increasingly they run a tight ship; they have to. All sorts of regulations are coming in: proper labelling, weights and measures, and so on. As for payment in kind, I really have very little experience so I would have to bow to the traditional expertise of Ridley. They are very successful and produce excellent products.'

Montgomerie began to breathe again.

'Sir Audrey White, have you anything to add?'

'Well I have a partnership at Mackeson's as Lady Cresswell knows. The brewing industry has faced many challenges down the years. One area I hope we will address today is the increased competition from abroad. We have to maintain our position in the market to satisfy our customers and safeguard jobs. We, like Rupe – I mean Viscount Ridley – permit our workers to drink as much as they like; some do and some don't. We're moderately successful, as I am sure you're well aware, with approximately 12 per cent share of the market. And I wholeheartedly refute Dent's view that beer induces slavery. It does nothing of the sort. I have drunk our product almost every day of my life and am sober as a judge.'

'Or think you are ...' said Dent.

Several flushed faces stared back at him. One or two looked irritated ... even angry.

'You see,' Dent continued, 'and I apologise if what I am about to say seems strange – the relationship between Man and alcohol is complex. Alcoholism is really just an extreme form of anxiety. There are, you see, two main parts of the brain: the lower or animal part which "acts"; and the higher, or human part, the cortex which "thinks". It is the friction between these parts, the doing and the thinking, which gives rise to the conflict temporarily alleviated by alcohol. And this phenomenon, as independent reports illustrate, is a growing problem. We—'

Lady Cresswell interrupted: 'Oh this is so frightfully interesting, Dr Dent. Does this mean when I want a sherry it's because I think too much?'

A ripple of laughter spread around the table. This pleased Lady Cresswell, who smiled and smoothed her bouffant hair.

'I'd like to know because my husband says I think too much. "There, there, my little squiffy," he says. "Have another sherry."'

The laughter grew when Sir Audrey called out: 'Don't all married men feel the same?'

Dent smiled patiently and waited for the music hall frivolity to die down.

'Well, in answer to your question, Lady Cresswell, anxiety can trouble all of us. Alcohol is indifferent to our circumstances. It is *we* who are changed by *it*. Depressing the front brain with alcohol is certainly one way of reducing our capacity for worry.'

Dent's remarks settled on the room like a wet blanket. Coutts glanced darkly across the table at Sir Audrey before introducing a more familiar narrative.

'Oh good heavens, Dent, are you one of these moralising do-gooders who thinks booze should be banned?'

It was Dent's turn to laugh. 'Not at all, I drink myself.'

Ridley thumped the table in frustration.

'Damn it, Monty, surely we don't have to listen to this new-fangled nonsense all morning? It's plain and simple. Alcohol is either beer or whisky, it's not a drug.'

Dent had seen this coming.

'I am sorry, but that is exactly what it is. Alcohol is a drug that changes our brains like heroin. The major differences are how it is procured and our attitude towards it. We may not buy it from the chemist or get it from the doctor but we use it to change our mood just like any mind-bending agent. What is so poorly understood is its impact on our health. Shall I continue?'

Montgomerie shifted uncomfortably.

'Well, Dent, this is all frightfully technical, how long will your explanation take?'

'I'll be as quick as I can,' said Dent, 'but unless the Committee can develop an understanding of alcohol and its effects how can we justify recommendations which may influence policy? After all, isn't this why we're here?'

Montgomerie felt sick. 'Yes, I suppose so,' he said miserably. 'But we have a lot to get through and we're busy people.'

'Me too,' added Dent.

Montgomerie loosened his tie further. His insides were melting; disaster loomed. Wherever he looked the cruel glint of the weasel's stare loomed. Beads of sweat appeared on his forehead. From where would salvation come?

'Hunt, you're a *highly* respected doctor. W-w-what d-do *you* think?'

Hunt straightened his back and grinned, revealing two rows of impeccably white teeth. He spoke in an offhand, slightly condescending tone.

'I'm of the opinion that addiction is not a disease. It is entirely due to a lack of willpower. Only the weak-minded suffer. You only have to look at the down-and-outs cluttering up Charing Cross every night. The police have the devil's own job clearing the streets. But instead of straightening out and getting a job they beg to buy drink. I ask you, why would any man do that when there's work to be had? Try and get a tradesman nowadays, it's virtually impossible. Quite simply this is a sign of how morally degenerate these people are. I am sure the Reverend Fogg agrees that the magistrates aren't helping. Tougher punishment is the only way; I'd birch them myself. Knock some sense into them.'

'So, like most of us, you think that they're simply not exercising responsibility?' ventured Montgomerie, weakly.

'Of course, any man can see that,' insisted Hunt.

'Well said!' chimed Lady Cresswell, throwing her head back as if she were posing for a photograph.

'Quite right!' said Ridley, slapping the table.

The Rev. Ernest Fogg raised his hand. His words were delivered with an eagerness which belied his age. 'I'm compelled to add that this is my firm opinion, too; and if I may say so, I speak for all of my parishioners, as well as myself. Temperance is what these unfortunates have lost sight of. Sobriety is the key to forbearance and much else besides. When I and the curate attend Pentonville and Holloway it is those who have lost sight of God who seek solace in the evils of wine and spirit. I see this time and time again.'

Dent shifted uncomfortably. 'So you'd like to see the use of alcohol banned?'

'Of course,' pitched the Reverend in a gaunt tone. 'It'd be of infinite benefit to us all.'

'And you'd extend that banning to the Eucharist?'

'Oh no, but that is an entirely different matter.'

'Is it? I once had to admit defeat in treating a priest who was unable to substitute wine for water. The church in its wisdom refused to allow this and sadly he died of alcohol poisoning. You see, Reverend Fogg, the abuse of alcohol is a consequence of *both* our hereditary traits *and* our environment, physical and psychological. It is a disease. I do not hear your parishioners asking cancer sufferers to pull their socks up. We like to think "just saying no" will solve the problem but the evidence suggests otherwise. In other words, quite apart from your evident lack of compassion, you're all talking rubbish.'

'What!?' huffed Hunt.

'Explain yourself, man,' demanded Sir Audrey.

Dent leant back and imagined that if he couldn't there'd be a duel on Hampstead Heath. He slowly gathered his thoughts.

'Some years ago I used to work in a hospital near one of the railway stations that Dr Hunt is referring to. And yes, he's right, every night the police used to bring in the "drunks". On one particular night a heavily pregnant girl arrived who went into labour more or less straightaway.' Dent paused to light a cigarette.

'In the morning we delivered a six-pound baby girl who cried morning, noon and night. The nurses attended to her but there didn't seem to be anything we could do until we discovered that the mother had taken surgical spirit to keep her quiet. The baby, you see, was born suffering from withdrawal because of her mother's drinking throughout pregnancy. Two weeks later the mother suddenly discharged herself. She vanished, taking her baby with her.'

'Oh how awful,' cried Lady Cresswell.

'A terrible story,' said Reverend Fogg, bowing his head.

'But not the end of it,' Dent forewarned. 'A year later the police returned the same mother and child to the hospital. The mother was again pregnant, intoxicated and gripping her one-year-old. When we attended to them, we realised that the child had just died but the mother had been too comatose to notice. I conducted a post-mortem and discovered that it had suffered from atrophic cirrhosis, a hepatic condition otherwise known as "hobnailed liver". A healthy liver is typically soft, a dark red. This one was yellow and pitted with nodules … typical of acute alcohol poisoning.'

Mrs Caxton's face blanched. She gasped.

'So, ladies and gentlemen, what we must ask ourselves is this: did this child "bring it upon herself"?'

Dent let the message sink in.

'And, assuming that *is* what you believe, would the sort of measures Dr Hunt favours have "straightened her out"?'

A dreadful silence invaded the room until it was broken by a sob from Mrs Caxton.

'Oh my God, I'm sorry.' She got to her feet and left, followed by Lady Cresswell, who signalled that she would attend to Mrs Caxton. Wendy had turned white and Montgomerie to stone. The weasel was poised to strike.

A clock in the corridor struck the hour. Somebody said it was lunchtime and everybody stirred apart from Montgomerie. He lurched suddenly as sharp pincer teeth snapped at his throat.

'Monty, MONTY, you alright? *Hello* Monty, chow time,' Ridley urged. 'Dunno about you Monty, but I need a stiff one after that. Meet in the bar, downstairs?'

'Ye-ess, thank you, Rupe ... Double Kümmel, thanks.'

'Coming up.'

Wendy approached Montgomerie and shook her head. He revived himself, calling after the departing Ridley. 'Look Rupert, I'm sorry but duty calls. I'll be along ... if I can.'

Wendy and Montgomerie collected their papers and returned to the office in silence. As they approached the door they saw the Health Minister striding towards them from the other end of the corridor.

Montgomerie gulped, beads of sweat breaking out all over his body.

'Get in there,' the minister barked. 'My office, immediately.'

'Don't tell me.' The minister shouted slamming the door. 'It's going badly, isn't it?'

'I tried to steer it our way,' Montgomerie blurted, 'but it's this Dent character. He's got an answer for everything. He'll recommend wholesale changes, I know he will. He's too well-informed and backs up everything with stories ... er, anecdotes. You cannot browbeat him and he's better informed than Hunt. He's a cave dweller by comparison ...'

The minister held up a hand, signifying that Montgomerie should shut up. He placed his hands on the tall marble mantelpiece and looked into the grate cradling a display of dried hydrangea and pine cones.

'It's worse than you know, Montgomerie. Worse than even *I* could have imagined.'

'What is?'

'Look at the names on this.' The minister produced a sheet of paper from his jacket.

Montgomerie looked at it, and then back at the minister.

'What's this sir, a cabinet reshuffle?'

'Oh bloody hell, Montgomerie, I must have sinned exceedingly in a previous life to end up with a clod like you. Those names are ex-patients of Dent or his friends, the Chessers; one of them is being treated right now, the PM's bloody brother! And you wanted to close down his clinic or threaten him with, what was it? "Unorthodox practices".'

Montgomerie let the paper fall from his sausage-like fingers.

'I had no idea.' He sighed.

'Exactly, you Neanderthal. "No idea" should be your fucking name: "No Idea Montgomerie", you dead-eyed, loathsome slug. "*Close down his clinic*",' the minister parodied in an effeminate voice before returning to sneering condescension. '*Half* the bloody cabinet! Half the bloody BBC; a *judge*! And while they're in there drying out with Dent, you fatuous toad, their mistresses are downstairs getting abortions!' The minister bent down and picked up the paper, pointing to one of the names. 'Look. LOOK! You empty vessel. Lunchtime, is it?' The minister rolled up the sheet of paper and shoved it into Montgomerie's half-open mouth.

'If you actually had a brain cell, Montgomerie, you'd be lethal. I've met sharper turnips. You've precisely ten man-minutes to come up with a solution because I give up.'

Montgomerie retrieved the rolled-up sheet of paper from the back of his mouth. Saliva dripped down his front. Not even being a fag at Harrow had induced this much misery. There was a knock on the door.

'NO!' roared the minister. He grabbed Montgomerie by the lapel. 'Pull yourself together, you slobbering blubber sack. Get out and be back with a strategy, you had ten minutes a minute ago, well now it's five! Go on, GO!'

As Montgomerie left Wendy came in. 'I have jotted down a brief résumé from this morning, Minister.' She did her best to sound light-hearted. 'It was a short but lively introduction.' She looked up, biting her lip.

'Let me see.'

'Here you are, sir.'

'This is going to be changed.' He pointed to the heading: 'Advisory Committee'. 'That's history,' he informed the bewildered Wendy.

'I see,' she said doubtfully.

'Wait till I've had another word with our resident moron.'

Wendy left ... as quietly as she could.

A deflated Montgomerie returned.

'Well? Come up with a solution, did we?' scoffed the minister.

Montgomerie said nothing. He was close to tears.

'Well, fortunately for you, Montgomerie, I have. We'll call this,' he waved his hand at Wendy's notes, 'an "*Interim* Advisory Committee" and Dent won't be invited when it's fledged.'

Montgomerie stirred himself: 'Er, won't he be suspicious; he's the only one who has anything to say.'

'What of it, he's a busy man ... all sorts of things to occupy him. His opinions may be relevant if this were a priority, which it isn't. Hopefully the drinks industry will modernise itself without coercion. It's defensive for a reason, they're behind the times. Today may have given them a taste of what's coming. In that sense today has served a purpose.'

The minister walked towards the window and looked down

Whitehall towards the Houses of Parliament. 'And in a month or so you can go to Dent and thank him for his contribution.' The minister turned to churn Montgomerie's guts with his eyeballs.

'Yes, that's right, no need to look so gormless. Go to his home and make your gratitude sound like an apology. Explain as best you can the virtues of political expediency. It'll be good for you, and he'll understand. He wasn't born yesterday.'

The minister laughed, unable to desist from the cruellest jibe of all. 'You never know, Montgomerie, if you ask him really nicely, he might offer to treat you!'

* * *

Three hours later Dent walked down Whitehall towards Trafalgar Square. He felt dispirited by a day that promised much but would deliver little. Indeed, the doctor was left with the clear impression that the problem of addiction would never be dealt with honestly by politicians as long as they valued commerce, even unethical commerce, above the nation's health. The Advisory Council on Alcohol and Drugs was a sham. He wondered if this realisation should be marked with a drink. He smiled ruefully and walked towards his regular watering hole: the Savage Club.

At the end of the bar he recognised Cleaver, a fellow member of the Society for the Study of Addiction and a rich medical entrepreneur. He ran a rest home for recovering alcoholics in the Midlands, another in the Cotswolds and was rumoured to be opening another in Richmond, West London. This concerned Dent since he knew that Cleaver used paraldehyde to wean people off alcohol. Years ago Dent had corresponded with the press that this was an intolerable practice as addiction to paraldehyde was far worse than the one it replaced and much harder to treat.

Cleaver saw Dent and immediately old enmities were resumed.

'Bit much isn't it, Dent,' he barked. 'You drinking beer. After all, you're always preaching about the sins of drink.'

Dent was wondering how to respond while Cleaver continued to harangue: 'I suppose you didn't think anyone from the Society would see you in here. They'd all be disappointed, perhaps shocked, to see one of their own contradicting their aims.'

'The aims of the Society,' said Dent, 'are primarily about scientific study and ultimately better education. We cultivate an open attitude towards the use of alcohol and there is absolutely no reason to assume that, in moderation, it does any lasting harm whatsoever. In fact it probably does a great deal of good as a culinary accompaniment, in its use at festivities, rites of passage and so on. Really, Cleaver, you should know better.'

Three regulars leaning on the bar between Cleaver and Dent nodded in approval but more in the hope that Cleaver would not take this lying down. They needn't have worried.

'I knew you'd take the Society downhill, Dent. That's why you can't get any more members, you so-called "progressives". Stupid and hypocritical more like. You should be sending out a message of absolute temperance! That's bloody crucial.' He stood up and faced the thickening crowd at the bar. 'And another outrage. Wasn't it you who got sponsorship for research from a bloody brewing company? I ask you!? Talk about consorting with the devil.'

Encouraged by murmurs of support, Cleaver punctuated every remark with a stamp of his foot. When he finally finished there were a few muffled cheers. Everybody looked expectantly at his adversary.

Dent looked up and responded in a quiet but clear voice.

'Why then, since you are so upset over the existence of alcohol, are you drinking it yourself?'

The room erupted in 'whoo's and ironic laughter. Cleaver's face spat fire:

'Damn and blast you. You effing well know I'd never do such a thing. Never! There isn't a drop of alcohol in this; it's bloody Cydrax.'

Dent drank up his pint and looked into the empty glass for a moment.

'The thing is, Cleaver, I point this out because it is critically important to your patients. For recovering alcoholics, the drinking of alcohol must be avoided as they have little or no tolerance. Doctors must be quite clear about this and should know where it is to be found. It is a popular misconception that there is no alcohol in some drinks. It seems you share this delusion. If you had bothered to move with the Society and not against it and if you had read the recent research you would be well aware that there is indeed a small amount of alcohol in Cydrax.'

Word had gone round the club that all the pre-dinner entertainment was to be had in the bar where Cleaver resembled a beef tomato, about to burst. Soon it was standing room only as people argued over who was right. Cleaver picked up the bottle and shouted at the gathered faces: 'Look, there's nothing on the label which says there's any alcohol in Cydrax. And if you look at this,' he reached over the bar and grabbed a bottle of Truman's Best Stout, 'it says quite clearly "five degrees proof". It has to. You're wrong, Dent, and I am not leaving here tonight without an apology.'

There were more cheers, egging Cleaver on. A book was quickly opened behind the bar and bets were placed. Cleaver was 2/1 on; Dent was evens.

Cleaver's claim, however, raised a technical problem and all manner of helpful and unhelpful proposals were ventured.

'I say, Cleaver old boy, aren't you a bit over the top?' asked one member.

'Tiddly?' probed another.

A wag with a piping voice briefly took centre stage and sauntered up to Cleaver. He adopted the posture of a bobby apprehending a 'drunk and disorderly'.

'Excuse me, sir. Can I trouble you to say "British Constitution"?'

This brainwave was met with numerous attempts as to how Cleaver might pronounce it if he tried. The game grew unruly when another member invited Cleaver to 'walk the white line without falling over'. Tables and chairs were moved aside as people offered their best attempts to follow a straight line along the carpet. Cleaver's ego exhibited bravura, on the surface he joked with the crowd, but underneath he boiled with rage. Everyone instinctively recognised a bully. This was Cleaver's comeuppance and ironically only Dent was reluctant to stick the boot in.

Eventually a senior surgeon from St Barts said that he would be happy to run a bottle of room temperature Cydrax down to the hospital lab and do a quick alcohol test and be back in thirty minutes with the result. Everyone agreed and two witnesses, one from each 'camp', left in a taxi with the surgeon and an unopened bottle of Cydrax. Dent felt increasingly uncomfortable at the fuss. Irrespective of the 'verdict' he wondered what impact the result would have on the fuming Cleaver, now drumming his fingers on the bar.

It was true that Dent had no respect for Cleaver's medical practices but because of his roles at the Society and as a family doctor he had a unique perspective on how policy and treatment had to interact to be effective. Dent also saw in his adversary many of the early signs of emotional frailty; his irascibility and self-importance, his inability to listen. Dent's instinct was to withdraw and not excite the dragooning culture remorselessly cultivated in the private school sector and perpetuated in London clubland. He deplored these tendencies and yet here he was at the heart of a typical episode which was likely to injure his nemesis. He longed for it all to be over.

Finally, after a wait of nearly an hour, the group returned and with vaudevillian absurdity the result was announced. The 'judge' stood on a chair. He was an accomplished actor and knew how to play to the gallery. With great solemnity he draped a linen dish cloth over his head.

'The ad hoc Judicial Committee' he started, clearing his throat, 'in the dispute "Cleaver *v.* Dent" wishes to thank the technical department at Barts for providing the use of its hydrometer, technical staff and laboratory. We have borne witness to an exacting scientific procedure conducted in a clinical setting and are now in a position to state categorically that we have arrived at a unanimous decision.'

'Get on with it!' somebody shouted.

'Silence in court! Ahem! I am able to declare beyond all doubt that Cydrax is between 1–2 degrees proof and that we, the judicial committee, find in favour of Dent!'

The room collapsed in a heady cocktail of laughter, mock cheers and boos. Bar the protagonists everybody had enjoyed the farce. Dent shifted uncomfortably as somebody slapped him on the back.

'Bravo, Dent! Well done!'

Since suffering TB Dent had always hated this treatment. He said nothing. At the other end of the bar Cleaver was being ridiculed, not so much for being wrong as for his pompous indignation. Trembling with fury he charged out of the building. Somebody heard him mutter that he was resigning. This was broadcast back to the bar to derisory cheers. Above the hubbub someone offered Dent 'one for the road'. 'A Cydrax?' someone suggested, to gales of laughter. The betting debts were settled and people started to drift off.

'Leaving early?' asked a brother Savage, on the steps leading into Carlton House Terrace.

'Self-preservation,' informed Dent, with a wry smile.

Outside he was glad of the clear air. He could have stayed for dinner but preferred to eat at home, away from the Savages or, as he openly referred to them, the 'Morlocks'. How would Uncle Louis have dealt with them, he wondered, or with Cleaver and Cydrax for that matter? Maybe if Louis had learnt to parody civilisation like Bertie Wells or Swift he'd have survived? *Castigat ridendo mores.*

He hailed a taxi: 'Addison Road, Kensington please.'

Fifteen minutes later he paid the cabbie while watching two men carry heavy furniture out of his front door.

'What's going on?' he asked.

'What's it look like, guvnor?'

Dent looked on helplessly as the men grunted their way into the street and heaved the chest of drawers onto the tailgate of a large removal lorry.

Dent entered his home and was greeted by a state of disarray and strange echoing sounds of a house stripped of soft furnishings. Two more men were struggling on the stairs with a bookcase. There was a note on his kitchen table... the one he'd carved himself alongside its matching benches and large chair. He sat down and leant against its tall solid back, against its carved relief of two intertwined eels... the ones always locked in a perennial struggle of opinion.

Dear John,

    I have had enough and feel this is for the best. The girls and I will be moving straight into Rudfyn, North Chase, our new home. The bank (tel: Western 8708) now own this one and have informed me that they will take possession at the end of the month: six days' time. Quite fortuitously I hear the Brenans are looking for residency in the neighbourhood and that No. 34, opposite, is vacant. I doubt very much Blair will mind and Rhoda not at all.

    I will be in touch as soon as we're settled.

    Alma

Dent felt the chill from the solid oak chair seep into him. He felt a twinge in his lungs and was reminded of the earlier slap on his back. 'That was bad,' he mumbled to himself, 'but better than a kick in the teeth.'

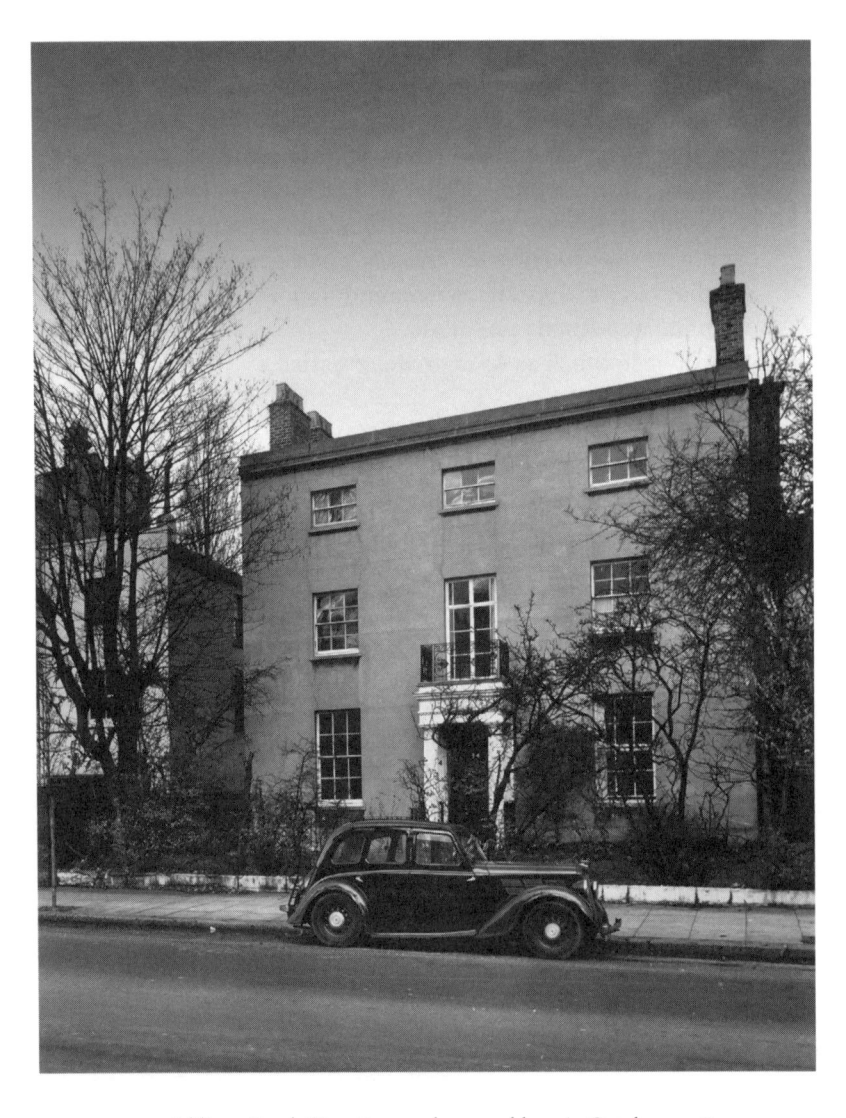

34 Addison Road, W14. Burroughs stayed here in October 1958.
The Dent/Brenan home for 20 years.
[©Collage, LPA, 2018]

18

When Lee Became Burroughs

> Am I the man to reproach Coleridge with this vassalage to opium? Heaven forbid! Having groaned myself under that yoke, I pity and blame him not. But undeniably, such a vassalage must have been created wilfully and consciously by his own craving after genial stimulation; a thing which I do not blame, but Coleridge *did*.
> – Thomas De Quincey
> *Confessions of an English Opium Eater*

On Sunday morning William Seward Burroughs returned to Addison Road but with purpose in his heart. He was still pinching himself over his transformation.

As before Peel rattled his chain, but Burroughs ignored him and reached confidently for the Beelzebub door knocker. He smiled wryly and knocked.

Rhoda answered, letting the door swing wide open. 'Ah, you'll be Mr Burroughs, do come in.'

'Hello, yes, thank you.'

'I am Rhoda Brenan … here, let me take your hat and coat … we're in the kitchen but John's finishing off upstairs. Come through.'

Burroughs walked into the warm kitchen, this time filled with activity. Three people were seated round the oak table kneading, peeling and chopping. Rhoda pulled back the large oak chair Burroughs had occupied on his first visit and introduced the latest arrival.

'Everybody, this is Mr Burroughs, he'll be with us for lunch. Blair

Brenan, my husband, Lydia, our daughter and Angus Wilson our other guest. Please, Mr Burroughs, make yourself comfortable... John should not be too long. Lunch should be ready in about an hour.'

Burroughs sat down and briefly made eye contact with the others, who returned his smile. As he leant back the phone rang in the hall. Rhoda went to answer it.

'Can I do anything?' Burroughs asked.

'We're well under control, thanks,' said Lydia, brightly.

'Yes,' said Wilson, 'I never do any cooking unless I end up here.' He laughed, raising his hands over a bowl of cooking apples and peel.

'All hands to the pump,' agreed Blair, holding up flour-dusted fingers.

'A co-op kitchen ensures a good appetite,' added Lydia.

'Oh, so that's what it is!' exclaimed Wilson. 'Not that I'm complaining. It's a plan that seems to work.'

'We're having roast beef with all the fixings,' said Blair. 'Apple pie to follow. A celebration of our culinary compatibility.'

'If nothing else,' added the American, with a grin. The other three laughed.

'Is that Burroughs?' Dent's voice boomed from the dumb waiter.

Lydia got up and lifted the screen. 'Yes,' she called up.

'And that was Stickler on the phone,' added Rhoda, returning from the hall. 'He's on his way over.'

'What, now?' came the voice from the wall.

'Yes.'

'Not a social call?'

'Doesn't sound like it. In fact he sounded cross. Muttered something about the journal being "intolerably late".'

'Oh dear. Never mind, send Burroughs up, we'll be as quick as we can.'

Rhoda closed the dumb waiter.

'You've been summoned by Zeus himself,' Wilson said.

'While we slave in the underworld,' added Blair, trying to sound miserable.

'We're like the three Furies,' threw in Lydia.

Rhoda ignored the banter, 'Mr Burroughs, you remember where to go?'

Burroughs nodded, went upstairs and tapped on Dent's consulting room door. Dent opened it and Ulysses ran in ahead of him. 'Two visitors!' laughed Dent. 'Do come in. Plenty of room.'

'You'll have another soon?' reminded Burroughs.

'Stickler, yes. Not to worry, that cannot be helped.' They shook hands.

'You think that about everyone, don't you?' Burroughs commented.

'Come again?' asked Dent.

'Those that want to be helped and those that don't.'

'Oh, I see. Yes, you're quite right.' The two men moved casually towards the back of the room. 'The damage that can be done by kicking in doors that do not want to be opened. That is why our little fireside chat...when was it...the week before last was critical...in getting us where we are today. Some think that care begins and ends with medicine or surgery. That is far from the case. I have to be sure that the patient is here of his own volition.'

'Too bad few have your understanding.'

'For any intervention to work we must treat the patient not the condition. But it's getting worse, Burroughs...everywhere I look...and patients indignant if their doctor cannot wave a wand. "I will carry on being the same drunken brute I always was but you have to make me better...now!" How can that work?'

'It cannot.'

'Change begets change, that is all.'

'I feel I've changed, in fact I know I have.'

'Good. Sleep well last night?'

'Yes.'

'Bit wobbly on your feet?'

'Not too bad, my strength is returning, and I got another one of your full English breakfasts this morning.'

'Did you enjoy it?'

'Yes, very much ... and another thing.'
'Yes?'
'I had a bath.'
'Voluntarily?'
'Ha! Yes.' Burroughs laughed and Dent joined in.
'Splendid, I'm delighted. But beware, there are traps out there.'

The two men sat down as before alongside the consultation desk jammed against the wall. Dent pushed a sheet of paper towards Burroughs. 'These are the medicines I know of that contain opiates. It is not comprehensive because new ones are coming out all the time. You're a traveller and people may pass them off as something else. If you are in any doubt throw it away. It is not worth taking the chance.'

'Because this might return me to where I was?'

'There is no "might" about this: it would. You must be absolutely clear about this. Your charts show you are now several days without any opiates at all. None. But the slightest amount will tip you back to where you were. Please be very careful. Look at you now. Your colour is good, no pain, sweats, cramps, or sickness. And you have an appetite. Try and remember where all this leads and use the knowledge. I repeat: you are still an addict ... you have had a treatment. At the moment you can function without these drugs, but your vulnerability to them remains and always will. Clear?'

Burroughs looked into the steel blue of Dent's eyes and saw the naked truth, simple and forthright. In an evil world full of rogues and idiots it was good to find an oasis of calm and honesty. He smiled and nodded in appreciation. Yet, as he looked around the room filled with universal treasures of mind and spirit, he realised that he had had a tremendous experience ... one filled with extraordinary colliding visions that he could both recall and mine. What if he fell off the wagon? Could apomorphine be revisited? He wouldn't mention this, that would be unseemly ... disrespectful.

'Yeah, I got it. I shan't forget,' he assured.

'When do you think you would like to leave the clinic? I think you should stay there tonight and we can decide tomorrow if you'd like.'

'You want me to skedaddle?'

WHEN LEE BECAME BURROUGHS

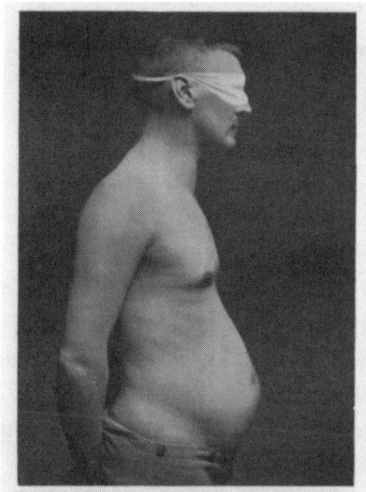

FIG. 17.—Here we see a man of early middle life whose abdomen has become pendulous and protuberant, due to excessive local fat deposit and faulty posture.

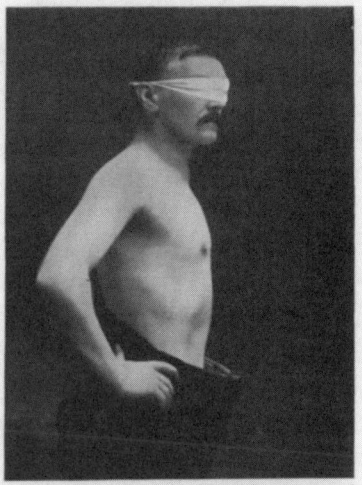

FIG. 18.—Shows the same subject after a course of treatment. Note the striking change in general contour and condition.

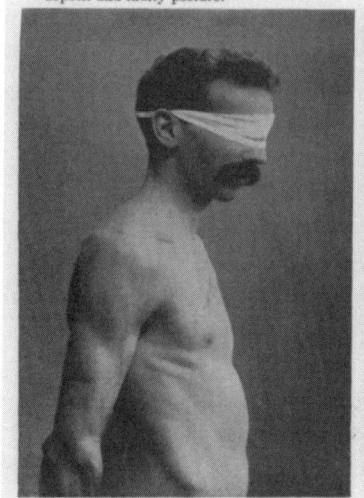

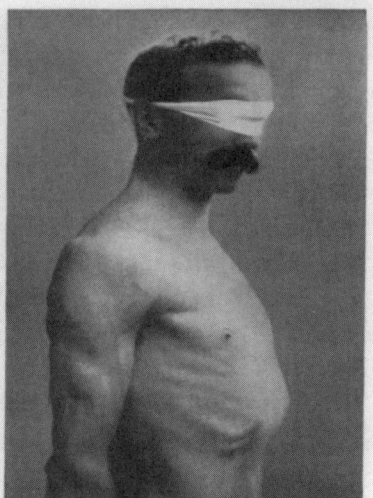

FIG. 1.—Shows the general external appearance of the body in faulty attitude, with dropped internal organs (Enteroptosis).

FIG. 2.—Shows the same subject with the errors corrected after a course of training by myself. Note the improved musculature and pose.

On Dent's recommendation Fred Hornibrook, the author of *The Culture of the Abdomen*, treated Burroughs. Fred also treated many other writers including H. G. Wells and Somerset Maugham.

[379]

'Not at all. You discharge yourself. Let me or Gibbie know. You're free to stay as long as you consider necessary... but you will be encouraged to leave.'

'I see, because that will be best for me.'

'Most definitely. When you return to your independence you'll be able to canalise good habits... apomorphine facilitates this, I am sure of it.'

'I think I get it. You mentioned pills... and exercises.'

'Yes, I will give you the same pills that you've already been taking, sub-emetics, dissolved under the tongue. Apomorphine has a negative tolerance... less is more. You know how to take it and that it helps you sleep. It is a somnambulant, not a tranquilliser. You should try to sleep without apomorphine... by getting into a routine but knowing that you have pills to fall back on will help.'

'And the exercises?'

'I have spoken to Fred Hornibrook on your behalf and he expects your call. He is a great believer in the body politic. A healthy body being the gateway to all manner of good things. I believe he is right. He and his wife specialise in abdominal exercises, they've written books about it. They're a lovely couple, you'll get along fine. Here's Fred's number, and address. Ring him anytime.'

'Thank you. Now, I'd like to pay your fee.'

'Yes, well... I have been thinking about this and I have a proposal.'

'Oh?' Burroughs sounded surprised.

'You can pay Gibbie and Hannah what you owe for your stay and their care; that is five pounds a day, each.'

'Yes, that's no problem.'

'But between you and I, how about we go quid quo pro?'

'How d'you mean?'

'Well, I may have mentioned I edit a journal...'

'John... John!' Rhoda's voice came from the wall.

'Excuse me a minute.' Dent got up and slid open the hatch. 'Yes?'

'That's the door, it'll be Stickler. What shall I do?'

'Send him up.'

'Are you sure?'

'Quite.'

Dent closed the shutter and turned to Burroughs. 'Look, Burroughs, I am sorry about this but if you wouldn't mind, could you just return to being Benway for a minute?'

'Er, sure, no problem.'

'*Dr* Benway,' Dent emphasised. 'I'd be so grateful…'

Stickler was huffing outside Dent's front door in a bubble of indignation. Yesterday and again that very morning he had drawn criticism from other members of the Committee of the Society for the Study of Addiction. 'Why,' they had wanted to know, 'have you been unable to bring Dent into line? Why,' they insisted, 'after your assurances, is the journal still not published?' Stickler was embarrassed and promised that this time Dent would not pull the wool over his eyes. On his short drive over from St John's Wood he had rehearsed his laying down of the law. He had emphasised each point by thumping the dashboard, drawing strange looks from a couple crossing Bayswater Road. 'I will not allow myself to be deflected, browbeaten or distracted by your games, Dent,' he had bellowed as he sped through Notting Hill Gate in his racing green Humber at nearly fifty mph. 'It is my duty to reflect the views of the Committee, and you must be left in no doubt whatsoever about who calls the tune.'

He hardly acknowledged Rhoda as he burst past her.

'Where's he hiding?' he steamed.

'Hello, Stickler,' greeted Rhoda, taken aback. 'Why don't you go straight on up…' she suggested sarcastically as he climbed the stairs as fast as his short legs would allow.

He strutted across the landing and rapped on the consulting room door. Dent opened it. 'Stickler! Do come in.' He marched in like a drill sergeant and spun on his heels.

'Now Dent,' he berated, 'I'm here to serve you an ultimatum. The Committee has had enough.'

'Excuse me, Stickler; can I introduce you…'

'No, you cannot…'

'Oh? Why? *You*...'

'Stop it, Dent. What of the journal, the bloody printers?'

'All done, everything's ready to roll.'

'Well ring them, tell them to go ahead.'

'Yes, of course, can you inform the Committee?'

'It's a Sunday!'

'Yes, I think you'll find the printers think that too.'

'Damn it, Dent, this is intolerable.'

'I agree, will you stop for lunch, because...'

'LUNCH! I'll see you in hell first...'

'Oh that's a shame because I was just discussing the journal...'

'The bloody journal that is going to be six weeks late!' Stickler's eyes pulsed, his fingers opened and closed in rapid, jerky movements.' 'Six weeks!' he repeated, raising his voice.

'Yes, Stickler, which is why I have decided to do exactly as you advised.'

'Eh? What's that?'

'You told me I should put to bed the papers in advance...to improve the workflow...' Dent hesitated and wondered if he was laying it on a bit thick. 'Our membership expects it,' he added, suppressing the urge to smile.

'But this one Dent, *THIS ONE*! Even if it came out today it would be a month late. Your lax approach is unforgivable.'

'Well it is certainly regrettable but,' Dent paused, like a poker player about to reveal a winning hand, '...that is precisely why the learned *Dr* Benway is here. A keen associate who, aware of our mission, has given up his valuable time to visit us today...all the way from America.' That last word hung in the air like a ripe plum.

Stickler was suddenly confused. He admired the Americans; he believed in the détente between Britain and America in the same way a four-year-old believes in Cinderella. Dent's temptation left him torn between continuing with his tirade or being gracious towards this stranger...a colleague...from the States.

'You see,' continued Dent, 'Dr Benway has a uniquely global perspective on the problem of addiction that can help us all, doctor *and* patient. Therefore, I am anxious to clinch the inclusion of his expertise for the journal as early as possible … just as you said I should.'

Dent's eyes shone over the top of his specs. 'Furthermore, Stickler, we get so few opportunities to share our ideals with our American cousins … the principles that make our little Society important? We simply cannot afford to remain isolated, can we?'

'America?' Stickler studied Burroughs for the first time. Dent's carefully chosen words had chimed with his dreamed-of ideal, one he coveted: the spirit of a scientific brotherhood with Britain's greatest ally. 'You, er, Dr B-B-Benway, you're from the States with experience of these matters …?'

'Sure, particularly in the neglected field of addiction,' confirmed Burroughs. A thin smile spread across his face … it was both there and not there, ghostlike.

'He has seen, for instance,' added Dent, quickly, 'how science can be tainted by too much commercial interference. It is crucial his beleaguered compatriots realise they are not alone in their struggle.'

Stickler took in a deep breath. 'Oh yes! That *is* critical.' He puffed out his chest, slipping a thumb into his waistcoat pocket. 'We in Britain certainly have an important contribution to make. I am delighted that our voice is being heard.' Stickler offered Burroughs the recondite nod that was immediately reciprocated.

Dent stood behind Burroughs. 'Dr Benway has also seen what goes on at Lexington, Kentucky. Have you heard about that?'

'Of course I have,' snorted Stickler, expanding his chest further. 'One of those fine fellows, a professor of biochemical research, told me all about it … very progressive place, you know … at the vanguard of modern science.'

Burroughs cleared his throat. 'You'll know, then, that Lexington is an addiction hospital provided by American Congress because of the complete failure of America's drug policies?'

'What's that? A "failure?"'

'Sure,' emphasised Burroughs. 'The federal prison system is so overcrowded with addicts they can't cope. But Lexington ain't worth a darn either. Did you know that there's a racial element to the research?

That very few treatments are voluntarily submitted to? Why do you think Lexington's real name is "*Prison* Hospital"?'

'Er, well, that does sound somewhat contradictory,' said Stickler, frowning.

'You can say that again,' the American drawled. 'Addicts are compulsorily detained; they're inmates, not patients. And let's be clear about this. There's a thirty foot perimeter fence with razor wire, armed guards and dogs! It's more of a concentration camp.'

Stickler raised his eyebrows. 'Good Lord! But the men, do they respond?'

'Hey, it ain't just for men. Plenty o' blocks for women too.'

'Alcoholics?'

'Mostly narcotics.'

'Well I never!' Stickler held his ruddy cheeks in his palms. 'That chap didn't say anything about that.'

'Why would he?' continued Burroughs. 'They say it's for research but who uses the information? Drug companies, and the CIA. So they know how best to control narcotics. The whole thing's a front.'

'Goodness gracious me!' Stickler shook his head.

'What you gotta do,' Burroughs continued, his voice beginning to whine like an air-raid siren, 'is make sure the same shocking travesty doesn't happen here … in Britain.'

Stickler, still holding his face, fell into the chair next to Burroughs. 'How right you are! That must never happen, never. You say Lexington is expanding?'

'Yeah.'

'How many beds, five hundred?' Stickler thought he'd overestimate.

'Two thousand, minimum.'

'Good Lord!'

'They're knocking up new wings all the time … just to stay on top.'

'Goodness gracious me!' Stickler's jaw dropped. 'My word, Dent, I hope you are getting this? Two thousand beds and still not enough. And opiates. How terrible!' He jerked his face to the ceiling as if in shock.

'Well,' said Dent, 'Lexington symbolises why Britain shouldn't

The Light of a New Day

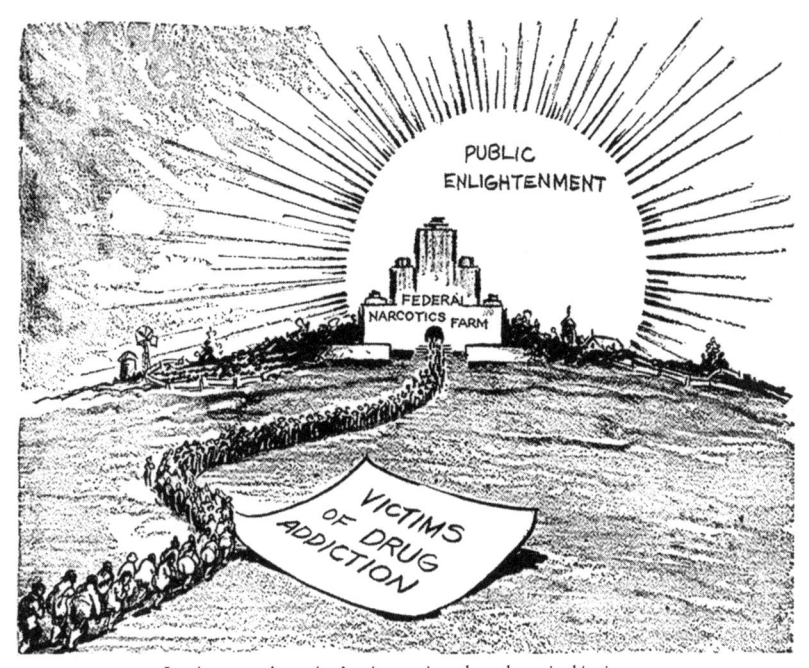

Lexington; America's pioneering drug hospital/prison, *Atlanta Georgian*, 4 March 1935.

embark on such a ruinous strategy. I am sure Dr Benway will spread the word.'

'It's one of the reasons I'm here,' rejoined Burroughs. 'Because of the complete breakdown of the situation in the States. You guys have a great deal to be proud of. The way you've contained the problem... kept it medical not political.'

'Agh,' Stickler perked up, 'but we're having the devil's own job, a battle.'

'You mustn't give in,' encouraged Burroughs, 'the big picture is what's critical.'

'Oh, rest assured,' Stickler boasted. 'There are only a couple hundred registered addicts in the whole of Britain. We know the importance of our position. And I am sure your American Congress will see sense and come round to our way of thinking.'

Dent was both saddened and amused by Stickler's blind faith. British doctors couldn't even influence each other, let alone Whitehall. What chance did they stand on Capitol Hill? Burroughs sensed that he should round off the discussion.

'Well, gentlemen, I'll naturally broadcast our shared ideals but if you permit me I'd also be most gratified to contribute to your journal with an article of my own. Good ole British values must be better understood Stateside, and boy!' Burroughs slapped his thigh, 'we certainly need strong leadership.'

Stickler beamed. Patriotic smugness had evaporated the last of his ire. 'Thank you, Dr Benway, a wider appreciation of the British system of containment certainly won't go amiss.'

'So you'll stay for lunch?' Dent repeated.

Stickler looked at his watch. 'Oh, gosh! Is that the time? No, sorry Dent, that is too kind. Normally I'd jump at the chance, but I promised my wife to take her out and even if I rush, I'm going to be late.' He got up and bowed in front of Burroughs. 'Doctor Benway, delighted to have made your acquaintance...keep up the good fight. Marvellous stuff.' They shook hands. 'And Dent, you'll ring the printers tomorrow, first thing?'

'Consider it done, and if you'd like to ring ahead...to your wife, use the phone downstairs, in the hall.' Dent opened the door and the two doctors parted cordially. Dent closed the door and went straight to the dumb waiter pushing his head and shoulders into the shaft. '*Rhoda*,' he whispered, 'Stickler's leaving, help him on his way, please ...thank you. We'll be down in five minutes.' Dent closed the hatch, sat down and eyed Burroughs. 'You're good at this, Burroughs, a deft performance, bravo!'

Burroughs threw his head back and laughed quietly, aware that Stickler could still be in the building...his doctor joined in.

They gradually settled down and turned their minds back to unfinished business. 'Now, where were we?'

'Your fee...' reminded Burroughs.

'Yes, and my offer. Well, everything I said to Stickler is true; I would like it if you would write an article about your experiences and consider ourselves quits as part of the bargain. We always hear from doctors but rarely from patients, or in your case a master addict. We need to hear these voices more than ever. Science cannot stop addiction and currently politicians are only making the disease burden worse. However, the stories from sufferers might make a difference... broaden everybody's horizons.'

'I accept, but won't you have to explain to Stickler my true identity?'

'Perhaps, but only if he asks. And if he does I will say that I had to ensure patient confidentiality.... He's a stickler for that sort of thing, is Stickler. He'll mumble away for an hour and twenty minutes saying, "Of course, you're quite right, jolly good show, by Jove"' The two men fell into another bout of the giggles.

'"Good Lord!"' mimicked Burroughs, lifting his glasses and rubbing his eyes.

'The only thing I am sure of is this.' Dent leant forward and placed a hand on Burroughs' knee. 'In my capacity as editor of the journal I can guarantee your inclusion.'

A burst of laughter thundered throughout the house... those in the kitchen looked knowingly towards the hole in the wall. Dent got up and gave Burroughs some old copies of the journal. 'Keep these for reference... and while you're at it feast your eyes on the esteemed contributors. Many with fewer letters in their names than after; the cream of the British scientific and medical communities. With their confirmed beliefs finally rubbing shoulders with an addict's understanding we might actually get somewhere.'

Burroughs took the journals. Dent sat back down and watched as his patient flicked through the pages, his eyes darting over the columns. The doctor was delighted by the level of engagement... it was the turnaround and reaction he had hoped for. He almost regretted what he would now have to say.

'However,' Dent's voice changed, 'there is a condition... a critical one.'

Burroughs looked up. 'Yes? And what's that?'

'It is quite simple. I will only accept and print your paper providing it appears under your birth name; William Burroughs.'

'Well, er... yes... but why?'

'It is simple. You have written about your life but under a pseudonym. This is a hedge, a temptation to be someone you are not. I do not care for mythologies; it goes against the grain. They rarely help and can often make things worse. I have treated or tried to treat many people who lead a Jekyll and Hyde existence; it is impossible. They can hold any number of positions.' Dent paused, thinking of the masterful way Burroughs had danced around Stickler. 'So, who are you? Jekyll or Hyde; Benway or Burroughs? This problem you have had will be easier to resist if you accept that it prevents you from being who you truly are...... your true self.'

'I see.'

'Remind me, what was your pseudonym?'

'Lee.'

'Wasn't he a military man?' Dent sounded almost derisory. 'Burroughs would be so much better. To my ear it'd sound indivisible from your one and true inner voice, one you can be proud of, no subterfuge.'

Burroughs thought better of telling Dent that Lee was actually his mother's maiden name. No need to muddy the waters.

'If you had an ugly venomous snake as a pet,' Burroughs asked, looking at Ulysses, 'would you name it after a general or a dictator?'

Dent thought for a second. 'I might call it Anslinger and mispronounce it.'

Burroughs guessed how and laughed.

'So,' Dent pressed, not wishing to be distracted, 'do you agree?'

'Yes, I have no objection. You're right about different personas. They can confuse things.'

'Well, I cannot tell you what to do with your other work, that is a matter for you. But your continued recovery will be made easier by being straight with yourself. I agreed to treat you because I recognised that you understood that being well is fundamentally a selfish act; it has to be for it to work.'

Burroughs nodded.

'And therefore to shield others from your feelings and true identity is to put their needs before your own. Ultimately if you can find a way to be yourself, no facade, that'll be one less anxiety and your people will find it easier to respect you ... no matter how difficult. And, dare I say, this will not only apply to family and friends but your readership too.'

Burroughs sucked air through his teeth. Maybe this was right ... his acting out had often been an avoidance strategy ... but a barrier to being clean? And his birth name, his father's with all that patrician WASP bullshit? Maybe he had to own it? Run with rather than from it ... perhaps? 'OK I get it, and I accept your condition: I have no objection to my name being used.'

'Good, and fair exchange is no robbery. We're quits.'

The two men relaxed into an easy silence ... the hiss of the fish tank once again drew Burroughs' attention. The languid fluttering of the Siamese fighting fish was still there, spectacular and incongruous. So too was Buddha's contemplative pose. He thought he should hold his hands in the same way but realised that he already was. Had this been unconscious or was he being inhabited by an unknown force?

'How much would your fee be if I hadn't accepted?' Burroughs thought out loud.

Dent smiled. 'Oh, a millionaire couldn't afford to pay.'

'It'd cost me that much?'

'Everything,' said Dent, with emphasis.

Burroughs watched Ulysses preening himself and thought of his obligation: an essay for this old croaker ... an immediate opportunity to hit the ground running as Kate had said ... and an obvious test of his resolve.

'When would you like my article?'

'When you're happy with it, not until.'

'Not to please Stickler?'

'No, write to please yourself, don't consider anyone. If you don't enjoy what you're doing nobody else will.'

'I won't forget,' said Burroughs, standing up and walking to the window. 'You have a big garden... with a fishpond.'

'Yes, family tradition. Always sink a pond wherever I live. I find it restful looking into water... but it is also the quickest and easiest way to introduce diversity to a garden. A monoculture, you see, is barren just like medical specialists. They never think outside their dull little empires.'

Burroughs nodded. 'Who is that man downstairs in the kitchen, the one with the bow-tie?'

'Wilson?'

'Yes.'

'A novelist, with a humanist streak, one of the Hampstead set.'

'Have you read him?'

'Oh yes. He's trying to move things along, but his style is a bit conventional and self-conscious for me. He met one of my daughters during the war, at Bletchley.'

'Bletchley?'

'Code-breaking, intelligence, that sort of thing. We don't talk about it, least, we're not supposed to. In fact the whole subject of war is fast becoming either taboo or myth. Most just say it was "terrible" without thinking. But that isn't my understanding, not at all. For instance, many people stopped coming to my surgeries. Their "aches and pains" disappeared.'

'I 'spose people had something real to be frightened about.'

'That's true but they also shared a unity of purpose.'

'To defeat fascism?'

'Yes, it was total war. Everybody had a lot of obviously right things to do and were all looking in the same direction... collaborating. And now our prize is this.' Dent threw his hand towards the window. '... A so-called democratic peace. In war we obeyed orders and policed ourselves. In peacetime we must criticise the views of others and this is a much harder job. Is it any wonder that those niggling doubts and anxieties come streaming back?' Dent didn't wait for an answer.

'Anyway, Wilson was at Bletchley with my daughter reading Japanese weather maps of all things, not that they were ever an item. No, Wilson is, as they say, "straight as a nine bob note". You don't mind queers do you?'

Burroughs was still wheezing with laughter as he led the old croaker onto the landing and down the stairs. Catching up with the speed of his internal renewal had amazed him but now, with the offer of something to write, he realised his external environment was also shifting alongside his expectations. Hope and virtue replacing fear and shame. He glided past the books stacked on Dent's stairs with a renewed appetite for the struggles ahead. It was doubtful his life would ever be on an even keel but suddenly, like a sailing ship emerging from the doldrums, there was a wind at his back and calmer waters ahead. He was also a little more trusting of his gift; his unique grace and presence and its rightful place within a magnificently tortured, unholy universe.

* * *

> 160 Holland Park Avenue.
> London W.11
> 16.1.1962

Dear Mr Burroughs,

 I know you will be sad to hear that John Dent died very suddenly on Jan 8th.
 It was a coronary thrombosis and he died as he would have liked sitting in his chair in the drawing room playing Patience.
 He had not been really well since we came here but the doctors kept giving very cheerful reports. I hoped my own fears were wrong.
 He was so fond of you and interested in your work. I wish there was any one like him to carry on his but I'm afraid there isn't.
 Do keep in touch with us and come and see us when you come to London if you feel inclined.
 I expect we will stay on here for the present anyway but after sharing everything for the last 23 years you can imagine the chaos we are in.

  Yours v sincerely,
  Rhoda Brenan

160 Holland Park
Avenue. W. 11
16. 1. 62.

Dear Mr Burroughs

I know you will be sad to hear that John Dent died very suddenly on Jan 8th. It was a coronary thrombosis & he died as he would have wished sitting in his chair in the drawingroom playing patience. He had not been really well since we came here but the doctors kept on giving very cheerful reports & I hoped my own fears were wrong.

He was so fond of you & interested in your work

I wish there was any one like him to carry on his but I'm afraid there isn't.

Do keep in touch with us & come & see us when you come to London. if you feel inclined. I expect we shall stay on here for the present anyway. but after sharing everything for the last 23 years you can imagine the chaos we are in.

Yours & sincerely
Rhoda Burman

July 15, 1983
PO Box 147
Lawrence, Kansas 66044
USA

Dear Baudron:
Many thanks for your communication and for your efforts in the apo-morphine cause. Doctor Dent who was the sanest and least paranoid of men, could not help but see a conspiracy on the part of the medical establishment, which is, in America at least, very much under control of the Narcotics Dept., to suppress the apo-morphine treatment for addiction. And I have a thick file of inquries, attempts to interest doctors and researchers, all ending in a dead end. Some of the inquirers even lost their jobs as a result of advocating at least a trial of the apomorphine treatment. It is also to be remembered that synthesis of the formulae could yield compounds with a much more potent regulatory activity and the nausea factor could be eliminated. Doctor Dent could not stress too heavily and too often that this is <u>not an aversion treatment</u>.

   I finally decided that a very potent vested interest does not want to know about a real cure for addiction any more than they want to know about a cure for cancer. So I am not surprised at the runaround you got from the experts. The alcoholic neurosis indeed, what rubbish. Doctor Dent said the alcoholic's nerurosis is that he drinks too much. Tell that to a psychiatrist.

   Doctors are, by and large drastically limited in outlook. They have read all there is to know on any subject and that is that. Anything outside their knowledge cannot be worth hearing about. So I really gave up years ago. Some doctors in Denmark still use the apo treatment but they clash with the psychiastrists. In my opinion a substantial number of psychiatrists should be broken down to veterinarians but that goes for the medical practice in general.

Interesting how large a part voice plays in psychosis. The patients who thought of words as parasitic entities. People who hear voices describe them as very loud and vibrant and they cannot believe that others do not hear the voices. They should be able to develop mikes sensitive enough to pick up subvocal speech.

William Burroughs

HARDY TREE

July 15, 1983
PO Box 147
Lawrence, Kansas 66044
USA

Dear Baudron:

Many thanks for your communication and for your efforts in the apo-morphine cause. Doctor Dent who was the sanest and least paranoid of men, could not help but see a conspiracy on the part of the medical establishment, which is, In America, at least, very much under control of the Narcotics Dept., to suppress the apo-morphine treatment for addiction. And I have a thick file of inquiries, attempts to interest doctors and researchers, all ending in a dead end. Some of the inquirers even lost their jobs as a result of advocating at least a trial of the apomorphine treatment. It is also to be remembered that synthesis of the formulae could yield compounds with a much more potent regulatory activity and the nausea factor could be eliminated.. Doctor Dent could not stress too heavily and too often that this is not an aversion treatment.

I finally decided that a very potent vested interest does not want to know about a real cure for addiction any more than they want to know about a cure for cancer. So I am not surprised at the runaround you got from the experts. The alcoholic neurosis indeed, what rubbish. Doctor Dent said the alcoholic's nerurosis is that he drinks too much. Tell that to a psychiatrist.

[396]

Doctors are, by and large drastically limited in outlook. They have read all there is to know on any subject and that is that. Anything outside their knowledge cannot be worth hearing about. So I really gave up years ago. Some doctors in Denmark still use the apo treatment but they clash with the psychitrists.. In my opinion a substantial number of psychiatrists should be broken down to veterinarias but that goes for the medical practice in general..

Interesting how large a part voice plays in psychosis. The patients who thought of words as parasitic entities. People who hear voices describe them as very loud and vibrant and they cannot beleive that others do not hear the voices. They should be able to develop mikes sesitive enough to pick up subvocal speech.

Letter reproduced with permission: ©Isabelle Aubert-Baudron, *The Time of the Naguals, Research, Tome 2* (Interzone Editions, ISBN 978-2-9531513-8-1)

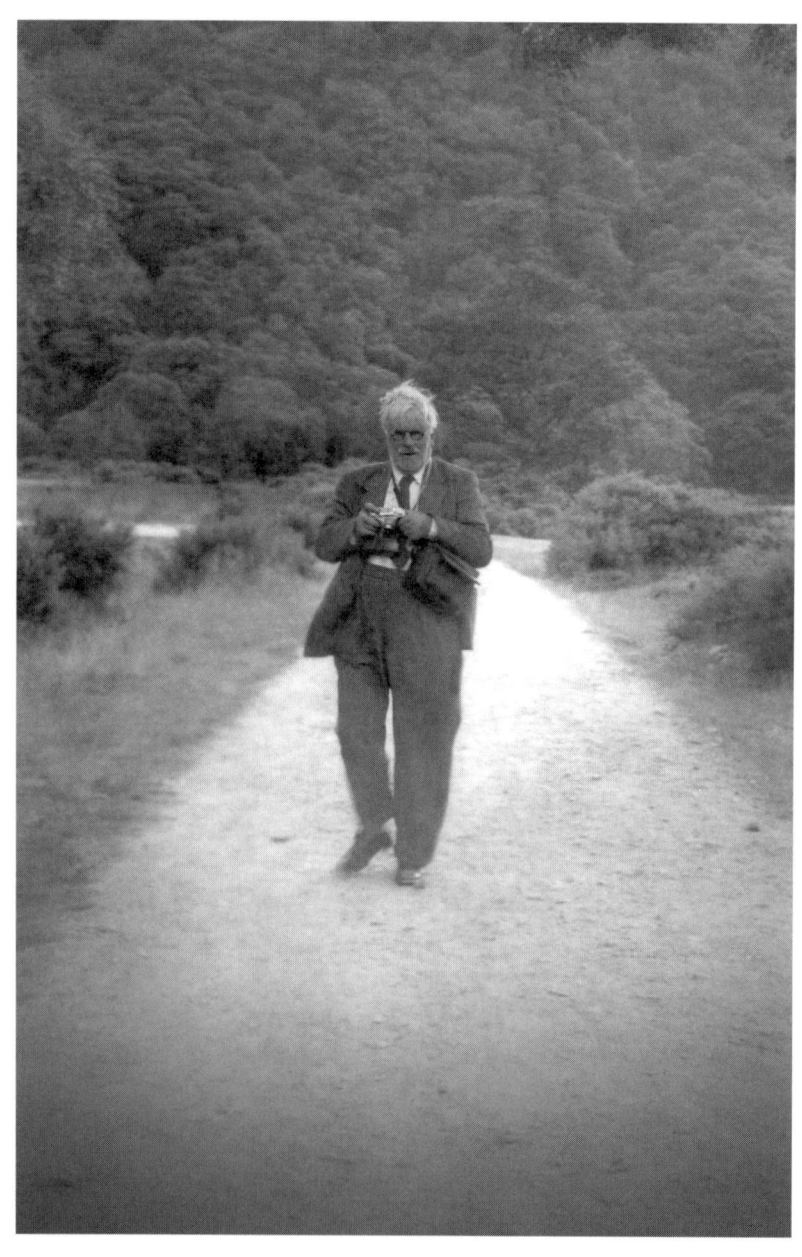

Dent on holiday, Co Wicklow, Ireland, 1956. [photo: Jane Yerbury Sweeney]

If a person can have his
mechanism sufficiently repaired…
… and then be encouraged to
struggle with his difficulties,
it is quite possible that he
will overcome them and
enjoy the struggle as
well as the victory.

– John Yerbury Dent
  Anxiety and its Treatment

First published 2019

Bracketpress
183 Dunkirk Rise College Bank Way Rochdale
Lancashire OL12 6UJ

All rights reserved
© J. Warwick Sweeney, 2019

The right of J. Warwick Sweeney to be identified as the author of this work has been asserted in accordance with Section 77 of the Copyright, Designs and Patents Act, 1988. No part of this publication may be copied, reproduced, stored in a retrieval system, or transmitted, in any form or by any means without the prior permission of the publisher, nor be otherwise circulated in any form of binding or cover other than that in which it is published and without a similar condition being imposed on the subsequent purchaser. While every effort has been made to trace the owners of copyright material reproduced herein, the publisher would like to apologise for any omissions and will be pleased to incorporate missing acknowledgments in any further editions.

Typesetting by Christian Brett

Printed and bound in England by
TJ International Ltd.
Padstow Cornwall PL28 8RW

ISBN 978-1-9996740-3-8

First edition